# Sources and Expressions of Resiliency in Trauma Survivors: Ecological Theory, Multicultural Practice

*Sources and Expressions of Resiliency in Trauma Survivors: Ecological Theory, Multicultural Practice* has been co-published simultaneously as *Journal of Aggression, Maltreatment & Trauma*, Volume 14, Numbers 1/2, 2007.

**Monographic Separates from the *Journal of Aggression, Maltreatment & Trauma*^TM^**

For additional information on these and other Haworth Press titles, including descriptions, tables of contents, reviews, and prices, use the QuickSearch

*Sources and Expressions of Resiliency in Trauma Survivors: Ecological Theory, Multicultural Practice,* edited by Mary R. Harvey, PhD and Pratyusha Tummala-Narra, PhD (Vol. 14, No. 1/2, 2006). *Examines the resiliency capacities of traumatized individuals and communitites.*

*Prevention of Intimate Violence,* edited by Sandra M. Stith, PhD (Vol. 13, No. 3/4, 2006). *A comprehensive overview of effective approaches in working to prevent intimate partner violence.*

*Ending Child Abuse: New Efforts in Prevention, Investigation, and Training,* edited by Victor I. Vieth, JD, BS, Bette L. Bottoms, PhD, Alison R. Perona, JD, MA, BS (Vol. 12, No. 3/4, 2006). *A collection of innovative approaches and aggressive strategies to end or significantly reduce child abuse in every community.*

*Trauma Treatment Techniques: Innovative Trends,* edited by Jacueline Garrick, CSW, ACSW, BCETS, and Mary Beth Williams, PhD, LSW, CTS (Vol. 12, No. 1/2, 2006). *"This collection SIGNIFICANTLY BROADENS THE UNDERSTANDING OF INNOVATIVE TECHNIQUES for the treatment of PTSD and associated conditions." (John P. Wilson, Co-founder and Past President, International Society for Traumatic Stress Studies, co-director, International Institute on Psychotraumatology).*

*Ethical and Legal Issues for Mental Health Professional: A Comprehensive Handbook of Principles and Standards,* edited by Steven F. Bucky, Joanne E. Callan, and George Stricker (Vol. 11, No. 1/2 and 3, 2005) *"It is safe to say that every psychotherapist will be confronted with ethical and legal problems in the course of his or her career. THIS BOOK SHOULD BE RETAINED ON THE SHELF OF EVERY MENTAL HEALTH PRACTITIONER. This is an exhaustive compendium written by a distinguished battery of attorneys and psychotherapists, each of whom is an expert in his or her field . . . . It should be used as a resource guide when problems arise in the course of one's practice." (Martin Fleishman, MD, PhD, Active Staff, St. Francis Memorial Hospital, San Francisco: Author of "The Casebook of Residential Care Psychiatrist")*

*The Trauma of Terrorism: Sharing Knowledge and Shared Care, An International Handbook,* edited by Yael Danieli, PhD, Danny Brom, PhD, and Joe Sills, MA (Vol. 9, No. 1/2 and 3/4, 2004 and Vol. 10, No. 1/2 and 3/4, 2005). *"This book pulls together key programs that enable society to cope with ongoing terrorism, and is thus a rich resource for both policymakers and those who aid terrorism's victims directly. It demonstrates the invaluable collaboration between government and private initiative in the development of a resilient society." (Danny Naveh, Minister of Health, Governement of Israel)*

# Sources and Expressions of Resiliency in Trauma Survivors: Ecological Theory, Multicultural Practice

Mary R. Harvey, PhD
Pratyusha Tummala-Narra, PhD
Editors

*Sources and Expressions of Resiliency in Trauma Survivors: Ecological Theory, Multicultural Practice* has been co-published simultaneously as *Journal of Aggression, Maltreatment & Trauma*, Volume 14, Numbers 1/2, 2007.

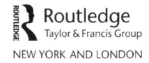

Routledge
Taylor & Francis Group

NEW YORK AND LONDON

Published by

The Haworth Maltreatment & Trauma Press, 10 Alice Street, Binghamton, NY 13904-1580 USA

Transferred to Digital Printing 2010 by Routledge
270 Madison Ave, New York NY 10016
2 Park Square, Milton Park, Abingdon, Oxon, OX14 4RN

*Sources and Expressions of Resiliency in Trauma Survivors: Ecological Theory, Multicultural Practice* has been co-published simultaneously as *Journal of Aggression, Maltreatment & Trauma*, Volume 14, Numbers 1/2, 2007.

The development, preparation, and publication of this work has been undertaken with great care. However, the publisher, employees, editors, and agents of The Haworth Press and all imprints of The
Haworth Press, Inc., including The Haworth Medical Press® and Pharmaceutical Products Press®, are
not responsible for any errors contained herein or for consequences that may ensue from use of materials or information contained in this work. With regard to case studies, identities and circumstances of
individuals discussed herein have been changed to protect confidentiality. Any resemblance to actual
persons, living or dead, is entirely coincidental.

The Haworth Press is committed to the dissemination of ideas and information according to the highest standards of intellectual freedom and the free exchange of ideas. Statements made and opinions
expressed in this publication do not necessarily reflect the views of the Publisher, Directors, management, or staff of The Haworth Press, Inc., or an endorsement by them.

Cover note: Panels of "Mary's Quilt," created by colleages and trainees of the Victims of Violence Program appears on the front cover courtesy of Mary Harvey.

### Library of Congress Cataloging-in-Publication Data

Sources and expressions of resiliency in trauma survivors : ecological theory, multicultural practice/
Mary R. Harvey, Pratyusha Tummala-Narra, editors.
      p. cm.
    "Co-published simultaneously as Journal of aggression, maltreatment & trauma, v. 14, no. 1/2
2007."
Includes bibliographical references and index.
ISBN 13: 978-0-7890-3462-5 (hard cover : alk. paper)
ISBN 10: 0-7890-3462-X (hard cover : alk. paper)
ISBN 13: 978-0-7890-3463-2 (soft cover : alk. paper)
ISBN 10: 0-7890-3463-8 (soft cover : alk. paper)
1. Psychic trauma. 2. Resilience (Personality trait) I. Harvey, Mary R. II. Tummala-Narra,
Pratyusha.
    [DNLM: 1. Psychic trauma 2. Stress Disorders, Post-Traumatic–therapy. 3. Cross-Cultural
Comparison. 4. Ecology 5. Survivors–psychology. W1 JO534BE v. 14 no 1/2 2007 / WM 170 S724
2007]
RC552.T7S68 2007
616.85′21–dc22
                                      2006026159

**Publisher's Note**
The publisher has gone to great lengths to ensure the quality of this reprint
but points out that some imperfections in the original may be apparent.

A Note About the Cover

The quilt was a gift to Mary Harvey, PhD on the occasion of her retire-
ment as Founding Director of the Victims of Violence Program. The
VOV Program is large and multifacedted. The idea of bringing the
program together to make a quilt as a means both of honoring Mary
and bringing our community together in common purpose began to
take hold. The stated vision was for each person to make a square representing Mary's relationship to them or to the program. Materials
were brought from home and included remnants from sewing projects, material from children's Halloween costumes and old clothes
and baubles collected over the years. On several occassions over the
summer of 2006, staff and trainees came together, not in a domain of
expertise but by taking risks together, creating something new together, working side by side, supporting vulnerabilities, admiring one
another's creativity, eating together, being playful, remembering,
bringing old scraps of material from each of their lives and representing their attachment to their work and to Mary, creating connections
that stitched together future working relationships while honoring the
past. The process, as much as the quilt itself, gave expression to the resilient capacities of the community that is the VOV.

*The* HAWORTH PRESS *Inc.*

## Abstracting, Indexing & Outward Linking

PRINT *and* ELECTRONIC BOOKS & JOURNALS

This section provides you with a list of major indexing & abstracting services and other tools for bibliographic access. That is to say, each service began covering this periodical during the the year noted in the right column. Most Websites which are listed below have indicated that they will either post, disseminate, compile, archive, cite or alert their own Website users with research-based content from this work. (This list is as current as the copyright date of this publication.)

Abstracting, Website/Indexing Coverage . . . . . . . . Year When Coverage Began

- **Academic Search Premier (EBSCO)\*\***
  <http://www.epnet.com/academic/acasearchprem.asp> . . . . . . . . 2006

- **CINAHL (Cumulative Index to Nursing & Allied Health
  Literature) (EBSCO)\*\*** <http://www.cinahl.com> . . . . . . . . . . . . 2000

- **CINAHL Plus (EBSCO)\*\*** . . . . . . . . . . . . . . . . . . . . . . . . . . . . . 2000

- **EMBASE Excerpta Medica (Elsevier)\*\*** <http://www.elsevier.nl> . 2000

- **EMBASE.com (The Power of EMBASE + MEDLINE Combined)
  (Elsevier)\*\*** <http://www.embase.com>. . . . . . . . . . . . . . . . . . . . . 2000

- **MasterFILE Premier (EBSCO)\*\*** <http://www.epnet.com/
  government/mfpremier.asp> . . . . . . . . . . . . . . . . . . . . . . . . . . . . 2006

- **Psychological Abstracts (PsycINFO)\*\*** <http://www.apa.org> . . . 2001

- **Social Services Abstracts (Cambridge Scientific Abstracts)\*\***
  <http://www.csa.com> . . . . . . . . . . . . . . . . . . . . . . . . . . . . . . . 1998

- **Social Work Abstracts (NASW)\*\*** <http://www.silverplatter.com/
  catalog/swab.htm> . . . . . . . . . . . . . . . . . . . . . . . . . . . . . . . . . 2001

- **Sociological Abstracts (Cambridge Scientific Abstracts)\*\***
  <http://www.csa.com> . . . . . . . . . . . . . . . . . . . . . . . . . . . . . . . 1998

- *Academic Source Premier (EBSCO)* . . . . . . . . . . . . . . . . . . . . . . . 2007

- *British Journal of Psychotherapy* . . . . . . . . . . . . . . . . . . . . . . . . . 2006

(continued)

(continued)

- *ILO/BIT-CIS Bulletin* ............................... 2000
- *Index to Periodical Articles Related to Law*
  *<http://www.law.utexas.edu>* ........................... 2000
- *IndexCopernicus <http://www.indexcopernicus.com>* .......... 2006
- *Internationale Bibliographie der geistes- und*
  *sozialwissenschaftlichen Zeitschriftenliteratur . . .*
  *See IBZ .......  <http://www.saur.de>* .................... 2000
- *JournalSeek <http://www.journalseek.net>* ................... 2006
- *Links@Ovid (via CrossRef targeted DOI links)*
  *<http://www.ovid.com>* ................................. 2005
- *National Criminal Justice Reference Service*
  *<http://www.ncjrs.org>* ................................. 2006
- *NewJour (Electronic Journals & Newsletters)*
  *<http://gort.ucsd.edu/newjour/>* ......................... 2006
- *OCLC ArticleFirst <http://www.oclc.org/services/databases/>* ..... 2006
- *Ovid Linksolver (OpenURL link resolver via CrossRef targeted DOI links)*
  *<http://www.linksolver.com>* ............................ 2005
- *PASCAL International Bibliography (c/o Institut de*
  *l'Information Scientifique et Technique) <http://www.inist.fr>* . . 1997
- *PILOTS Database (Published International Literature On*
  *Traumatic Stress) <http://www.ncptsd.org>* ................. 1997
- *Prevention Evaluation Research Registry for Youth (PERRY)* ...... 2001
- *PSYCLINE <http://www.psycline.org>* ....................... 2006
- *PTSD Research Quarterly <http://www.ncptsd.org>* ............. 2000
- *Referativnyi Zhurnal (Abstracts Journal of the All-Russian Institute*
  *of Scientific and Technical Information-in Russian)*
  *<http://www.viniti.ru>* ................................. 1998
- *Risk Abstracts (Cambridge Scientific Abstracts) <http://csa.com>* ... 2006
- *SafetyLit <http://www.safetylit.org>* ......................... 2006
- *Scopus (See instead Elsevier Scopus)*
  *<http://www.info.scopus.com>* ........................... 2005
- *Social Care Online (formerly CareData)*
  *<http://www.elsc.org.uk>* ............................... 1998

(continued)

- *Sociedad Iberoamericana de Información Científica (SIIC) <http://www.siicsalud.com/>* . . . . . . . . . . . . . . . . . . . . . . 2006
- *SocIndex (EBSCO)* . . . . . . . . . . . . . . . . . . . . . . . . . . . . . . . . . . . . . 2006
- *SocINDEX with Full Text (EBSCO)* . . . . . . . . . . . . . . . . . . . . . . . 2007
- *TOC Premier (EBSCO)* . . . . . . . . . . . . . . . . . . . . . . . . . . . . . . . . . . 2007
- *Violence and Abuse Abstracts (Sage)* . . . . . . . . . . . . . . . . . . . . . 2001
- *Women, Girls & Criminal Justice Newsletter (Civic Research Institute)* . . . . . . . . . . . . . . . . . . . . . . . . . . . . . . 2004

## Bibliographic Access

- **Cabell's Directory of Publishing Opportunities in Psychology <http://www.cabells.com>**
- **MediaFinder <http://www.mediafinder.com>**
- **Ulrich's Periodicals Directory: The Global Source for Periodicals Information Since 1932 <http://www.bowkerlink.com>**

*Special Bibliographic Notes related to special journal issues (separates) and indexing/abstracting:*

- indexing/abstracting services in this list will also cover material in any "separate" that is co-published simultaneously with Haworth's special thematic journal issue or DocuSerial. Indexing/abstracting usually covers material at the article/chapter level.
- monographic co-editions are intended for either non-subscribers or libraries which intend to purchase a second copy for their circulating collections.
- monographic co-editions are reported to all jobbers/wholesalers/approval plans. The source journal is listed as the "series" to assist the prevention of duplicate purchasing in the same manner utilized for books-in-series.
- to facilitate user/access services all indexing/abstracting services are encouraged to utilize the co-indexing entry note indicated at the bottom of the first page of each article/chapter/contribution.
- this is intended to assist a library user of any reference tool (whether print, electronic, online, or CD-ROM) to locate the monographic version if the library has purchased this version but not a subscription to the source journal.
- individual articles/chapters in any Haworth publication are also available through the Haworth Document Delivery Service (HDDS).

This section provides you with a list of major indexing & abstracting services and other tools for bibliographic access. That is to say, each service began covering this periodical during the the year noted in the right column. Most Websites which are listed below have indicated that they will either post, disseminate, compile, archive, cite or alert their own Website users with research-based content from this work. (This list is as current as the copyright date of this publication.)

Abstracting, Website/Indexing Coverage . . . . . . . . . Year When Coverage Began

- **Academic Search Premier (EBSCO)**
  <http://www.epnet.com/academic/acasearchprem.asp> . . . . . . . . 2006

- **CINAHL (Cumulative Index to Nursing & Allied Health
  Literature) (EBSCO)** <http://www.cinahl.com> . . . . . . . . . . . 2000

- **CINAHL Plus (EBSCO)** . . . . . . . . . . . . . . . . . . . . . . . . . . . . . 2000

- **EMBASE Excerpta Medica (Elsevier)** <http://www.elsevier.nl> . 2000

- **EMBASE.com (The Power of EMBASE + MEDLINE Combined)
  (Elsevier)** <http://www.embase.com> . . . . . . . . . . . . . . . . . . . . 2000

- **MasterFILE Premier (EBSCO)** <http://www.epnet.com/
  government/mfpremier.asp> . . . . . . . . . . . . . . . . . . . . . . . . . . . . 2006

- **Psychological Abstracts (PsycINFO)** <http://www.apa.org> . . . 2001

- **Social Services Abstracts (Cambridge Scientific Abstracts)**
  <http://www.csa.com> . . . . . . . . . . . . . . . . . . . . . . . . . . . . . . . . 1998

- **Social Work Abstracts (NASW)** <http://www.silverplatter.com/
  catalog/swab.htm> . . . . . . . . . . . . . . . . . . . . . . . . . . . . . . . . . . . 2001

- **Sociological Abstracts (Cambridge Scientific Abstracts)**
  <http://www.csa.com> . . . . . . . . . . . . . . . . . . . . . . . . . . . . . . . . 1998

- *Academic Source Premier (EBSCO)* . . . . . . . . . . . . . . . . . . . . . . 2007

- *British Journal of Psychotherapy* . . . . . . . . . . . . . . . . . . . . . . . . 2006

(continued)

## ABOUT THE EDITORS

**Mary R. Harvey, PhD,** is Founding Director of the Victims of Violence Program of the Cambridge Health Alliance and Associate Clinical Professor of Psychology in the Department of Psychiatry at Harvard Medical School. A clinical and a community psychologist, she is a Fellow of the American Psychological Association and of APA's Division 27 (Society for Community Research and Action), and a member and former Board Member of the International Society for Traumatic Stress Studies (ISTSS). In 1996, ISTSS honored her as a recipient of the society's Sarah Haley Award for outstanding service to traumatized populations. She is the co-author (with Mary P. Koss) of *The Rape Victim: Clinical and Community Interventions* (Sage, 1991) and the author and co-author of numerous theoretical, empirical, and clinical publications. Her private clinical practice is located in Cambridge, MA.

**Pratyusha Tummala-Narra, PhD,** is a clinical psychologist, and the Founding Director (1997-2003) of the Asian Mental Health Clinic at the Cambridge Health Alliance/Harvard Medical School. While on faculty at the Cambridge Health Alliance, she was a supervisor and research associate in the Victims of Violence Program, and Interim Director for psychology and psychology training (2002-2003). From 2003-2005, Dr. Tummala-Narra was Co-Director of the Trauma and Loss Program and Director of Clinical Outreach in the Center for Mental Health Outreach, both at Georgetown University Hospital in Washington, DC. More recently, she was a Visiting Scholar at the University of Michigan Psychological Clinic, where she supervised psychology interns and post-doctoral fellows. She is currently Adjunct Professor at the Michigan School for Professional Psychology and works with clients in private practice in Farmington Hills. She is also a Teaching Associate at the Cambridge Health Alliance/Harvard Medical School, and the Chairperson of the Multicultural Concerns Committee in Division 39 (Psychoanalysis) of the American Psychological Association. Her scholarly publications and presentations concern the areas of psychological trauma, multicultural psychology, and related psychodynamic perspectives.

# Sources and Expressions of Resiliency in Trauma Survivors: Ecological Theory, Multicultural Practice

## CONTENTS

About the Contributors                                                      xix

Preface                                                                      xxv
   *Judith L. Herman*

Acknowledgments                                                            xxix

INTRODUCTION

Sources and Expression of Resilience in Trauma Survivors:
   Ecological Theory, Multicultural Perspectives                          1
   *Mary R. Harvey*
   *Pratyusha Tummala-Narra*

SECTION ONE: UNDERSTANDING RECOVERY
   AND RESILIENCY: THEORY

Towards an Ecological Understanding of Resilience in Trauma
   Survivors: Implications for Theory, Research, and Practice              9
   *Mary R. Harvey*

Conceptualizing Trauma and Resilience Across Diverse
   Contexts: A Multicultural Perspective                                  33
   *Pratyusha Tummala-Narra*

SECTION TWO: ASSESSING RESILIENCE: MULTIPLE
   DIMENSIONS, MULTIPLE APPROACHES

The Multidimensional Trauma Recovery and Resiliency
   Instrument: Preliminary Examination of an Abridged Version    55
   *Belle Liang*
   *Pratyusha Tummala-Narra*
   *Rebekah Bradley*
   *Mary R. Harvey*

The Story of My Strength: An Exploration of Resilience
   in the Narratives of Trauma Survivors Early in Recovery    75
   *Shannon M. Lynch*
   *Amy L. Keasler*
   *Rhiannon C. Reaves*
   *Elizabeth G. Channer*
   *Lisa T. Bukowski*

Where the Whole Thing Fell Apart: Race, Resilience,
   and the Complexity of Trauma    99
   *Lynn Sorsoli*

SECTION THREE: MULTICULTURAL ASSESSMENT
   OF TRAUMA, RECOVERY AND RESILIENCE

Interpersonal Violence, Recovery, and Resilience
   in Incarcerated Women    123
   *Rebekah Bradley*
   *Katrina Davino*

Exposure to Violence and Expressions of Resilience in Central
   American Women Survivors of War    147
   *Angela Radan*

Exploration of Recovery Trajectories in Sexually Abused
   Adolescents    165
   *Isabelle Daigneault*
   *Mireille Cyr*
   *Marc Tourigny*

Assessing Trauma Impact, Recovery, and Resiliency
   in Refugees of War                                              185
      *Nancy Peddle*

SECTON FOUR: ECOLOGICALLY INFORMED
   INTERVENTION

Trauma and Resilience: A Case of Individual Psychotherapy
   in a Multicultural Context                                       205
      *Pratyusha Tummala-Narra*

Group Therapy as an Ecological Bridge to New Community
   for Trauma Survivors                                            227
      *Michaela Mendelsohn*
      *Robin S. Zachary*
      *Patricia A. Harney*

Revolutionizing the Clinical Frame: Individual and Social
   Advocacy Practice on Behalf of Trauma Survivors                 245
      *Carol Gomez*
      *Janet Yassen*

Fostering Resilience in Traumatized Communities:
   A Community Empowerment Model of Intervention                    265
      *Mary R. Harvey*
      *Anne V. Mondesir*
      *Holly Aldrich*

Resilience and Post-Traumatic Recovery in Cultural
   and Political Context: Two Pakistani Women's Strategies
   for Survival                                                     287
      *Shahla Haeri*

Epilogue                                                            305
      *Mary R. Harvey*
      *Pratyusha Tummala-Narra*

Appendix A: Multidimensional Trauma Recovery
   and Resiliency Scale (MTRR-99) Clinical Rating Form          307

Appendix B: Multidimensional Trauma Recovery
   and Resiliency Interview (MTRR-I) (Short Form,
   2000 Version)                                                315

Index                                                          319

# ABOUT THE CONTRIBUTORS

**Holly Aldrich** is an independently licensed clinical social worker and founding Coordinator of the Center for Homicide Bereavement, a service of the Victims of Violence Program. She is also a former Coordinator of the Community Crisis Response Team and has worked extensively with traumatized communities in Massachusetts, Alaska, New York, and Eastern Europe. In addition, Ms. Aldrich provides training and supervision to clinical and community practitioners throughout Massachusetts and has a private clinical practice in Cambridge.

**Lisa T. Bukowski** received a Bachelor of Science Degree in Psychology at Western Illinois University and is pursuing a graduate degree in school counseling at Northern Illinois University. Her interests are in adolescent development and clinical practice.

**Rebekah Bradley, PhD,** is Assistant Professor in Department of Psychiatry and Behavioral Science at Emory University in Atlanta, GA. She is also a licensed clinical psychologist. She completed her PhD at the University of South Carolina in Clinical/Community Psychology and her internship at the Cambridge Hospital, Department of Psychiatry, Harvard Medical School. Her research focuses on the impact and treatment of interpersonal violence, particularly in low SES and racial and ethnic minority populations. In addition she focuses on personality pathology in the areas of: classification, measurement, and etiological factors.

**Elizabeth G. Channer** completed a Master's Degree in General Psychology at Western Illinois University. Her interests are in qualitative methodology, violence against women, and the meaning of work.

**Mireille Cyr, PhD,** is Full Professor at the department of psychology at the Université de Montréal and one of the founding members of CRIPCAS. Dr. Cyr's main interests in research include: reactions and adaptations of non-offending mothers as well as their interactions with their sexually-abused children, factors related to sexual intergenerational transmission, the investigation of various sequelae of sexual abuse in children and adolescents and children's characteristics influencing their accounts under investigative interview. Her work has been published in French and English and presented to audiences in Canada, the United States, and Europe.

**Isabelle Daigneault, PhD,** is a post-doctoral Fellow at the Sexology Department of the Université du Québec à Montréal. She is also a licensed clinical psychologist since 1996. She completed her PhD in Psychology and a clinical Master's degree at the Université de Montréal. Since 1997, her research has included treatment outcome studies of sexually abused adolescents and implementation studies of group treatments for parents of sexually abused children. She has also been a consulting member with the advisory committee on sexual abuse in Montreal's youth centers (CPS) and is a member of the *Centre de recherche interdisciplinaire sur les problèmes conjugaux et les agressions sexuelles* (CRIPCAS is a research center dedicated to sexual assaults and marital problems).

**Katrina Davino, PhD,** is a licensed clinical psychologist in private practice in Atlanta, GA. In addition, she serves a consultant to the Laboratory of Personality and Psychopathology, Emory University. She completed her PhD at the University of South Carolina in Clinical/Community Psychology and her internship at the University of Massachusetts Medical School. Her clinical work and research focuses on the impact and treatment of interpersonal violence. Her clinical work integrates interpersonal theories with cognitive behavioral components and she specializes in the treatment of PTSD and personality and eating disorders.

**Carol Gomez** has worked as an advocate, community organizer, domestic violence counselor, educator, and community researcher both in the US and in Malaysia. She is Founding Director of MataHari–Eye of the Day and its project–The Trafficking Victims Outreach and Services network in Massachusetts and New England and sits on the Governor's Commission on Domestic Violence and Sexual Assault, the South Asian Health Advisory Board, and the Asian Pacific Islander Women's Social Justice Project. She is a member of the Boston chapter of INCITE! Women of Color Against Violence, and she is the former coordinator of the Victim Advocacy and Support Team (VAST) of the Victims of Violence Program where she served as Co-Director of the interagency SafetyNet Program for trafficked and exploited persons. Ms. Gomez offers to national and international audiences education, training and consultation on violence prevention, immigrant care, modern-day slavery, violence against women, advocacy, and anti-oppression, coalition building.

**Shahla Haeri, PhD,** is Director of Women's Studies Program and Associate Professor of Cultural Anthropology in the Department of Anthropology at Boston University. She has conducted research in Iran, Pakistan, and India, and has written extensively on religion, law, and gender dynamics in the Muslim world. She is the author of *No Shame for the Sun: Lives of Professional Pakistani women* (Syracuse University Press in the US, and

Oxford University Press in Pakistan, 2004), and *Law of Desire: Temporary Marriage, Mut'a, in Iran* (1989, 1993). She has been awarded several post-doctoral fellowships, including one at the Women's Studies in Religion Program, Harvard Divinity School (2005-2006), Fulbright (1999-2000, 2002-2003), St. Anthony's College, Oxford University (1996), Social Science Research Council (1987-1988), Pembroke Center for Teaching and Research on Women, Brown University (1986-1987), and the Center for Middle Eastern Studies, Harvard University (1985-1986).

**Patricia Harney, PhD,** is Associate Director of Psychology at the Cambridge Health Alliance, Harvard Medical School. She also maintains a psychotherapy practice in Cambridge, MA. She has clinical expertise in the area of trauma and has published several papers on the assessment and treatment of trauma.

**Amy L. Keasler** completed a Master's Degree in Clinical/Community Mental Health Psychology at Western Illinois University. Her research and practice interests include therapeutic alliance, processes of change, and family influences on development.

**Belle Liang, PhD,** is Associate Professor in the Department of Counseling and Developmental Psychology at the Lynch School of Education at Boston College and a licensed clinical psychologist. Her research focuses on community interventions for underserved, minority populations, including Asian adolescents and multi-ethnic trauma survivors. She is involved in the design of preventive interventions based on developmental and cultural theory, and in the development of new tools for assessing complex social experiences and relationships

**Shannon M. Lynch, PhD,** is Assistant Professor in the Department of Psychology at Idaho State University and a research associate with the Victims of Violence Research Project. Previously, she was at Western Illinois University. She obtained her PhD in Clinical Psychology from the University of Michigan and completed a postdoctoral fellowship at the Victims of Violence Program in Massachusetts. Her research is focused on violence against women and survivors' use of resources to cope with and to recover from traumatic events.

**Michaela Mendelsohn, PhD,** is a clinical and research psychologist at the Victims of Violence Program of the Cambridge Health Alliance, and a Clinical Instructor at Harvard Medical School. Her clinical practice focuses on the assessment and treatment of trauma-related disorders, and her research contributions include studies of the effects of political violence on children and youth, gender and social attitudes towards trauma victims, and group treatment of complex trauma.

**Anne Mondesir** is a licensed clinical social worker and Coordinator of the Community Crisis Response Team of the Victims of Violence Program. Her community work includes extensive interaction with police departments, youth service, and criminal and juvenile justice programs in the Greater Boston area.

**Nancy Peddle, PhD,** educated in early childhood development at Bank Street College (MS) and in human organization and development at Fielding Graduate Institute (MA, PhD), is the CEO of LemonAid Fund, aiding individuals who experienced violence change their lives and those of their communities. Peddle's expertise has taken her to over 20 countries focusing on trauma and violence and participatory research. She was the first Director of the International Society for the Prevention of Child Abuse and Neglect and a Research Fellow at Prevent Child Abuse America.

**Angela Radan, PhD,** is a psychologist at the Latino Mental Health Program and Coordinator of the Political Trauma Services Network, both at the Cambridge Health Alliance. A native of Costa Rica, Dr. Radan is the recipient of a Distinguished Service Award from the Costa Rican Psychological Association in recognition of her 20 years of service to the community. She was instrumental in establishing her country's first services for battered women. In 1989, she became a Fulbright Scholarship recipient and came to the U.S. to continue her graduate studies at Tufts University and Boston College. Her interests are focused in the area of human rights and mental health of immigrants and refugees.

**Rhiannon C. Reaves** completed a Master's Degree in Clinical/Community Mental Health Psychology at Western Illinois University. Her interests are in clinical psychology, specifically trauma and PTSD.

**Lynn Sorsoli, EdD,** directs a longitudinal study of the relationship between television consumption and adolescent sexuality at the Center for Research on Gender and Sexuality at San Francisco State University, where she also co-directs the post-doctoral training program. She completed her doctorate at Harvard's Graduate School of Education in 2003. In her dissertation, which focused on the connection between disclosure and psychological health, she examined the experiences women feel reluctant to share in their relationships, including traumatic experiences, the ways they convey these experiences, and the ways they have come to understand the power of relationships and the potential for personal disclosure. More recently, she has explored the disclosure experiences of male survivors of childhood sexual abuse and the ways these experiences can be complicated by their understandings of masculinity; and she has just begun to study the "coming out" experiences of lesbian, gay, and transgendered youth.

**Marc Tourigny, PhD,** is Professor of Psychoeducation in the Department of Specialized Education at the University of Sherbrooke (Canada) and also a member of CRIPCAS. He has been studying the problem of child maltreatment since 1985. One of his recent research projects was the first Quebec Incidence Study of Reported Child Abuse, Neglect, Abandonment, and Serious Behavior Problems (QIS). He has also worked extensively on treatment outcome studies of sexually abused children.

**Janet Yassen, LICSW,** is Crisis Services Coordinator of the Victims of Violence Program, the Cambridge Health Alliance. She is also co-founder of the Boston Area Rape Crisis Center. Ms. Yassen has lectured and consulted nationally and internationally about trauma and has written about crisis intervention as well as secondary traumatic stress. In addition to her work at the Victims of Violence Program, she maintains a private practice of individual and group therapy, supervision, consultation and training.

**Robin Zachary, LICSW,** is Coordinator of Group Services at the Victims of Violence Program of the Cambridge Health Alliance and a clinician in the VOV Program. Her clinical work is highlighted by her development and supervision of early and later-stage group treatment models for complexly traumatized survivors, including those with major dissociative disorders and those who struggle with issues of self-care and self harm. Her private clinical practice is in Brookline, MA.

# Foreword

Judith L. Herman

Only the very fortunate go through life without ever encountering either natural disaster or human violence. Consider, for instance, a large scale, random sample study of US citizens (Kessler, Sonnega, Bromet, Hughes, & Nelson, 1995), conducted during a time of peace and prosperity. The authors found that even in this privileged country, the majority of the population had been exposed at least once, at some point in their lives, to fire or flood, accident or assault, combat or rape–the kind of horrific event that can lead to a traumatic stress disorder. The same study found that almost 8% of the population actually developed post-traumatic stress disorder (PTSD). Eight percent is a remarkably high prevalence figure for a psychiatric disorder, but one might argue that the truly remarkable finding of this study is the number of people who did *not* develop PTSD. The great majority of people exposed to a traumatic stressor recovered spontaneously. Few received professional help; most of the people who recovered relied on their own inner resources and the help of families, friends, and supports available within their own communities.

Resiliency, the natural capacity of survivors to heal, is too often overlooked, too little studied. Yet no recovery is possible without it, and all of our therapeutic interventions build upon it. Resiliency is not a vague or mystical entity. Its dimensions can be defined, observed, even reli-

[Haworth co-indexing entry note]: "Foreword." Herman. Judith L. Co-published simultaneously in *Journal of Aggression, Maltreatment & Trauma* (The Haworth Maltreatment & Trauma Press, an imprint of The Haworth Press, Inc.) Vol. 14, No. 1/2, 2007, pp. xxxi-xxxiii; and: *Sources and Expressions of Resiliency in Trauma Survivors: Ecological Theory, Multicultural Practice* (ed: Mary R. Harvey, and Pratyusha Tummala-Narra) The Haworth Maltreatment & Trauma Press, an imprint of The Haworth Press, Inc., 2007, pp. xxv-xxvii. Single or multiple copies of this article are available for a fee from The Haworth Document Delivery Service [1-800-HAWORTH. 9:00 a.m. - 5:00 p.m. (EST). E-mail address: docdelivery@haworthpress.com].

Available online at http://jamt.haworthpress.com

ably measured (see Section Two, this volume). Its outlines are clearly recognizable across cultures. The collection of articles in this publication offers the basis for a new understanding of resiliency, as it is manifested in many different groups of people, both those who seek professional help and those in greater numbers who do not. Applying basic concepts of ecological theory as outlined by the editors in Section One of the volume, the authors delineate the features of resiliency as they appears in diverse populations (see Section Three, this volume).

This work is also the product of a particular ecosystem, the Victims of Violence Program in the Department of Psychiatry at Cambridge Health Alliance. Twelve of the authors are current or former fellows or staff at the Program. Located within a public-sector teaching hospital affiliated with Harvard Medical School, the Victims of Violence Program honors the twin missions of its home institution: (a) to offer the widest range of public services accessible to all and (b) to contribute to new knowledge and understanding of public health problems. This issue offers a detailed description of the broad array of therapeutic modalities developed by the Victims of Violence Program, from individual and group psychotherapy to victim advocacy and community intervention (see Section Four, this volume).

A special note about the editors: Mary Harvey is the Director of the Victims of Violence program, which we co-founded more than 20 years ago. As both a clinical and community psychologist who always thinks in terms of the social matrix of healing practice, she has provided the steady leadership, both intellectual and pragmatic, that has allowed the program to expand and flourish over the years. Pratyusha Tummala-Narra began her affiliation with the program as a post-doctoral fellow, and went on to become a full staff member and a program leader in her own right, founding the South Asian Mental Health Clinic at Cambridge Health Alliance before moving on to her present academic affiliation at the University of Michigan. We like to think that the Victims of Violence Program fosters the kind of collaborative partnership that maintains its liveliness even at long distance; certainly this editorial collaboration would be a testament to the lasting connections forged within the program.

Having been present at the Program's birth, and having participated in its growth and development, I take special pride and pleasure in presenting to the reading public the fruits of a long and rewarding collaboration.

# REFERENCE

Kessler, R. C., Sonnega, A., Bromet, E., Hughes, M., & Nelson, C. B. (1995). Posttraumatic stress disorder in the National Comorbidity survey. *Archives of General Psychiatry, 52*(12), 1048-1060.

# Acknowledgments

To our families:
   Oliver, Eric and Chie, Abigail, Maggie and Jonanthan, Vinod, Keshav and Ishan, Sabita and Madhusudana Rao Tummala, Pradyumna and Anita, Venkat, Neel, and Sai . . .

To our colleagues at the Victims of Violence Program and the Cambridge Health Alliance who are, after all, too many to name . . .

To the authors who contributed their work to this volume . . .

And, to the survivors who shared their stories so that these works could be written . . .

Thank you, thank you so very much.

*Mary R. Harvey*
*Pratyusha Tummala-Narrra*

# INTRODUCTION

# Sources and Expression of Resilience in Trauma Survivors: Ecological Theory, Multicultural Perspectives

Mary R. Harvey
Pratyusha Tummala-Narra

**SUMMARY.** There is growing recognition among trauma researchers, clinicians, and human rights activists of the need for greater understanding of the nature, impact, and mediators of traumatic exposure among trauma survivors from diverse cultures and contexts and a growing interest in the phenomenon of resiliency and the possibility of recovery in the aftermath of traumatic exposure. This introduction briefly describes the

Address correspondence to: Mary R. Harvey, PhD, Victims of Violence Progam, 26 Central Street, Somerville, MA 02143.

[Haworth co-indexing entry note]: "Sources and Expression of Resilience in Trauma Survivors: Ecological Theory, Multicultural Perspectives." Harvey, Mary R., and Pratyusha Tummala-Narra. Co-published simultaneously in *Journal of Aggression, Maltreatment & Trauma* (The Haworth Maltreatment & Trauma Press, an imprint of The Haworth Press, Inc.) Vol. 14, No. 1/2, 2007, pp. 1-7; and: *Sources and Expressions of Resiliency in Trauma Survivors: Ecological Theory, Multicultural Practice* (ed: Mary R. Harvey, and Pratyusha Tummala-Narra) The Haworth Maltreatment & Trauma Press, an imprint of The Haworth Press, Inc., 2007, pp. 1-7. Single or multiple copies of this article are available for a fee from The Haworth Document Delivery Service [1-800-HAWORTH, 9:00 a.m. - 5:00 p.m. (EST). E-mail address: docdelivery@haworthpress.com].

articles that comprise this volume, emphasizing their status both as individually unique and worthwhile contributions to this literature and as a collection of works that speak powerfully to the promise of multi-cultural research and practice and to the need for a theoretical framework able to account for wide variations in individual expressions of psychological trauma, trauma recovery, and resilience. For us as co-editors of this volume, that framework resides in the ecological perspective of community psychology and in the attention to culture and context inherent in ecological theory. doi:10.1300/J146v14n01_01 *[Article copies available for a fee from The Haworth Document Delivery Service: 1-800-HAWORTH. E-mail address: <docdelivery@haworthpress.com> Website: <http://www.HaworthPress.com> © 2007 by The Haworth Press, Inc. All rights reserved.]*

**KEYWORDS.** Trauma, resilience, culture, context, ecological theory

Violence, abuse, tragedy, and catastrophe know no national boundaries. Indeed, they make themselves at home in nations, cultures, homes, and communities throughout the globe. As a result, there is growing recognition in the traumatic stress studies field–and among clinicians, social scientists, and human rights activists worldwide–of the need for greater understanding of the nature, impact, and mediators of traumatic exposure and response among trauma survivors from diverse cultures and contexts.

To date, much of the literature on psychological trauma has been characterized by a relative overemphasis on the diagnosis of PTSD, a relative under-emphasis on a broader spectrum of traumatic disorders, including what Judith Herman (1992) has referred to as "complex PTSD," and too little attention to contextual mediators of individual and community responses to traumatic exposure. Fortunately, there is evident in the emerging literature not only a needed interest in culture and context, but an equally great and growing interest in the phenomenon of resiliency and the possibility of recovery in the aftermath of traumatic exposure: recovery as a result of clinical intervention, yes, but also recovery as a result of the many internal and external resources that trauma survivors are able to craft and call upon in widely diverse environments.

The articles that comprise this volume are presented not only as individually unique and worthwhile contributions to this emerging literature, but also as a collectivity of works that together speak to the promise of multi-cultural research and practice and to the need for a theoretical framework capable of accounting for the variations in individual expressions of psychological trauma, trauma recovery, and resilience that are witnessed throughout the world and in diverse contexts. For us, that framework resides in the ecological perspective of community psychology and in the attention to culture and context inherent in ecological theory.

In preparing this volume and in selecting the articles presented here, we have been guided by multiple goals, namely: (a) to offer an ecological framework for understanding the multiple sources and expressions of resiliency that trauma survivors may bring to the challenge of trauma recovery, (b) to consider the applicability of this framework to the lives of trauma survivors, treated and untreated, from culturally, politically, and economically diverse social contexts, (c) to examine the cross-cultural utility of an ecologically informed approach (and companion assessment tools) to assessing trauma impact, recovery, and resilience in survivors from diverse contexts, and (d) to consider the implications of this framework for clinical practice, community intervention, and social change in the wake of violence. We thank the authors who have contributed to this volume, for we believe that they have helped us realize each of these goals.

We also want to note the process involved in compiling this volume, which reflects our shared interest in trauma recovery and resilience, and our shared clinical experience with diverse populations. In our vision for this volume, we recognize a growing need to integrate various clinical and empirical perspectives in better understanding the process of recovery in trauma survivors.

This volume is divided into four sections. The first of these is entitled, simply *"Theory."* Harvey's lead article examines the theoretical perspectives, values, and research contributions of community psychology, particularly as these can inform our understanding of resilient responses to traumatic exposure and provide guidelines for effective, multi-level interventions to foster resilience in trauma survivors and their communities. She derives from this analysis five premises of an ecologically informed understanding of the resilience that trauma survivors from diverse environments may exhibit as they "transact" their recovery. The services, program components, and research activities of the Victims of Violence (VOV) Program, which she co-founded with her colleague Judith Herman some 20 years ago, are presented as case examples of ecological theory in action. Next, Tummala-Narra examines the role of culture and cultural context, not only as sources of resilience and supports to trauma recovery, but also as sources of very different and sometimes culturally specific definitions of "trauma," "resilience," and "recovery." Drawing on research concerning the role of race, culture, and class and underscoring the ways in which theory, research, and practice with trauma survivors have too often failed to attend to the overarching role of culture, she emphasizes the need for multiculturally informed inquiry and practice and the centrality of multicultural awareness in an ecological understanding of trauma. Finally, she offers a case example from her own clinical practice to illustrate the possibilities for recovery and healing available to patients of multiculturally aware practitioners.

Articles in the second section are grouped together under the title *"Assessing Resilience: Multiple Dimensions, Multiple Approaches."* Each of the papers that comprise this section makes use of assessment tools developed in the context of the VOV's Trauma Recovery and Resiliency Research Project, namely the Multidimensional Trauma Recovery and Resiliency Scale (MTRR-99) and Interview (MTRRI), designed as companion measures to assess trauma impact, recovery, and resilience on each of eight domains of psychological functioning and to operationalize the trauma recovery criteria described by Harvey's (1996) ecological framework. Developed for use with both clinical and community samples of trauma survivors, the MTRR-99 permits quantitative comparisons of trauma survivors at different stages of recovery and/or with different types of trauma histories. The MTRR-I can be administered to trauma survivors who are receiving or have received clinical care and to those who have had little or no clinical care. The interview can be rated using the MTRR scale (Harvey et al., 2003) and its narrative material can be analyzed for insights into the complex processes by which trauma survivors struggle to overcome and make meaning of their experience (Harvey, Mishler, Koenen, & Harvey, 2000).

The papers that comprise this section illustrate the multiple assessment approaches made possible by the MTRR measures. Liang, Tummala-Narra, Bradley, and Harvey examine the psychometric properties of the MTRR-99, an abridged (and psychometrically improved) version of original MTRR scale (Harvey et al., 2003), and consider its utility with both clinical and non-clinical samples of trauma survivors. Next, Lynch, Keasler, Reaves, Channer, and Bukowski leave quantitative analysis behind and probe a group of MTRR-I narratives for greater understanding of the strengths that complexly traumatized survivors may evince even early in the recovery process. Finally, Sorsoli mines the layered intricacies of a single narrative for greater understanding of the intersection between race, resilience, and complex trauma. The English language versions are of both measures, and instructions to the reader for accessing non-English translations of them, are presented as Apendices A and B to this volume.

Sorsoli's paper provides a bridge to the papers presented in the third section of this volume, titled *"Multicultural Assessment of Trauma, Recovery and Resilience."* Over the past decade, the MTRR measures have found their way into the hands of clinicians and researchers around the country and indeed around the globe. They have been translated into Spanish, French, Portuguese, and Japanese and have been used in studies of both treated and untreated survivors from five countries and diverse settings. The papers found here are representative of the range of researchers, research participants, and research contexts that are contributing to our own growing understanding of the ecological forces influencing risk and resiliency among trauma survivors and their communities.

Together, these papers also make evident both the need for and the promises of cross-cultural research involving shared constructs, common tools, and diverse methodologies. Bradley and Davino, for example, utilized the MTRR-I and the MTRR-99 as well as other measures to inquire into the resilient capacities of incarcerated women, many of them African American, whose lives in prison followed upon years of exposure to violence and abuse outside of prison. Their paper, among other things, provides support for the correspondence of MTRR findings with more familiar measures of trauma-engendered psychopathology, and also for the ability of the MTRR measures to detect expressions of strength and resilience across the indexed domains that are seldom if ever tapped by other measures. Radan translated the MTRR-I into Spanish and used it to conduct in-depth interviews with Central American women, all of whom had survived war in their homelands (and, many of them, violence in their new land) and most of whom had never received clinical treatment as a result of their experiences. Rating their interviews using the MTRR-99, she found evidence of considerable resilience across multiple domains. She also found at least some descriptions reflective of culturally familiar adaptations to trauma among Latina women to be missing in the MTRR-99 items and suggests that future versions of the measure make room for the inclusion of culture-specific items in the indexed domains. Daigneault, Cyr, and Tourigny translated the MTRR measures into French and conducted initial and follow-up interviews with French-speaking Canadian ado-

lescents who had come to the attention of child protective services because of documented intrafamilial sexual abuse. This paper, like Radan's,
considers the applicability of the ecological framework and the cross-
cultural utility of (and modifications needed in) the MTRR measures.
And, finally, Peddle, using the English version of the MTRR-I, describes adaptations she made to the MTRR-I protocol in order to allow
family members of culturally diverse refugees who had experienced
torture and political violence to co-participate in qualitative interviews.
What is exciting to us about all of these papers is the extent to which
they have found the premises of an ecological framework and a multidimensional conception of trauma recovery and resilience to resonate
with their own experiences of the very different groups of trauma survivors with whom they have worked. Equally exciting are the prospects
for future collaborations among the authors whose work is represented
here and the possibilities for shared cross-cultural work on and with the
MTRR measures.

The final section of this volume is entitled "*Ecologically Informed
Intervention.*" Five papers comprise this section. Together they speak to
the need for theory to serve as a viable foundation for individual, community, and societal interventions to foster and mobilize resilience in
the aftermath of trauma. Tummala-Narra begins with a clinical case discussion and a detailed consideration of how dynamically formulated individual psychotherapy that is informed by ecological theory and is
attentive to complex influences of culture and context can identify and
help to mobilize the resilient capacities of traumatized patients.
Mendelsohn, Zachary, and Harney consider the role of group psychotherapy and the contributions of ecological theory and a "stages by dimensions" approach to the design and conduct of stage-specific groups.
Next, Gomez and Yassen describe the individual and social advocacy
practices that define the Victim Advocacy and Support Team (VAST)
of the VOV Program, providing case examples of individual advocacy
to support personal safety and empowerment, on the one hand, and social advocacy to bring about social change and systems reform, on the
other. Harvey, Mondesir, and Aldrich follow these papers with a description of the VOV's Community Crisis Response Team and its community empowerment model of intervention along with a case example
that illustrates the role of ecological theory in the design and conduct of
community-level interventions. Each of the forgoing papers make reference to work that is done at the VOV Program, where the ecological
framework guides not only the conduct of clinical care, but also the design and implementation of community interventions and social change

strategies. Together they confirm the value of ecological theory and multicultural analysis as foundations for trauma-focused intervention at multiple ecological levels.

The final paper in this section is by cultural anthropologist Shahla Haeri, who is not from VOV and who examines from an anthropological perspective the resilience expressed in the survival strategies and public demeanor of two Pakistani women, one who had been physically tortured while in police custody but denied having been raped and the other who, with her family, came forward to acknowledge her rape and demand social and political restitution. In her analysis of the contextual nuances of each woman's struggle, Haeri relates the ethnographic methodology of cultural anthropology to the ecological understanding of trauma and resilience with which we began this volume, thus bringing us full circle and confirming not only the cross-cultural viability of this perspective but also its potential for multidisciplinary analysis. Perhaps most importantly, her paper reminds us that as survivors struggle to craft individually resilient strategies in complex social and cultural contexts, they also call upon others to recognize their struggle as a search not only for personal healing and but also for social justice: justice that can only be achieved by social action and political reform.

## REFERENCES

Harvey, M. R. (1996). An ecological view of trauma and trauma recovery. *Journal of Traumatic Stress, 9*, 3-23.

Harvey, M., Mishler, E., Koenen, K., & Harney, P. (2000). In the aftermath of sexual abuse: Making and remaking meaning in narratives of trauma and recovery. *Narrative Inquiry, 10*(2), 291-311.

Harvey, M. R., Liang, B., Harney, P. A., Koenen, K., Tummala-Narra, P., & Lebowitz, L. (2003). A multidimensional approach to the assessment of trauma impact, recovery and resiliency: Five psychometric studies. *Journal of Aggression, Maltreatment & Trauma, 6*(2), 87-109.

Herman, J. L. (1992). *Trauma and recovery.* New York: Basic Books.

doi:10.1300/J146v14n01_01

# SECTION ONE:
# UNDERSTANDING RECOVERY
# AND RESILIENCY:
# THEORY

# Towards an Ecological Understanding of Resilience in Trauma Survivors: Implications for Theory, Research, and Practice

Mary R. Harvey

**SUMMARY.** The ecological perspective of community psychology offers needed understanding of diverse sources and expressions of resilience among trauma survivors. Investigations by community psychologists into the nature of wellness-enhancing interventions and empowering social

Address correspondence to: Mary R. Harvey, PhD, The Victims of Violence Program, 26 Central Street, Somerville, MA 02143

[Haworth co-indexing entry note]: "Towards an Ecological Understanding of Resilience in Trauma Survivors: Implications for Theory, Research, and Practice." Harvey, Mary R. Co-published simultaneously in *Journal of Aggression, Maltreatment & Trauma* (The Haworth Maltreatment & Trauma Press, an imprint of The Haworth Press, Inc.) Vol. 14, No. 1/2, 2007, pp. 9-32; and: *Sources and Expressions of Resiliency in Trauma Survivors: Ecological Theory, Multicultural Practice* (ed: Mary R. Harvey, and Pratyusha Tummala-Narra) The Haworth Maltreatment & Trauma Press, an imprint of The Haworth Press, Inc., 2007, pp. 9-32. Single or multiple copies of this article are available for a fee from The Haworth Document Delivery Service [1-800-HAWORTH, 9:00 a.m. - 5:00 p.m. (EST). E-mail address: docdelivery@haworthpress.com].

change can inform trauma-focused interventions at individual, community, and societal levels. Here, works by selected community psychologists are reviewed. The ecological view of trauma, recovery, and resilience guiding work at the Victims of Violence (VOV) Program, the range and reach of VOV's clinical and community interventions, and elements of its trauma recovery and resiliency research project illustrate the implications and relevance of these works. Five premises of an ecological understanding of resilience in trauma survivors are discussed.

doi:10.1300/J146v14n01_02   *[Article copies available for a fee from The Haworth Document Delivery Service: 1-800-HAWORTH. E-mail address: <docdelivery@haworthpress.com> Website: <http://www.HaworthPress.com> © 2007 by The Haworth Press, Inc. All rights reserved.]*

**KEYWORDS.** Trauma, resilience, ecological theory, community psychology

The field of community psychology, and particularly what Kelly (1968, 1986) and Trickett (1984, 1997) have called the "ecological analogy" of community psychology, have much to offer those of us who are seeking to understand and promote resilient responses to human suffering. In its emphasis on the interdependence of individuals and communities, its focus on the prevention of harm and promotion of wellness, and its interest in the empowering possibilities of ecologically informed intervention, community psychology has generated theoretical frameworks and research paradigms relevant to the study of psychological resilience in trauma survivors (Harvey, 1996; Norris & Thompson, 1995).

This article begins with a brief summary of the range and scope of traumatic events that human beings suffer worldwide and an equally brief review of research documenting the psychological price paid by many exposed to these events. These literatures serve as preludes to more recent developments in the traumatic stress studies field, including its growing interest in sources and expressions of resilience in trauma survivors. The history and tenets of community psychology, and works by selected community psychologists, are reviewed in terms of their contributions to the understanding of resilience and the design of interventions to foster resilience in both individuals and their communities. The ecological view of psychological trauma, recovery, and resilience guiding the work of the Victims of Violence (VOV) Program, the range and reach of VOV's clinical and community interventions, and elements of its trauma recovery and resiliency research project are offered as case illustrations of these contributions.

## THE EPIDEMIOLOGY OF HUMAN SUFFERING

A fair reading of the epidemiological literature of the past 30 years would confirm that huge numbers of individuals in this country and around the world have suffered, or will at some point in their lives suffer, violence, abuse, atrocity, and catastrophe. These experiences are not randomly distributed. Gender, age, income, race, class, and cultural context have a great deal to do with who is at greatest risk of different types of violence. In the United States, as in most other countries, for example, an alarming number of women and children live at substantial risk of physical and sexual violence within their own homes and most intimate relationships (Tjadeen & Thoennes, 1998, 2000). There is by now considerable evidence that abuse in childhood sets the stage for future abuse (Follette, Polusny, Bechtle, & Naugle, 1996) and that violence against women and children has become a public health problem of pandemic proportions (United Nations, 2003).

In the United States, men are more likely to become victims of violence at the hands of strangers (Tjaden & Thoennes, 1998). Around the world, in countries and cultures afflicted by civil strife and international warfare, men are also more likely to encounter the horrors of war as armed combatants. Women and children, the very old and the very young, endure the many other hardships of war (Goldstein, 2001; Graca Machel/United Nations, 1996), becoming "collateral damage" as battle fields invade civilian populations and noncombatant men, women, and children are forced to flee war-torn homelands for uncertain status as refugees. Increasing numbers of children have been witness to genocide, commandeered into armed conflicts as "child soldiers," and forced to recruit and even execute other children (Garbarino, Kostelny, & Dubrow, 1991; Mendelsohn & Straker, 1998; Myers-Walls, 2003). In the context of war, women and girls are subject to repeated rape and treated as "trophies" of war by conquering soldiers and occupying forces. Among them are those who, having been violated by enemy combatants, are ostracized by their communities and abandoned by their families (Gingerich & Leaning, 2004; McKay, 1999).

Apart from these atrocities are a host of natural and manmade disasters affecting entire communities. Earthquakes, floods, and hurricanes annually combine with incidents of school and community violence, industrial catastrophes, and acts of terror and revenge to ensure that here at home and on a worldwide stage, human suffering is broad in scope, diverse in nature.

## THE PSYCHOLOGICAL AFTERMATH OF TRAUMA

Over the course of these same 30 years, researchers and clinicians have drawn convincing links between the extreme events to which human beings are exposed and the symptoms of psychological distress and characterological impairment that can follow such exposure (Ballenger et al., 2004; Bedard, Greif, & Buckley, 2004; Herman, 1992).

That a significant number of men and women in combat suffer immediate, delayed, and ongoing symptoms of PTSD is by now well-established (Figley, 1978; Gallers, Foy, Donahoe, & Goldfarb, 1988; Schnurr, Lunney, Sengupta, & Waelde, 2003). Equally well-documented is the psychological harmfulness of criminal victimization (Kilpatrick, Saunders, Veronen, Best, & Von, 1987), rape (Burgess & Holmstrom, 1974; Koss, 1993), child abuse and incest (Briere & Elliot, 2003; Herman, 1981), disaster (Barron, 2004; Norris, Friedman, & Watson, 2002a, 2000b), and exposure to prolonged and recurrent trauma (Herman, 1992), including the extreme violations of political violence, terrorism, and torture (Goldfield, Mollica, Pesavento, & Farone, 1988; Resnick, Galea, Kilpatrick, & Vlahov, 2004; Turner, 2004) and trafficking and prostitution (Farley et al., 2003). In toll, this research has yielded significant advances in the understanding of PTSD and other posttraumatic disorders, including what Judith Herman (1992) has called "complex PTSD," and led to a rethinking of diagnostic labels, a reexamination of the etiology of emotional disorders, and a search for effective, trauma-focused treatments (Foa, Keane, & Friedman, 2000; Weiss, Saraceno, Saxena, & van Ommeren, 2003).

## NEW DIRECTIONS IN TRAUMA RESEARCH

### An Interest in Untreated Survivors

Community studies of populations exposed either to natural disasters or to violence of human design suggest that individuals differ considerably in their vulnerability to symptom development and the extent to which their early onset symptoms persist (McFarlane & de Yehuda, 1996; Norris, 1992; Norris et al., 2002a). Those who do become symptomatic differ in the nature, duration, and intensity of their symptoms, their interpretations of their experience, and the avenues they pursue to secure symptom relief. These differences reflect a complex interplay of many influences, including: the nature and chronicity of the events to which they have been exposed; demographic factors such as age, race, class, and gender; neurobiological mediators of hardiness and vulnerability; the influence and stability of relevant social, cultural, and political contexts; and any number of ecological factors that support or impede access to natural support, comforting beliefs, and trauma-informed clinical care (Green, Wilson, & Lindy, 1985; Harvey, 1996; Hernandez, 2002; McFarlane & de Yehuda, 1996).

In the face of these findings, it is important that future research not only document the range and extremity of traumatic exposure among untreated survivors, but also determine who within these populations is and is not at risk of symptom development (Yehuda, 2004). Equally important is the development of public health strategies to support positive coping and extend solace and support to those individuals and groups who are unlikely to receive professional care.

## An Interest in Multicultural Influences and the Role of Context

A full understanding of the resilience that trauma survivors may bring to the challenge of trauma recovery requires that clinicians and researchers attend to the influence of cultural and contextual mediators of traumatic response (Hernandez, 2002; Tummala-Narra, 2001 and both articles in this volume). While symptoms of PTSD have been found among trauma survivors of both genders, all ages, and diverse racial, ethnic, and cultural groups, it is also true that particular events (e.g., incest, rape, or spousal abuse) and symptoms (e.g., dissociation, somatic complaints, ataques nervios) may have quite different meanings in different cultural contexts (Radan, this volume). Cultural and community values exert profound influence over a victim's willingness to disclose (or not) a particular incident of violation or abuse (Haeri, this volume), for example, and cultural interpretations of the events to which they have been exposed shape survivors' own understandings of these events (Tummala-Narra, "Conceptualizing trauma," this volume). Finally, cultural groups may differ considerably in their definitions of what is and is not resilient (Hobfoll, Jackson, Hobfoll, Pierce, & Young, 2002).

## An Interest in Resilience

Within the larger body of untreated trauma survivors, and indeed among survivors who do access professional care, are large numbers of individuals who do not develop complete or persistent PTSD despite their experience (Norris et al., 2002a; Yehuda, 2004) and an indeterminate number who seem not only to survive but even to thrive (Tedeschi & Calhoun, 1995; Wild & Pavio, 2003). These groups have created an interest in identifying origins and indices of risk and resilience in trauma survivors (Harvey, 1996; McFarlane & de Yehuda, 1996) and in what has been labeled "positive" or "adversarial" growth posttrauma (Tedeschi & Calhoun, 1995; Linley & Joseph, 2004).

With few exceptions (e.g., Wild & Pavio, 2003), the "resilience" literature and the "positive" or "adversarial" growth literature seldom cross-reference one another. Implied in both, however, is a consensus that resilience is evident when a given event has little or no deleterious impact, presumably because the individual is able to mobilize internal resources that existed pre-trauma, while positive or adversarial growth is manifest post-trauma in a higher level of functioning that has been wrested from a struggle to overcome the devastation of trauma. These distinctions blur, however, as investigators cite as evidence of resilience the ability of some survivors to transform their experience post-trauma (Grossman, Cook, Kepkep, & Koenen, 1999; Higgins, 1994) and as studies of positive or adversarial growth confirm the relevance of attributes that clearly existed pre-trauma (Linley & Joseph, 2004). While both constructs could benefit from further clarification, it seems likely that some degree of resilience pre-trauma is requisite for posttraumatic growth, and that posttraumatic growth is itself a sign of resilience.

Recently, Bonanno (2004) has questioned the approach that trauma researchers have taken to the study of psychological resilience, suggesting that their immersion in the struggles of trauma survivors who clearly require clinical care have led them to view resilience ". . . either as a pathological state or as something seen only in rare and exceptionally healthy individuals" (p. 20). Locating his critique in the spirit of Seligman's and Csikszentmihalyi's (2003) call for a "positive psychology," he suggests that resilience is common, not rare; that individuals pursue multiple pathways to resilience; and that future research must identify the full range of outcomes people suffer and achieve posttrauma.

In fairness, it is important to note that, with few exceptions, most trauma researchers would agree that it is typically a minority (though often a sizeable minority) of survivors who develop severe and long-lasting symptoms (Ballenger et al., 2004). Indeed, according to Yehuda (2004), "The normal path is recovery, which is facilitated by a supportive environment" (p. 35). Needed is knowledge about how to create and sustain such environments.

Like many authors, Bonanno (2004) seems to regard resilience as an all-or-none phenomenon (i.e., one is either resilient or not resilient, affected or not affected). How then do we classify the incest survivor who in the daytime performs exceedingly well at a challenging job where she enjoys amicable relationships with her colleagues, but at night may be afraid to sleep because of recurrent nightmares in which she relives the many horrors of her childhood? She functions well during the work-week, but is isolated, anxious, and lonely on the weekends. Is she resilient? Is she impaired? Is it possible she might be both? Clinical practice and recent research suggest that resilience is a multidimensional phenomenon and that she is indeed both complexly traumatized and resilient (Lynch, Keasler, Reaves, Channer, & Bukowski, this volume). Similarly, how are we to classify the illegal immigrant who makes it out of a war-torn homeland, across dangerous borders and into the United States where s/he is able to secure employment and send money home, but is beset by symptoms of depression, anxiety, and PTSD? Research with war refugees (Peddle, this volume; Radan, this volume) suggests that this person, too, is both resilient and distressed, and that resilience co-occurs with even severe distress.

When resilience is defined as multidimensional (Harvey, 1996), it becomes possible to see trauma survivors as simultaneously suffering and surviving, and to suggest that both trauma recovery and the process of posttraumatic growth require the survivor to somehow access his or her resilient capacities. The need now is to augment research on the psychopathology of trauma with investigations into developmental and contextual mediators of resilient response and the nature of interventions able to foster resilience in traumatized individuals and their communities.

## THE CONTRIBUTIONS OF COMMUNITY PSYCHOLOGY

Complementing these relatively recent inquiries into the nature and nurture of resilience in trauma survivors is a long-standing interest among community psychologists in the promotion of wellness, the influence of context on psychological functioning, and the empowering possibilities of ecologically informed intervention at individual, community, and societal levels.

## Community Psychology: A Brief History

The field of community psychology was formally "birthed" at Swampscott (MA) in 1965 when 39 participants gathered to consider the future of psychology in the then-growing community mental health movement. Those in attendance questioned the mental health field's preoccupation with individual psychopathology, its bias towards person-centered analysis and intervention, and its neglect of environmental variables (Caplan & Nelson, 1973). Determined that psychology had a role to play in addressing and ameliorating such social ills as poverty, racism, oppression, and discrimination, participants in the Swampscott Conference went on to generate new conceptual frameworks, engage in social action and social action research with oppressed and marginalized community groups, and promote individual, community, and social change by means of multi-level, competency-oriented interventions (Heller & Monahan, 1977).

Since Swampscott, community psychologists have brought to bear on the field's continuing development the tenets of liberation psychology (Watts & Serrano-Garcia, 2003), the overarching goal of social justice (Fondacaro & Weinberg, 2002; Prilletiensky, 2001), and the premises of feminist theory and research (Bond & Mulvey, 2000; Koss & Harvey, 1991; Riger, 2001). They have also generated theoretical frameworks and research paradigms for examining the reciprocal influences of persons and contexts. Particularly relevant to the understanding of resilience is the ecological perspective guiding these inquiries (Harvey, 1996; Kelly, 1968; Norris & Thompson, 1995; Trickett, Kelly, & Vincent, 1985).

## The Ecological Perspective of Community Psychology

Community psychologists share with field biologists the premise that organisms live (i.e., survive, thrive, or decline) in interdependence with their environments. The ecological analogy incorporates a "resource perspective," assuming that human communities, like other living environments, evolve adaptively and can be described in terms of their development, preservation, and exchange of community resources (Hobfoll & Lilly, 1993; Kelly, 1986). These resources include the people who comprise a community's membership and the qualities they bring to bear on community development; the formal and informal settings that define community membership and both nurture and proscribe competencies, values, and beliefs vital to community life; and the events that mark, celebrate, and sometimes challenge a community's identity vis a vis the larger world (Koss & Harvey, 1991). Healthy and health-promoting community ecosystems are characterized by an abundance and diversity of these resources and by multiple opportunities to participate in and influence community life (Heller & Monahan, 1977).

An implication of the ecological perspective is that resilience is transactional in nature, evident in qualities that are nurtured, shaped, and activated by a host of person-environment interactions. Resilience is the result not only of biologically given traits, but also of people's embeddedness in complex and dynamic social contexts, contexts that are themselves more or less vulnerable to harm, more or less amenable to change, and apt focal points for intervention. Moreover, within these contexts, individuals are not simply the passive recipients of contextual forces; rather they are "agentic, capable of negotiating and influencing, as well as being influenced by context" (Riger, 2001, p. 75).

*Pathways to wellness: Guidelines for health-promoting preventive intervention.* The engagement of persons and contexts creates possibilities for enhancing both individual and community wellness. Studying these engagements, community psychologist Emory Cowen (1994) has identified five "pathways to wellness" and corresponding opportunities for wellness-promoting interventions throughout the lifespan and at multiple ecological levels. The pathway he calls "forming wholesome early attachments," for example, is salient early in childhood and recognizes the importance of early, family-focused interventions to nurture positive parent-child attachments. A second pathway, "acquiring age- and ability-appropriate competencies," gains importance later when intervention programs in settings relevant to developing youth can offer compensatory wellness-support to children who have not received adequate care and nurturance earlier in life. "Exposure to settings that favor wellness outcomes," pathway three, highlights the need to create a variety of social milieus in which diverse individuals and groups can develop a sense of belongingness, relatedness, and self-esteem. "Having the empowering sense of being in control of one's fate," pathway four, and "coping effectively with stress," pathway five, are relevant to wellness outcomes across groups and developmental stages. However, empowering interventions may be particularly vital to the well-being of oppressed, disadvantaged, and marginalized groups, while interventions to promote positive coping may be crucial in the face of stress and adversity.

For Cowen (1994), these pathways constitute "mutually enhancing elements in an elaborate system" (p. 159). Interventions to foster positive attachments in early childhood support the child's acquisition of age-appropriate competencies later in childhood, and access to settings that promote competence, agency, and empowerment will play an important role in preparing individuals to cope with stress and adversity.

*The power of social contexts.* Community psychologist Rudolf Moos (2002, 2003) and his colleagues have spent decades studying the ways in which individuals and social contexts influence one another and what attributes of social context might underlie the beneficial effects of intervention. These attributes, he suggests, can be categorized into three broad dimensions that have salience across multiple settings: (a) Relationship dimensions include such attributes as participants' support of one another and the degree of spontaneity and open expression among them; (b) Personal growth and goal orientation dimensions include the extent to which the context provides opportunities for personal growth; and (c) system maintenance and change dimensions include qualities such as clarity of purpose and responsiveness to change. Moos' (2003) research further suggests that intervention programs function as transient social contexts and can be assessed on these same dimensions. Supportive relationships and group cohesion among intervention participants, reasonably high expectations for personal growth, clear goals, and a moderate degree of structure are associated with positive intervention outcomes, for example. However, while the more enduring contexts of family, school, workplace, and established community setting exert both powerful and relatively long-lasting impacts on individual health and well-being, even highly effective interventions will have short-lived influence without post-intervention support from familiar social and cultural contexts (Moos, 2002, 2003).

The literature of community psychology is replete with investigations into the attributes of effective intervention programs (see, e.g., Durlak & Wells, 1997; Harvey, 1985; Paster, 1980). Invariably, these studies confirm that: (a) the beneficial influence of interventions depends heavily on their knowledge of and responsiveness to contextual influences, and (b) the durability of an intervention's influence depends on if and how its effects are incorporated into the life and culture of more enduring social contexts. At the level of individually-focused interventions, mutual self-help groups have proven effective vehicles for providing on-going support to participants in time-limited clinical interventions (Moos, 2003). In a similar vein, stage-specific group treatment may offer to trauma survivors an "ecological bridge" to new and safer community (Mendelsohn, Zachary, & Harney, this volume). At the level of local community, sound knowledge of existing resources and the "match" achieved between intervention resources and a target community's resource needs are essential to intervention success (Sandler, 2001). Equally important is a collaborative relationship with community members who can help to sustain the beneficial effects of intervention (Paster, 1980). The empowerment model of community crisis response (Harvey, Mondesir, & Aldrich, this volume), for example, is one that seeks to augment the resources of traumatized communities and to link the short-term goal of timely, collaborative trauma-focused response with the longer term goal of community capacity-building.

*The influence and nuances of cultural mediators.* An ecological perspective includes the supposition that culture matters and that attentiveness to nuances of culture, race, and ethnicity is essential to the design of health-promoting interventions. Community psychologist Ed Trickett (1996) refers to a "diversity of contexts" in recognition of the many and varied cultural contexts within which individuals develop and are socialized, and to "contexts of diversity" in recognition of the fact that broad generalizations about race, class, and culture are not helpful. Instead, phenomena such as ethnic identity are "potentially fluid, negotiated in the differing settings of importance, and intimately connected to the complex interdependence of cultural history, current circumstance and future aspiration" (Trickett, 1996, p. 218).

In applying an ecological perspective to the understanding of resilience in diverse cultural contexts, Tummala-Narra ("Conceptualizing trauma," this volume) notes that prevailing views of resilience are generally shaped by middleclass and Western values of individual autonomy and achievement, values that may not resonate across cultures and may not reflect culturally salient views of positive response to adversity. Hobfoll et al. (2002) suggest that across cultural contexts, expressions of agency and mastery may rely on different loci of control (i.e., the self in many Western cultures, the family or the community in others). Interventions to foster resilience in non-mainstream cultural contexts must be alert to these differences.

Developing ecologically relevant and effective interventions requires attention not only to differences *between* but also to differences *within* racial, cultural, and ethnic groups, and consideration of the ways in which these differences are expressed, highlighted, concealed, and negotiated in various social contexts (Kelly, 1986; Trickett, 1996; Tummala-Narra, "Conceptualizing trauma," this volume). Other factors influencing the efficacy of interventions in specific cultural contexts include the meaning of an intervention to participants, its relevance and appropriateness to participants and settings, the cultural validity of its underlying constructs, and cultural and contextual factors affecting the durability of its impact over time (Trickett, 1997).

*Transforming social environments.* Contextual forces can impede as well as foster individual and community well-being. Because social problems are often deeply embedded in relatively intransigent social environments and long-standing cultural practices, community psychologist Kenneth Maton (2000) emphasizes the importance of intervention programs that have as their goal the transformation of social environments. He identifies four dimensions of social environments that are amenable to change and four corresponding intervention goals: (a) capacity-building to reform the instrumental attributes of a social environment (e.g., core activities, problem-solving capacities, leadership); (b) group empowerment to restructure social environments and alter power relationships and resource distribution among social groups; (c) relational community building to develop new relational norms for social environments and ensure an array of opportunities to a diverse citizenry; and (d) culture-challenge to address aspects of prevailing cultural norms that contribute to the persistence of social problems.

Interventions to pursue these goals can be initiated at multiple ecological levels. At the individual level, for example, culture challenge may involve asking individuals to rethink familiar understandings and abandon long-standing biases. At the community level, it may require activism to create new community settings or to reform existing ones, and at the societal level, participation in movements for social reform and social justice. Each of Maton's (2000) goals has relevance to the design of interventions to support the resilient capacities of trauma survivors and their communities. Each is represented, too, in the clinical, community, and research activities of the Victims of Violence Program.

## THE VICTIMS OF VIOLENCE PROGRAM

The Victims of Violence Program (VOV) is an adult outpatient trauma clinic located in a multi-site urban public health system that serves a diverse client population, including large numbers of economically disenfranchised citizens and growing numbers of immigrants and political refugees from Africa, Asia, Latin America, Haiti, and the Mid-

dle East. Initiated in 1984 with start-up funds from local city government, VOV was established as a training program of the hospital's
academically affiliated Department of Psychiatry in 1985. Since then,
its mission in the hospital, in the network of health care services in
which it is located, and in the larger community has been to develop
comprehensive mental health services for crime victims and crime victimized communities

## Services and Service Components of the VOV

VOV's services include crisis intervention and response, psychological assessment and longer-term clinical care, and a wide array of
groups. Clinical care at VOV is guided by an ecological view of psychological trauma (Harvey, 1996; Yassen & Harvey, 1998) and a "stages by
dimensions" understanding of trauma recovery (Lebowitz, Harvey, &
Herman, 1992; Mendelsohn et al., this volume). This framework emphasizes the importance of attending to lives in context and the need for
clinical care with trauma survivors to focus, first, on securing and maintaining personal safety and, then, on forming new, more empowered relationships with others.

Since its inception, VOV has secured grant funding[1] to create and
sustain new resources for communities and community settings afflicted
by violence. VOV's Community Crisis Response Team (CCRT), initiated in 1988, translates an ecological view of psychological trauma
(Harvey, 1996) into a protocol for timely intervention in diverse contexts (Harvey et al., this volume). Its Victim Advocacy and Support
Team (VAST), initiated in 2000, brings the lessons of grass roots activism to bear on clinical care and clinical training (Gomez & Yassen,
this volume), and its more recently initiated Center for Homicide Bereavement (CHB) integrates clinical and community care for individuals and families bereaved by homicide.

## An Ecological View of Psychological Trauma, Trauma Recovery, and Resilience

VOV's varied services and program components reflect the organizing influence of an ecological view of psychological trauma and trauma
recovery (Harvey, 1996). Drawing directly upon the ecological perspective of community psychology, this framework proposes that individual differences in traumatic response (and, indeed, in risk of
traumatic exposure) are the result of complex interactions among per-

son, event, and environmental factors. Interdependent and reciprocal interactions among these factors set the stage for more or less resilient and agentic responses to traumatic exposure, help to determine the quality and availability of informal sources of social support and underlie both access to and comfort with professional care.

The ecological model includes a definition of trauma recovery that is hallmarked by achievements in eight domains of psychological functioning (Harvey, 1996; also see Liang, Tummala-Narra, Bradley & Harvey, this volume). Resilience is understood to be a multidimensional phenomenon. A survivor may be seriously impaired in one or more domains typically impacted by trauma and yet evince remarkable strengths in others. Resilience is also conceptualized as an active process by which individual survivors are able to access strengths in some domains in order to secure recovery in others. An important goal of psychotherapy with trauma survivors is to recognize and help the survivor mobilize his or her resilient capacities.

Recognizing that most trauma survivors will not turn to psychotherapy (or any other highly specialized form of professional care), the ecological framework also acknowledges the importance of environmental interventions to foster wellness and enhance resilience among untreated trauma survivors and their communities. At VOV, environmental interventions towards these ends include not only the CCRT, VAST, and the CHB, but also year-round staff involvement in anti-violence coalitions, public education campaigns, and human rights activism.

### Ecologically Informed Intervention and Research at the VOV

The ecological framework provides theoretical foundation for clinical care, community intervention, and research at VOV.

*Clinical assessment and clinical care.* Clinical intervention at VOV begins with an assessment that attends not only to signs and symptoms of distress but also to attitudes and values prevailing in the larger society and in the client's cultural context and home community. It asks the clinician to inquire not only about the behavior of family members and friends, but also about the actions of medical, mental health and social service providers, criminal justice personnel, and religious and community figures. One goal of this assessment is insight into the ways in which clients' location in complex ecological networks shapes their experience of and adaptive (and/or maladaptive) coping with trauma. Another is that assessment set the stage for care that will foster safer connections with others and new, more empowered action in the world outside of therapy.

*Community intervention, social advocacy, and social action.* Within VOV the aims of community-wide interventions are guided by respect for ecological context. The goals of community intervention are to address the community's vulnerability and promote community healing, not by replacing or overwhelming but rather by augmenting and enhancing existing community resources. These aims infuse all VOV services but are perhaps most clearly recognized in the outreach, consultation, and intervention strategies of the CCRT and in VAST's integration of individual and social advocacy practices. Both programs are described in depth in articles included in this volume (Harvey et al.; Gomez & Yassen).

*Ecologically-informed research on resilience in trauma survivors.* The ecological model suggests that full understanding of psychological trauma, recovery, and resilience requires research with both treated and untreated survivors and the delineation of factors relevant to recovery in both populations. Research at VOV, therefore, incorporates attention to the experience of trauma survivors from diverse contexts and at various points in the recovery process, as well as inquiry into the cross-cultural applicability of constructs and assessment tools developed in the context of our Trauma Recovery and Resiliency Research Project. Within this project, the multidimensional definition of trauma recovery and resilience (Harvey, 1996) has been operationalized in the form of two assessment tools: the Multidimensional Trauma Recovery and Resiliency scale (the MTRR-99) and companion interview, the MTRR-I.[2] These measures can aid clinicians in their search for a nuanced understanding of the strengths that trauma survivors bring with them to psychotherapy (Lynch et al., this volume; Tummala-Narra, "Trauma and resilience," this volume), and can be used with treated and nontreated survivors in studies of resilience in racially, culturally, and linguistically diverse survivors (Bradley & Davino, this volume; Daigneault, Cyr, & Tourigny, this volume; Radan, this volume;).

## *DISCUSSION*

The literature of community psychology, the contributions of the community psychologists whose work has been reviewed here, and the now twenty-year history of VOV highlight the relevance of ecological theory to the understanding of resilience in trauma survivors and the salience of ecological considerations in the design and conduct of interventions to nurture and mobilize the resilient capacities of trauma survivors and their communities.

## An Ecological View of Resilience in Trauma Survivors: Five Premises

Five premises, each with corresponding implications for ecologically informed intervention and each supported by the theory and practice of community psychology, offer a new and deeper understanding of psychological resilience in trauma survivors. Each has been instrumental in shaping theory, practice, research, and training at the VOV.

- Resilience is best understood as both transactional and contextual, arising from the reciprocal engagement of persons and contexts. Persons and contexts, individuals and communities, groups and societies, survivors and ecosystems are appropriate focal points for interventions to foster resilience among those at risk.
- Resilience is also a multidimensional phenomenon, expressed in relative degrees across multiple domains of psychological functioning. Expressions of resilience can co-exist with symptoms of even severe psychopathology. A goal of clinical intervention is to help the survivor mobilize his/her resilient capacities. A goal of social and community intervention is to develop social contexts that can foster wellness and sustain multiple modes of resilience among those at risk and those who have already suffered harm.
- Whether initiated at individual, community, or societal level, interventions to promote and sustain resilience must enhance the relationship between person and context. Communities characterized by a wide diversity of resources and multiple opportunities for community members to influence community life are ideal contexts for persons to become resilient. Contributing to the development of such contexts is or ought to be an explicit goal of social and community interventions to promote resilient functioning.
- Attention to cultural context and nuance is an important determinant of intervention efficacy; culture challenge may be an important component of meaningful intervention.
- Finally, even highly effective interventions will rely for lasting impact on their becoming embedded in and familiar to more enduring social settings and community contexts. Attention to the possibili-

ties for ensuring lasting impact and enduring change are important features of intervention design and conduct.

## VOV and the Ecological Perspective of Community Psychology

In many ways, VOV is a unique intervention program located in an equally unique social context. In other respects, it can be viewed as an evolving example of ecological theory in action. From the perspective of community psychology, VOV can be viewed as follows:

*An exemplar of ecologically informed intervention.* VOV began life not only as a new clinical service for trauma survivors, but also as a self-conscious commitment to enhancing the victim service resources of our local community, altering the ecology of a relatively traditional psychiatric setting and changing the ecological relationship between crime victims and the larger community. In its 20-year history, the program has evolved from a small, poorly funded, and quite marginalized intervention program into an elaborate set of service, training, and research activities and into a relatively well-established community setting. The challenge now is for VOV to remain a source of innovation and itself become a context amenable to change.

*A partner with and consultant to other community resources.* Heeding Moos' (2003) advice that intervention programs depend for lasting impact on the support of enduring social contexts, VOV staff have maintained and further developed strong ties with the grassroots feminist organizations that nurtured us twenty-plus years ago. We have also developed strong and reciprocal relationships with victim advocacy, human rights, and anti-violence programs throughout the greater metropolitan area as well as with other psychiatric settings serving trauma survivors. We have exchanged consultation, training, and other resources with these organizations and groups and worked with them to form a collaborative network we are all able to call upon for political and social support. And in our engagement with others in the traumatic stress studies field, we have been able to benefit from and contribute to national and international dialog concerning the needs of trauma survivors and the possibilities of clinical and community intervention on their behalf.

*A sponsor of capacity-building interventions and new community resources.* The CCRT (Harvey et al., this volume), VAST (Gomez & Yassen, this volume), and CHB are emblematic of VOV's efforts to develop new community resources, contribute to the development of new competencies and capacities in traumatized individuals and communities and to, in Cowen's (1994) language, create new and needed wellness-enhancing settings. Each of these services is located in the community, not the hospital; each is an integral component of VOV; and each is making a unique contribution to the changing ecosystems of both hospital and community.

*A setting characterized by increasing diversity and attentiveness to issues of race, class, and culture.* Like many feminist programs, VOV began life as an undertaking of white, middle-class professional women. Over the years, attentiveness to the limitations of a racially and culturally homogeneous organization, a value for diversity and strategic decisions in terms of staff hiring, program development, and trainee recruitment have enabled VOV to become increasingly diverse. Today, our multiracial, multicultural, and multidisciplinary staff is a much closer "match" to the population we serve. It includes men as well as women and a range of linguistic capabilities that were unimagined by us when we began. These changes have not occurred free of tensions and misunderstandings, and the work is certainly not done. However, the benefits of diversity are clear in range of services we are able to provide, the multicultural competencies we are developing, and our own growing comfort with our diversity

In sum, VOV's origins and evolution, its varied service, research, and training activities, and its engagements with health care system, local community, and larger society are indicative of the potent contributions that community psychology can make to helpful and timely trauma-focused clinical care, to culturally relevant social and community interventions, to ecologically informed research with trauma survivors from diverse social and cultural contexts, and to a new and needed understanding of the resilience that trauma survivors and traumatized communities can bring to bear on the process of trauma recovery.

## CONCLUDING REMARKS

Maton (2000) describes the women's movement as illustrative of the power, possibilities, and reciprocal influences of integrated social transformation strategies. It is important to note, then, that VOV traces its origins and much of its continuing passion for social justice to the women's movement. Feminism has shaped our understandings of violence, gender, and culture, given direction to our personal, professional, and political aspirations, and supported our own resilience in the face of recurrent exposure to violence and abuse. In our partnerships with local feminist organizations and our international ties to feminist colleagues and activists, VOV staff participate in local, national, and international campaigns for societal transformation. It is through our engagement with these that we are constantly reminded of the enormous resilience that trauma survivors are able to craft from supportive social and cultural contexts.

## NOTES

1. The Community Crisis Response Team, Victim Advocacy and Support Team, and Center for Homicide Bereavement of the Victims of Violence Program are supported by federal Victim of Crime Act funds awarded by the Massachusetts Victim Witness Assistance Board. The Victim Advocacy and Support Team receives additional grant support from the Office of Victim of Crime for services to victims of domestic and international trafficking.

2. The English-language versions of the MTRR-99 and the MTRR-I are included in this volume. Spanish and French translations of the MTRR-I can be obtained from the authors of papers included in this volume: Angela Radan, PhD (Spanish), and Isabelle Daigneault (French). The Japanese translation can be obtained by contacting Dr. Kuniko Muramoto, PhD, at kunikomura@mub.biglobe.ne.jp

## REFERENCES

Ballenger, J. C., Davidson, J. R. T., Lecrubier, Y., Nutt, D. J., Marshall, R. D., Nemeroff, C. B. et al. (2004). Consensus statement update on posttraumatic stress disorder from the international consensus group on depression and anxiety. *Journal of Clinical Psychiatry, 65*(Suppl. 1), 55-62.

Barron, R. A. (2004) International disaster mental health. *Psychiatric Clinics of North America, 27,* 505-519.

Bedard, M., Greif, J. L., & Buckley, T. C. (2004) International publication trends in the traumatic stress literature. *Journal of Traumatic Stress, 17*(2), 97-101.

Bonanno, G. (2004). Loss, trauma and human resilience: Have we underestimated the human capacity to thrive after extremely aversive events? *American Psychologist, 59*(1), 20-28.

Bond, M. A., & Mulvey, A. (2000) A history of women and feminist perspectives in community psychology. *American Journal of Community Psychology, 28*(5), 599-629.

Bradley, R., & Davino, K. (2007). Interpersonal violence, recovery and resilience in incarcerated women. *Journal of Aggression, Maltreatment & Trauma, 14*(1/2), 123-146.

Briere, J., & Elliott, D. M. (2003) Prevalence and symptomatic sequelae of self-reported childhood physical and sexual abuse in a general population sample of men and women. *Child Abuse and Neglect, 27,* 1205-1222.

Burgess, A. W.. & Holmstrom, L. L. (1974). Rape trauma syndrome. *American Journal of Psychiatry, 131*, 981-986.

Caplan, N., & Nelson, S. D. (1973). On being useful: the nature and consequences of psychological research on social problems. *American Psychologist, 28*, 299-211.

Cowen, E. L. (1994). The enhancement of psychological wellness: Challenges and opportunities. *American Journal of Community Psychology, 22*(4), 149-177.

Daigneault, I., Cyr, M., & Tourigny, M. (2007). Exploration of recovery trajectories in sexually abused adolescents. *Journal of Aggression, Maltreatment & Trauma, 14*(1/2), 165-184.

Durlak. J. A., & Wells, A. M. (1997). Primary prevention mental health programs for children and adolescents: A meta-analytic review. *American Journal of Community Psychology, 25*(2), 115-152.

Farley, M., Cotton. A., Lynne, J., Zumbeck, S., Spiwak, F., Reyes, M. et al. (2003). Prostitution and trafficking in nine countries: An update on violence and post-traumatic stress disorder. In M. Farley (Ed.), *Prostitution, trafficking and traumatic stress* (pp. 33-74). Binghamton, NY: Haworth Press.

Figley. C. R. (1978). Psychosocial adjustment among Vietnam veterans: An overview of the research. In C.R. Figley (Ed.), *Stress disorders among Vietnam veterans* (pp 57-70). New York: Brunner/Mazel.

Foa, E. G., Keane, T., & Friedman, M. J. (Eds.) (2000). *Effective treatments for PTSD: Practice guidelines from the International Society for Traumatic Stress Studies.* New York: Guilford.

Follette. V. M.. Polusny, M. A., Bechtle, A. E., & Naugle, A.E. (1996). Cumulative trauma: The impact of child sexual abuse, adult sexual assault, and spouse abuse. *Journal of Traumatic Stress, 9*, 25-35.

Fondacaro, M. R., & Weinberg, D. (2002). Concepts of social justice in community psychology: Toward a social ecological epistemology. *American Journal of Community Psychology, 30*(4), 473-492.

Gallers. J., Foy, D. W., Donahoe, C. P., & Goldfarb, J. (1988). Post-traumatic stress disorder in Vietnam combat veterans: Effects of traumatic violence exposure and military adjustment. *Journal of Traumatic Stress, 1*(2), 181-192.

Garbarino, J., Kostelny, K.. & Dubrow, N. (1991). *No place to be a child: Growing up in a war zone.* Lexington, MA: D.C. Heath and Company.

Gingerich. T., & Leaning. J. (2004). *The use of rape as a weapon of war in the conflict in Darfur, Sudan: Prepared for U.S. Agency for International Development/OTI.* Program on Humanitarian Crises and Human Rights, François-Xavier Bagnoud Center for Health and Human Rights, Harvard School of Public Health, Boston, MA.

Goldfield, A. E., Mollica, R. F., Pesavento, B. H., & Farone, S. V. (1988). The physical and psychological sequelae of torture: Symptomatology and diagnosis. *Journal of the American Medical Association, 259*(18), 2725-2729.

Goldstein, J. (2001). *War and gender: How gender shapes the war system and vice versa.* New York: Cambridge University Press.

Gomez. C., & Yassen, J. (2007). Revolutionizing the clinical frame: Individual and social advocacy practices in the care of trauma survivors. *Journal of Aggression, Maltreatment & Trauma, 14*(1/2), 245-263.

Graca Machel/United Nations Study. (1996). *The impact of armed conflict on children.* New York: United Nations.

Green, B., Wilson, J. P., & Lindy, J. (1985). Conceptualizing post-traumatic stress disorder: A psychosocial framework. In C. R. Figley (Ed.), *Trauma and its wake: The study and treatment of post-traumatic stress disorder* (pp. 53-69). New York: Bruner/Mazel.

Grossman, F. K., Cook, A. B., Kepkep, S. S., & Koenen, K. C. (1999). *With the phoenix rising: Lessons from ten resilient women who overcame the trauma of childhood sexual abuse.* San Francisco: Jossey-Bass.

Haeri, S. (2007). Resiliency and post-traumatic recovery in cultural and political context: Two Pakistani women's strategies for survival. *Journal of Aggression, Maltreatment & Trauma, 14*(1/2), 287-304.

Harvey, M. R. (1985). *Exemplary rape crisis programs: A cross-site analysis and case studies.* Rockville, MD: National Institutes of Mental Health, U.S. Department of Health and Human Services.

Harvey, M. R. (1996). An ecological view of psychological trauma and trauma recovery. *Journal of Traumatic Stress, 9*(1), 3-23.

Harvey, M. S., Mondesir, A., & Aldrich, H. (2007). Fostering resilience in traumatized communities: A community empowerment model of intervention. *Journal of Aggression, Maltreatment & Trauma, 14*(1/2), 265-285.

Heller, K., & Monahan, J. (1977). *Psychology and community change.* Homewood, Ill: The Dorsey Press.

Herman, J. L. (1981). *Father-daughter incest.* New York: Basic Books.

Herman, J. L. (1992). *Trauma and recovery.* New York: Basic Books.

Hernandez, P. (2002). Trauma in war and political persecution: Expanding the concept. *American Journal of Orthopsychiatry, 72*(1), 16-25.

Higgins, G. O. (1994). *Resilient adults: Overcoming a cruel past.* San Francisco, CA: Jossey-Bass.

Hobfoll, S., & Lilly, R. (1993). Resource conservation as a strategy for community psychology. *Journal of Community Psychology, 21*, 128-148.

Hobfoll, S. E., Jackson, A., Hobfoll, I., Pierce, C. A., & Young, S. (2002). The impact of communal-mastery versus self-mastery on emotional outcomes during stressful conditions: A prospective study of Native American women. *American Journal of Community Psychology, 30*(6), 853-871.

Kelly, J. G. (1968) Towards an ecological conception of preventive intervention. In J. W. Carter (Ed.), *Research contributions from psychology to community mental health* (pp 3-57). New York: Behavioral Publications.

Kelly, J. G. (1986). An ecological paradigm: Defining mental health consultation as a preventive service. *Prevention in Human Services, 4*(3/4), 1-35.

Kilpatrick, D. G., Saunders, B. E., Veronen, L. J., Best, C. L. & Von, J. M. (1987). Criminal victimization: Lifetime prevalence, reporting to police, and psychological impact. *Crime and Delinquency, 33*, 479-489.

Koss, M. P. (1993). Rape: Scope, impact, interventions and public policy responses. *American Psychologist, 48*, 1062-1069.

Koss, M., & Harvey, M. (1991). *The rape victim: Clinical and community interventions* (2nd ed.). Newbury Park, CA: Sage.

Lebowitz, L., Harvey. M. R.. & Herman, J. L. (1992). A stage by dimension model of recovery from sexual trauma. *Journal of Interpersonal Violence, 8,* 378-391.

Liang. B.. Tummala-Narra. P., Bradley, R. & Harvey. M. R. (2007). The multidimensional trauma recovery and resiliency instrument: Preliminary examination of an abridged version. *Journal of Aggression, Maltreatment & Trauma, 14*(1/2), 55-74.

Linley, P. A., & Joseph, S. (2004). Positive change following trauma and adversity: A review. *Journal of Traumatic Stress, 17*(1), 11-21.

Lynch. S. M., Keasler. A. K., Reaves, R. C., Channer, E. G., & Bukowski, L. T. (2007). The story of my strength: An exploration of resilience in the narratives of survivors of trauma. *Journal of Aggression, Maltreatment & Trauma, 14*(1/2), 75-97.

Maton. K. (2000). Making a difference: The social ecology of social transformation. *American Journal of Community Psychology, 28*(1), 25-57.

McFarlane, A. C.. & de Yehuda, R. (1996). Resilience, vulnerability and the course of posttraumatic reactions. In B. A. van der Kolk, A. C. McFarlane, & L. Weisaeth (Eds.), *Traumatic stress: The effects of overwhelming experience on mind, body and society* (pp. 155-181). New York: Guilford Press.

McKay, S. (1999). The effect of armed conflict on girls and women. *Journal of Peace Psychology, 4,* 399-413.

Mendelsohn. M., & Straker, G. (1998). Child soldiers: Psychosocial implications of the Graca Machel/UN study. *Peace and Conflict: Journal of Peace Psychology, 4,* 399-413.

Mendelsohn, M., Zachary, R. & Harney, P. A. (2007). Group therapy as an ecological bridge to new community for trauma survivors. *Journal of Aggression, Maltreatment, and Trauma, 14*(1/2), 227-243.

Moos. R. H. (2002). The mystery of human context and coping: An unraveling of clues. *American Journal of Community Psychology, 30*(1), 67-88.

Moos. R. H. (2003). Social contexts: Transcending their power and their fragility. *American Journal of Community Psychology, 31*(1/2), 1-15.

Myers-Walls, J. (2003). Children as victims of war and terrorism. *Journal of Aggression, Maltreatment, and Trauma, 8*(1/2), 41-62.

Norris. F. H. (1992). Epidemiology of trauma: Frequency and impact of different potentially traumatic events on different demographic groups. *Journal of Consulting and Clinical Psychology, 60,* 409-418.

Norris, F. H.. Friedman, M. J., & Watson, P. J. (2002a). 60,000 disaster victims speak: I. An empirical review of the empirical literature, 1981-2000. *Psychiatry, 65*(3), 207-239.

Norris, F. H., Friedman, M. J., & Watson, P. J. (2002b). 60,000 disaster victims speak: II. Summary and implications of the disaster mental health research. *Psychiatry, 65*(3), 240-260.

Norris. F. H., & Thompson, M. P. (1995) Applying community psychology to the prevention of trauma and traumatic life events. In J. Freedy & S. Hobfall (Eds.), *Traumatic stress: From theory to practice* (pp. 49-71). New York: Plenum Press.

Paster, V. S. (1980). Organizing primary prevention programs with disadvantaged community groups. In D. Klein & S. Goldston (Eds.) *Primary prevention: An idea whose time has come* (pp. 85-89). Rockville, MD: National Institute of Mental Health, U.S. Department of Health and Human Services.

Peddle, N. (2007). Assessing trauma impact, recovery, and resiliency in refugees of war. *Journal of Aggression, Maltreatment & Trauma, 14*(1/2), 185-204.

Prilletiensky, I. (2001). Value-based praxis in community psychology: Moving toward social justice and social action. *American Journal of Community Psychology, 29*(5), 747-778.

Radan, A. (2007). Exposure to violence and expressions of resilience in Central American women survivors of war. *Journal of Aggression, Maltreatment & Trauma, 14*(1/2), 147-164.

Resnick, H., Galea, S., Kilpatrick, D., & Vlahov, D. (2004). Research on trauma and PTSD in the aftermath of 9/11. *PTSD Research Quarterly, 15*(1), 1-7.

Riger, S. (2001). Transforming community psychology. *American Journal of Community Psychology, 29*(1), 69-81.

Sandler, I. (2001). Quality and ecology of adversity as common mechanisms of risk and resilience. *American Journal of Community Psychology, 29*(1), 19-61.

Schnurr, P. P., Lunney, C. A., Sengupta, A., & Waelde, L. C. (2003). A descriptive analysis of PTSD chronicity in Vietnam veterans. *Journal of Traumatic Stress, 16*(6), 545-533.

Seligman, M. E. P., & Csikszenthmihalyi, M. (2003). Positive psychology: An introduction. *American Psychologist, 55*(1), 5-14.

Tedeschi, R. G., & Calhoun, L. G (1995). *Trauma and transformation: Growing in the aftermath of suffering.* Thousand Oaks, CA: Sage Publications.

Tjaden, P., & Thoennes, N. (1998). *Prevalence, incidence and consequences of violence against women: Findings from the National Violence Against Women Survey.* Washington, DC: Department of Justice and Centers for Disease Control and Prevention.

Tjaden, P., & Thoennes, N. (2000). *Event, nature and consequences of intimate partner violence: Findings from the National Violence Against Women Survey.* Washington, DC: Department of Justice and Centers for Disease Control and Prevention.

Trickett, E. J. (1984). Towards a distinctive community psychology: An ecological metaphor for the conduct of community research and the nature of training. *American Journal of Community Psychology, 12*, 261-269.

Trickett, E. J. (1996). A future for community psychology: The contexts of diversity and the diversity of contexts. *American Journal of Community Psychology, 24*(2), 209-234

Trickett, E. J. (1997). Ecology and primary prevention: Reflections on a meta-analysis. *American Journal of Community Psychology, 25*(2), 197-206.

Trickett, E. J., Kelly, J. G., & Vincent, T. A. (1985). The spirit of ecological inquiry in community research. In E. Susskind & D. E. Klein (Eds.), *Community research: Methods, paradigms and applications* (pp. 283-333). New York: Praeger.

Tummala-Narra, P. (2001). Asian trauma survivors: Immigration, identity, loss and recovery. *Journal of Applied Psychoanalytic Studies, 3*(3), 243-258.

Tummala-Narra, P. (2007a). Conceptualizing trauma and resilience across diverse contexts: *A multicultural perspective. Journal of Aggression, Maltreatment & Trauma, 14*(1/2), 33-53.

Tummala-Narra, P. (2007b). Trauma and resilience: A case of individual psychotherapy in a multicultural context. *Journal of Aggression, Maltreatment, & Trauma, 14*(1/2), 205-225.

Turner, S. (2004). Emotional reactions to torture and organized state violence. *PTSD Research Quarterly, 15*(2), 1-7.

United Nations. (2003). *Special report on violence against women.* New York: Author.

Watts, R. J., & Serrano-Garcia, I. (2003). The quest for a liberating community psychology: An overview. *American Journal of Community Psychology, 31*(1/2), 73-79.

Weiss, M.G., Saraceno, B., Saxena, S., & van Ommeren, M. (2003). Mental health in the aftermath of disasters: consensus and controversy. *Journal of Nervous & Mental Disease, 191*(9), 611-615.

Wild, N. D., & Pavio C. (2003). Psychological adjustment, coping and emotion regulation as predictors of posttraumatic growth. *Journal of Aggression, Maltreatment & Trauma, 8*(4), 97-119.

Yassen, J., & Harvey, M. (1998). Crisis assessment and interventions with victims of violence. In P. M. Kleespies (Ed.), *Emergencies in mental health practice: Evaluation and management* (pp. 117-144). New York: Guilford Publications.

Yehuda, R. (2004). Risk and resilience in posttraumatic stress disorder. *Journal of Clinical Psychiatry, 65*(Suppl. 1), 29-36.

doi:10.1300/J146v14n01_02

# Conceptualizing Trauma and Resilience Across Diverse Contexts: A Multicultural Perspective

Pratyusha Tummala-Narra

**SUMMARY.** This paper offers a multicultural understanding of trauma and resilience as experienced in the lives of individuals from diverse cultural and racial backgrounds. The research and clinical literature on resilience has focused largely if not exclusively on individual personality traits and coping styles, and has neglected to explore all possible sources and expressions of resilience in individuals and groups. For many ethnic minorities, traditional notions of resilience, shaped largely by middle class European and North American values, may not capture culturally more familiar modes of positive adaptation to adverse and traumatic experience. This paper explores the concept of resilience as a multi-determined phenomenon, and considers the implications of this perspective for clinical research and intervention with ethnic minorities. doi:10.1300/J146v14n01_03 *[Article copies available for a fee from The Haworth Document Delivery Service: 1-800-HAWORTH. E-mail address: <docdelivery@haworthpress.com> Website: <http://www.HaworthPress.com> © 2007 by The Haworth Press, Inc. All rights reserved.]*

Address correspondence to: Pratyusha Tummala-Narra, PhD (E-mail: ushatummala@yahoo.com).

[Haworth co-indexing entry note]: "Conceptualizing Trauma and Resilience Across Diverse Contexts: A Multicultural Perspective." Tummala-Narra, Pratyusha. Co-published simultaneously in *Journal of Aggression, Maltreatment & Trauma* (The Haworth Maltreatment & Trauma Press, an imprint of The Haworth Press, Inc.) Vol. 14, No. 1/2, 2007, pp. 33-53; and: *Sources and Expressions of Resilience in Trauma Survivors: Ecological Theory, Multicultural Practice* (ed: Mary R. Harvey, and Pratyusha Tummala-Narra) The Haworth Maltreatment & Trauma Press, an imprint of The Haworth Press, Inc., 2007, pp. 33-53. Single or multiple copies of this article are available for a fee from The Haworth Document Delivery Service [1-800-HAWORTH, 9:00 a.m. - 5:00 p.m. (EST). E-mail address: docdelivery@haworthpress.com].

Available online at http://jamt.haworthpress.com
doi:10.1300/J146v14n01_03

**KEYWORDS.** Resilience, ethnic minorities, immigrants, racial trauma

Contemporary roots of resilience theory and research can be identified in studies of schizophrenia, poverty, and trauma in the 1970s and 80s, and in the field of developmental psychopathology (Cicchetti & Garmezy, 1993). Within this literature, little attention has been directed toward the experience of trauma, recovery from trauma, and resilience in the face of traumatic exposure in racially and ethnically diverse populations.

An ecological view regards community values, beliefs, and traditions as pivotal influences on individual responses to and recovery from violence, abuse, and other traumatic events (Harvey, 1996). This paper explores the nature of traumatic experience and resilience across cultural and racial contexts, and considers how understanding of these phenomena is enhanced by ecological and multicultural frameworks. Trauma is defined as inclusive of a broad range of experiences that share the threat of violation and have implications for the individual's relationship with his/her larger community or life context. A culturally relevant definition of resilience, the experience of trauma in ethnic minority communities, expressions of resilience, and some implications for trauma recovery are discussed.

## *DEFINING RESILIENCE IN TRAUMA RESEARCH*

Resilience in coping with traumatic events has been multiply defined; for example, as the ability to return to one's original functioning following exposure to a stressful or traumatic event, successful adaptation under challenging circumstances, and a trait of character or personality that enables positive adaptation to adversity and the timely attainment of psychological milestones (e.g., academic achievement, social acceptance among peers, formation of identity; Masten & Coatsworth, 1998; Werner-Wilson, Zimmerman, & Whalen, 2000). These definitions underscore the importance of the individual's innate or learned capacities to overcome the adverse effects of traumatic exposure, but fail to consider the interdependence of individual capacities, salient attributes of family and community, and/or larger cultural belief systems.

More recently, several researchers and clinicians have suggested that risk and resiliency cannot be understood apart from context (Grossman,

Cook, Kepkep, & Koenen, 1999; Harvey, 1996, this volume; Hobfall, Jackson, Hobfall, Pierce, & Young, 2002). They further caution that resilience is not a static trait, but rather an unfolding process in which new vulnerabilities and strengths emerge during developmental, societal, and cultural transitions throughout one's life and during periods of acute stress and trauma (Cicchetti & Garmezy, 1993; Laney, 1996).

## *Cultural Bias in Resiliency Research*

Despite the increased emphasis on social context in the study of resilience, defining resilience operationally in research continues to be problematic. First, measurement of resilience in much of the trauma literature continues to rely on the use of self-report scales to measure variables (i.e., educational attainment, signs of mental illness, socioeconomic status, hardiness) that may not be relevant across cultural contexts, and may contribute very little to the task of more accurately defining resilience in those contexts (Gold, Engdahl, Eberly, Blake, Page, & Frueh, 2000; King, King, Foy, Keane, & Fairbank, 1999; Werner-Wilson et al., 2000). Self-report scales typically do not measure such distinctions.

Second, there is a lack of concordance among measures used across resiliency research, and some measures assess outcome in only certain aspects of recovery. For instance, some measures focus on the ability of children to develop social competence with peers, while others assess academic achievement in children (Lyons, 1991; Masten & Coatsworth, 1998). The constructs assessed by these measures may be further problematic with respect to their cultural relevance across diverse populations. The problem of defining resiliency, as evident in these measures, is further complicated by the challenge of defining violence across cultural groups (Hamby, 2000). Cousineau and Rondeau (2004), in their review of transnational studies of family violence, emphasize the dilemma of cultural relativism in defining violence, where some actions seen as violent by people outside a particular culture may yet be encouraged within the culture, as in the case of defining physical "discipline" versus "abuse" across different cultural contexts.

Third, the populations examined in most studies are largely homogenous, the majority being white Americans. In a meta-analytic study of risk factors for post-traumatic stress disorder in adults exposed to trauma, for example, Brewin, Andrews, and Valentine (2000) noted that while race appeared to be a weak predictor of PTSD across the studies reviewed, it was also true that race had been coded only dichotomously (i.e., White vs. non-White minority groups). The studies chosen for the meta-analysis included 77 English-language articles published since 1980, which assessed symptoms of PTSD as delineated by the DSM. The researchers found that gender, age, and race predicted PTSD with varying success across different populations, and that it was not possible to identify a set of pre-trauma indicators of PTSD of equal validity across different groups. Thus, it remains unclear as to how intra- and inter-racial and ethnic differences might contribute to trauma recovery and/or to expressions of resilience in the aftermath of trauma. It is also unclear how particular racial and ethnic groups may differ in terms of their own definitions of what is and is not resilient. In addition, the meta-analysis included only studies that assessed risk factors for PTSD in a manner consistent with the DSM-III, DSM III-R, or DSM-IV, thus limiting the generalizability of the findings for survivors whose trajectories may not entail PTSD symptoms. This is particularly poignant since most exposed individuals do not develop PTSD as defined by the DSM (American Psychiatric Association, 1994).

## *DEFINING RESILIENCE WITHIN AND ACROSS CULTURAL CONTEXTS*

Resilience from a cross-cultural perspective involves examination of multiple phenomena, including individual development, community impact, and cultural systems of thought. A wide range of individual characteristics contribute to resilience in the face of trauma (Apfel & Simon, 2000; Harvey et al., 2003; Masten & Coatworth, 1998), and developmental changes have important effects on how an event influences an individual's life. Individual adaptations to traumatic experience depend to some degree on life circumstances and developmental stage. A study of narratives of female sexual abuse survivors by Harvey, Mishler, Koenen, and Harney (2000) highlights the importance of "turning points" in survivors' understandings of their experiences–at different stages in their recovery, and as prompted in part by life transitions. While both individual attributes and developmental transitions are important contributors to resilience and coping, both are also influenced by salient qualities of family, social support network, and community and by prevailing cultural beliefs and values.

## The Role of Community in Resiliency

Communities can serve as sources of resilience by providing individuals with needed resources, or can serve as sources of additional turmoil and distress. Indeed, traumatic events can often disrupt support networks at the same time that they are most needed (Harvey, 1996; Koss & Harvey, 1991; Lyons, 1991). Traumatic events and the ways in which the larger community understands and responds to these events can actually undermine an individual's access to and reliance upon traditional support networks. This seems to have been the case, for example, when the disclosures of children who were being sexually abused by parish priests were ignored by family and church, and, later still, when their delayed complaints were scorned by church officials who opted to protect abusive priests from public scrutiny. Today, as many of the now-adult children who were abused come forward in search of recognition and restitution, they and their families find themselves unable to attend church, participate in religious ceremony, and/or rely on the church for moral guidance and support (Harris, 2003; Shepard, 2003). In other instances, religious institutions may play a critical role in building survivors' resilience. For example, a priest or rabbi may provide spiritual guidance for survivors who come to question previously held religious beliefs and/or offer a sense of community in the face of isolation.

## Cultural Beliefs and Resilience

Cultural attitudes and ideals play an important role in fostering and helping to maintain resilience in the aftermath of trauma. Conceptions of the self in relationship to the external world and of the nature of traumatic experience vary considerably across cultures. A particular trait or circumstance that is seen as promoting resilience in one cultural context may actually be seen as a liability in a different cultural context. For example, in cultures where individualism and individual accomplishment are highly valued, such as the United States and Western Europe, personal autonomy and achievement, self-expression, and a strong sense of personal boundaries are upheld as ideal, particularly among the middle class. On the other hand, in cultures (e.g., Chinese, Indian, Turkish) with a collectivistic orientation, the interdependence of self and other and an emphasis on the importance of preserving and affirming relationships with family and community are highly valued (Roland, 1996). In these latter cultures, an individual's reliance on coping strategies that

exclude family wishes and obligations as guides for coping with interpersonal violence, such as rape or domestic violence, can be experienced as isolating to the individual and stressful to both the individual
and his/her communities of reference. This point is highlighted in a
prospective study of 103 Native American women conducted by
Hobfall et al. (2002), who found that participants high in communal-
mastery experienced less increase in depressive mood and anger when
faced with high stress circumstances than participants who were low in
communal-mastery. Their findings support the notion that within more
collectivist cultures, a sense of shared efficacy, or communal-mastery,
may be more central to people's resiliency in the face of stress and adversity.

## TRAUMA IN RACIALLY DIVERSE COMMUNITIES

Deeper understanding of the ways in which culture and community
foster recovery and resilience in racially and ethnically diverse populations of trauma survivors requires understanding of the kinds of traumatic events these populations may suffer specifically because of
race, ethnicity, and/or culture. Several epidemiological studies have
addressed the global prevalence of different types of violence (De
Girolamo & McFarlane, 1996; Krug, Dahlberg, Mercy, Zwi, & Lozano,
2002; Marsella, Bornemann, Orley, & Ekblad, 1994). Other recent
studies indicate prevalence rates for physical and sexual violence
against women, and related cultural and social barriers to help-seeking
in the case of domestic violence across different countries, such as Canada, Europe, and Israel (Eisikovits, Winstok, & Fishman, 2004; Kury,
Obergfell-Fuchs, & Woessner, 2004; Rinfret-Raynor, Riou, Cantin,
Drouin, & Dube, 2004; Shirwadkar, 2004). Findings from these studies
emphasize the influence of traditional attitudes towards women and violence, increasing poverty, and a reluctance to report violence due to
cultural and religious beliefs in legitimizing and/or perpetuating violence.

Despite growing research on violence in different countries, research
on interpersonal violence in developing countries has been less well
documented. Transnational and cross-cultural studies on intimate
partner violence outnumber those on other forms of family violence
(i.e., child abuse, elder abuse; Cousineau & Rondeau, 2004), and most
traumatized groups within these countries have not been studied. Of
135 studies conducted on the prevalence of PTSD across cultures, only

8 (6%) focused on developing countries, despite the fact that these countries are more commonly the sites of natural disasters and wars (De Girolamo & McFarlane, 1996).

Within the United States, a parallel problem exists, where the prevalence of violence (e.g., in ethnic minority communities across different socioeconomic contexts) has received relatively little attention. Generally, research in this area has focused on the prevalence of PTSD in ethnic and racial minority populations or on demographic variables related to risk of exposure to violence. These studies suggest that stress related to minority status, such as racial prejudice, may increase the risk for developing PTSD, and that women of color are often at particular disadvantage with respect to safety and securing access to care.

## *Experience of Trauma in Diverse Communities*

The way in which trauma is experienced by the individual or community and the way it should be approached from a clinical standpoint is highly influenced by cultural history. Ignoring the realities of cultural bias and racism in the experience of trauma undermines our ability to recognize resilient capacities within individuals and communities. It is important to remember that the diagnosis of PTSD was formulated in Western cultures that generally value the aim of individual control of one's circumstance and destiny. Indeed, the notion that PTSD occurs as a normal response to abnormal conditions implies that, under normal circumstances, individuals do or should have control over their fate (deVries, 1996). Little research has been conducted, however, in cultural contexts where a belief in fate as determined by an external spiritual force is prevalent, and where an individual's ability to accept his or her apparent fate may be highly valued. In other words, the very definition of what experiences are "normal" and what constitutes a "normal" response to trauma and/or evidence of recovery from trauma is determined by one's larger cultural system.

The fields of cross-cultural psychology, community psychology, and anthropology have noted the pervasive role of culture as a mediator of the experience and expression of emotion (Haeri, this volume; Harvey, 1996, this volume; Markus & Kitayama, 1994). Cultural variations in the experience of trauma are evident, for example, in the experience of many Salvadoran refugees who report attaques nervios, a somatic response involving feelings of anxiety, fear, and anger, and calor, an experience of intense heat that extends through one's body (Jenkins, 1996). In Central American and in many other societies, somatic experiences, such as headaches and gastric distress, may be perceived as more acceptable or understandable expressions of anxiety, sadness, and anger than the verbal expression of these feelings to family or community members. In other instances, spiritual and cultural beliefs can buffer traumatic experience and may encourage individuals to endure suffering more silently for the larger good of the community.

## Misdiagnosis and Trauma

Trauma that is racially based takes many forms. Within the mental health field, a particularly insidious type of racially-based trauma lies in the frequent misdiagnosis of the clinical presentations and symptoms of patients from racial or ethnic minority groups. Studies indicate, for example, that African American patients struggling with symptoms of anxiety are often mistakenly diagnosed with psychotic disorders, in part due to differences in describing their symptoms (Frueh, Hamner, Bernat, Turner, Keane, & Arana, 2002). In one recent study of African American and Caucasian American combat veterans diagnosed with PTSD, Frueh et al. found that the African American veterans endorsed more items suggestive of psychosis than did Caucasian American veterans, although no significant differences were found between the groups on a more general self-report measure of disturbed thinking. The African American veterans also endorsed higher levels of dissociation. In interpreting their findings, the researchers noted that the psychotic symptoms reported by the African American veterans may have actually been indicative of dissociative symptoms related to re-experiencing traumatic combat events. These findings are reminiscent of the classic study on social class and mental illness by Hollingshead and Redlich (1958), which documented the unequal, class- and race-based distribution of mental health diagnoses and treatment, including the over-diagnosis of mental illness and decreased access to care among poor African Americans. It appears that while the problem of misdiagnosis may be increasingly recognized in the clinical and research literature, little change has taken place in actual clinical assessment and practice.

Misdiagnosis also may stem, in part, from the distorted images of ethnic minorities that are prevalent within the culturally mainstream reference groups of most U.S. medical practitioners. Image distortion can contribute to a further sense of helplessness and mistrust of mental health assessment and intervention in ethnic minorities. Daniel (2000) highlighted the image of African American women as "mentally unstable," during the Clarence Thomas-Anita Hill hearings, as a way of maintaining the status quo, suggesting that therapists must expand their "cognitive and affective lenses" (p. 133) if they are to hear the traumatic racial memories of African American women. The paucity of and distortion of public images have potentially damaging effects for other minority groups in the mental health system, as well. Thus, the label of "model minority" applied to Asian Americans promotes a paradoxical sense of academic and professional accomplishment, and the perpetuation of stereotypes of Asian Americans as "silent," "passive," "powerless" individuals who dare not question white mainstream authority (Eng & Han, 2000).

## *Effects of Racial Trauma*

Racial violence and oppression is typically experienced across generations and becomes both a personal and shared experience. Trauma that occurs in the context of social upheaval can create discontinuity and unpredictability both on an individual and community level. African Americans, for example, have endured a history of slavery followed by prolonged physical and psychological oppression. Their experience has been referred to as the "second American holocaust," the first being that directed against Native Americans (Helms & Cook, 1999). Daniel (2000) noted the profound extent to which actual and threatened physical and psychological violence has been aimed against African Americans for centuries. Ongoing incidents of racism often trigger individuals' memories of racial trauma that they previously experienced. These incidents further evoke collective memories of racial trauma that were experienced by other African Americans, some of whom may be from a previous generation.

Other examples of collectively experienced racial trauma include the genocide of Native Americans, the Nazi Holocaust, and the forced internment of Japanese Americans during the Second World War. These experiences have had profound implications not only for the individual's identity, adjustment, and relationship with the external world, but also for the culture as a whole and, according to numerous researchers, for generations to come. It appears that a racial or ethnic community's collective memory of past traumas helps to create a "second generation" of survivors (Kogan, 1993). In the case of the Nazi Holocaust, for example, children of holocaust survivors may consciously or unconsciously absorb their parents' experience, and the effects may be transmitted even to children born long after the original trauma (Danieli, 1998). Thus, although many holocaust survivors and their children demonstrate external markers of success (e.g., academic or occupational achievement), they may nonetheless suffer profound internal challenges to adaptation.

## Impact of Racial Trauma on Sense of Self

As with other types of traumatic experience, racial trauma can have a profound impact on an individual's sense of self, identity formation, relationships with others, and perceptions of mental health care (Sorsoli, this issue). Racially driven trauma is distinct from other forms of interpersonal trauma (Tummala-Narra, 2005) and poses particular challenges to an individual's development of a positive bicultural or biracial identity. In addition, this type of trauma has the effect of dehumanizing one's sense of security in and identification with larger social structures.

Loo (1994) discusses a case study of a Chinese American veteran of the Vietnam War who was born and raised in the U.S., drafted into the Army at age 19, and served as a helicopter crew chief and door gunner. Over 20 years later, he sought treatment for PTSD. During the war, he had not only been exposed to messages that contradicted his identity as an Asian American, but also had been forced to acquire racial labeling, involving statements such as "gook" and "hate Asians, kill Asians" (p. 641). Further, he had often been mistaken for the enemy by his comrades, leading to heightened states of vigilance and hyperarousal. This "double assault" (p. 641) eventually led to his increased isolation and to intense conflict between the increasingly dehumanizing identity as an American soldier and a growing emotional and cultural connection he felt toward Vietnamese people, creating an affective split or disconnection.

Racial trauma compounds the effects of other forms of interpersonal trauma as connoted in the notions of "double assault" (Loo, 1994) and "soul wound" (Braveheart-Jordan & DeBruyn, 1995). For example, Native Americans have been noted to be victims of violent crimes at a rate of 124 per 1,000, over 2.5 times the national average, and Native American women are affected by violent crimes (98 per 1,000) more frequently than women of any other ethnic minority group in the U.S. (Walters & Simoni, 2002). Historic traumas, such as boarding schools, coercive migration, and non-Native custodial care placements have contributed to further exposure to interpersonal violence, such as childhood abuse and neglect, and related psychological distress, such as substance abuse, depression, and PTSD.

Individuals who are immigrants to the U.S. face similar, and somewhat different challenges than those who are indigenous to the country (i.e., Native Americans) or those forced into migration (i.e., African Americans, exiles). The experience of being a minority may be a surprisingly new and disorienting experience for many immigrants, as they cope with anti-immigrant sentiments (Akhtar, 1999). In the face of different forms of hostility, many immigrants struggle with forming a positive sense of self and with forming trusting relationships with those outside of their immediate communities. A recent example of such a struggle occurred in the context of the terrorist attacks on the World Trade Center and the Pentagon on September 11, 2001, when many Middle Eastern Americans and South Asian Americans faced violence and discrimination that contrasted sharply with their images of themselves as Americans prior to September 11 (Tummala-Narra, 2005).

## MULTICULTURAL EXPRESSIONS OF RESILIENCE

Understanding the unique trajectories of trauma recovery in individuals from diverse cultural contexts entails the consideration of resilience as a culturally shaped phenomenon. Harvey (1996) suggests four conceptually distinct recovery pathways through which individuals cope with traumatic experiences, including, first, those who either do or do not receive clinical care and, within each of these categories, those who either do or do not recover from these experiences. Cultural factors then help to determine which survivors seek and benefit from clinical care and which seek recovery in the context of culturally familiar social networks. In addition, she proposes that recovery from trauma involves multiple domains of psychological functioning (Harvey, 1996; Harvey et al., 2003). While recovery for trauma survivors of any cultural background may involve change in these domains, the specific ways in which individuals mobilize their internal and external resources to achieve recovery will vary significantly with cultural context. Several articles in this volume represent inquiries into origins and expressions of resilience among trauma survivors from diverse cultural backgrounds and contexts (e.g., Bradley & Davino; Daigneault, Cyr, & Tourigny; Radan).

### Resilience and Reshaping of Individual Cultural Identity

Recovery from trauma in diverse contexts often involves the task of redefining oneself, in part due to how the trauma is defined in the cultural context with which one identifies. Child-rearing practices in many

ethnic minority communities entail teaching children about strategies to
cope with potential hostility aimed against them by mainstream culture.
Socializing with others in one's own racial and/or cultural group serves
an important protective function for children to build a sense of safety
and security with respect to their own racial and cultural identifications.
This is often an important component of one's racial and cultural identity development (Helms & Cook, 1999). Several researchers and clinicians have discussed the dual existence of ethnic minorities, which
involves the adaptation to two or more cultural contexts (Miller &
MacIntosh, 1999; Roland, 1996). This adaptation can involve the co-
existence of two or more dissonant parts of one's experience, as seen in
the case of many bilingual individuals who associate different affective
experiences with their native and more recently acquired languages
(Foster, 1996).

While these experiences of shifting from one world to the other can
cause deep anguish and confusion, they can also be a source of resilience.
The ability to move from one context to another allows for cognitive and
emotional flexibility that can significantly enhance the recovery progno-
sis of traumatized individuals. The following case vignette describes a
client with whom I worked in individual psychotherapy for 18 months.
The case of Juhi illustrates the complications and benefits of belonging
to more than one cultural context.

*Juhi*

Juhi is a 23-year-old Indian American woman who was sexually assaulted by a male acquaintance when she was 20 years old. Juhi sought
psychotherapy after being encouraged by a friend to cope with her depression and traumatic memories. She was born in India, lived in England until age 10, and then moved to the U.S. with her family. Her
parents worked in a small business and interacted primarily with other
Indian immigrants both in England and the U.S. While growing up, she
became a devout Hindu with the guidance of her parents, who visited
the temple a couple of times a week.

While she felt close to her family, she also began to feel increasingly
inhibited in speaking with them about her personal life, particularly in
her early teens. Her most closely guarded secret involved her sexuality.
She did not disclose her lesbian identity to her parents until she was 22
years old, when they began to question her about meeting a man to
marry. Her parents reacted initially with anger, and then mostly with

confusion. They had expected her to marry a man, and homosexuality was another foreign element of their larger immigration experience.

Juhi had struggled with "fitting in" most of her life, and she had hoped that she would meet more friends outside of her Indian American community while attending college. She did form close friendships, and became more involved in a primarily white lesbian community. A couple of years later, she was assaulted by a male acquaintance whom she met through a classmate. She was badly bruised and with the help of some friends, received medical care and reported the assault to police. After the assault, Juhi found herself more withdrawn from her family and her friends, experiencing depressed mood, anxiety, and feelings of isolation.

In psychotherapy, she explored her feelings about the assault and its aftermath. She recalled that she wanted to tell her family about what happened to her, but felt this was not possible due to the silence around issues of sexuality and rape in her community. She struggled with not feeling understood by either her longstanding Indian American community or her newly formed American community.

Juhi explained that she felt "strong and healthy" in certain ways when she was with her family, and in other ways when she was with her college friends. She connected her ability to survive under difficult and changing circumstances with being an immigrant, an experience she shared only with her family and other Indians, and her ability to broaden aspects of her individuality, which included her sexuality and an understanding of trauma, with her friendships outside of her family. She spoke in therapy of needing to "refuel" herself by being in both worlds to cope with the rape and to feel grounded.

Juhi's case illustrates the dramatic shifts in redefining various aspects of one's identity, and particularly one's multicultural self, in the face of trauma. Juhi's ability to participate in both cultural worlds provided her with the opportunity to engage with different aspects of her traumatic and other stressful experiences. Juhi's resilience is expressed in her ability to participate in both cultural worlds, her refusal to be defined by or isolated from either, and in her ability to draw upon critical resources in each. An important task of recovery involves the re-integration of cultural identity through building awareness of how the traumatic experience challenges and/or reifies one's cultural identifications. This is a process that is an essential component of defining one's multicultural self.

# HEALING FROM TRAUMA IN DIVERSE CONTEXTS

## Collective Resilience and Hope

While clinical perspectives on trauma tend to emphasize the problematic and/or pathological effects of trauma on individuals' functioning, ecological and multicultural perspectives have underscored the importance of individuals' capacities to process trauma, both internally and within family and community systems, in potentially transformative ways. Collective resilience refers to the construction of coping processes within a particular social and political context. Under conditions of social and political oppression, communities play a critical role by deconstructing oppressive social ideologies and reconstructing trusting relationships. It is through these mechanisms that hope is engendered on a community level (Hernandez, 2002).

The ways in which hope is produced under traumatic or stressful circumstances are evident in both brief and prolonged types of trauma. For many ethnic minorities, a critical strategy for surviving racial violence and oppression involves preserving a strong attachment to their communities by relying first on the resources those communities have to offer. For many immigrants, the process of migration carries with it not only a sense of apprehension, but also a sense of optimism and hope for new possibilities for their families (Radan, this volume; Peddle, this volume). The shared experience of hope within a community for a better future mobilizes individuals and groups to endure and often recover from the effects of traumatic experiences.

## Role of Family Support

Consistent support from one's family is an important form of collective resilience. Resilience in the family context involves belief systems that shape the meaning of adversity, views of positive outcomes, understandings of family cultural history in the context of social and economic resources, and communication processes such as emotional expression and problem solving (Hernandez, 2002). Several studies have indicated the importance of social support from significant others, such as immediate and extended family members, as a protective factor in trauma recovery among ethnic minority women (Banyard, Williams, Siegel, & West, 2002). The family also acts as a conduit for spiritual beliefs that may help traumatized individuals to develop protective coping mechanisms. Research on the effects of spiritual beliefs on psychosocial adjustment indicates the positive role that spirituality may play across various ethnic minority communities in the U.S., including Native American, African American, Asian American, Latino American, immigrant, and refugee populations (Holtz, 1998; Walters & Simoni, 2002).

*Group Movements and Social Change*

Collective resilience also takes form in group movements for social change, and may ultimately lead to the transformation of individual and group trauma. There are numerous illustrations of social change and transformation in the face of trauma across cultural contexts, including peace-building efforts and human rights activism. Examples include the Truth and Reconciliation Commission of South Africa, focused on seeking social justice for an entire nation; the United States Holocaust Memorial Museum, which allows individuals to bear witness to past atrocities against Jews and other minority groups during the Nazi Holocaust; the mothers and grandmothers of the Plaza de Mayo in Buenos Aires, who since the 1970s have demanded to know what happened to their children who were murdered by paramilitary forces; and RAHI, an organization in Northern India developed to build social awareness of sexual abuse and incest.

Bloom (1998) highlights the notion that an individual's identification with the group is a core component of one's sense of personal identity. The group's role in the recovery from trauma entails issues of justice, accountability, and transformation. Addressing these issues is often critical for individuals to confront the realities of trauma, and ultimately "break" from their traumatic past. Group movements, therefore, offer validation and a sense of hope for both individuals and whole communities. For the mothers and grandmothers of the Plaza de Mayo, a primary objective remains the silent protesting of the death of their children, rather than seeking compensation (Bloom, 1998). Their movement has raised consciousness across the globe about the injustice inflicted by paramilitary forces, and perhaps more importantly provided these women with a sense of resilience both on individual and collective levels.

*Artistic Creation*

Traumatic experience can also be transformed through artistic creation. Groups of young artists who share a similar ethnic background,

recently formed across the U.S., have focused their artistic efforts on issues of trauma and social justice. For instance, several members of a
Boston based group, the South Asian American Theatre (SAATH), produced a play about an Indian American woman who was battered and
eventually killed by her husband. The play provided an opportunity for
other South Asians to discuss domestic violence within their ethnic
community, without feeling personally threatened or exposed. Similarly, various films produced in the past decade have brought forth issues of domestic violence, sexual abuse, rape, and political and racial
violence (i.e., *Beyond Rangoon* [Boorman, 1995]; *A Time to Kill*
[Schumacher, 1996]; *Monsoon Wedding* [Nair, 2001]). Increasingly,
works by several immigrant and first generation writers, such as Amy
Tan and Jumpa Lahiri, and African American writers, such as Toni
Morrison and Maya Angelou, have become increasingly noted and accessible in mainstream U.S. culture. These authors highlight issues of
interpersonal violence, race, and immigration in their writings, giving
validity to many readers' own traumatic experiences within a particular
cultural setting. The opportunity that these forms of artistic creation
provide with respect to a contextual perspective on trauma can be criti-
cally important to many ethnic minorities' recovery from trauma.

## Psychotherapy

Psychotherapy can be a meaningful contribution to the recovery from
trauma for individuals of diverse backgrounds (Tummala-Narra, this
volume). Burstow (2003) pointed out that trauma occurs in layers,
where each trauma experienced by an individual is compounded by another trauma, which is associated with one's group identity and historical trauma. In light of the impact of one's cultural context on the
processing and healing of trauma, it is critical that therapists address
both internal (i.e., intrapsychic) experience and external (i.e., family,
community) ramifications of individual and collective traumatic experiences. The modification of traditional psychotherapeutic approaches is
an important consideration in working with ethnic minorities, as resiliency is defined in distinct ways across and within cultural groups. This is
particularly salient in light of the fact that people of color in the U.S.
tend to underutilize counseling and psychotherapy services (Sue & Sue,
1999). Increased awareness of one's own cultural values and assumptions, increased knowledge about culturally different ethnic groups in
the U.S., and the awareness of the influence of systemic forces in the

provision of treatment are necessary for effective psychotherapeutic interventions with ethnic minorities (Sue et al., 1998).

## CONCLUSION

A culturally informed, ecological understanding of trauma and resilience requires the exploration of multiple phenomena, including existing cultural bias in research with ethnic minorities, definitions of resilience across cultural groups, the role of family, ethnic, and/or religious community, and cultural beliefs in shaping individual resiliency. The experience of race-related trauma, such as misdiagnosis in mental health care systems, racism, and racially based violence on individual and group levels, has significant impact on individuals' sense of cultural and racial identity and trust in larger social structures (i.e., mainstream culture, government, health care systems). Expressions of resilience are influenced by one's identifications with a cultural group, relationships with family, and interactions with mainstream culture. Recovery from trauma entails an appreciation of the diverse nature of expressions of resilience, as well as the various ways in which healing occurs. It is critical that these forms of healing respect the unique trajectory of recovery involving both challenges and strengths faced by an individual within a specific sociocultural context.

## REFERENCES

Akhtar, S. (1999). *Immigration and identity: Turmoil, treatment, and transformation.* Northvale, NJ: Jason Aronson, Inc.

American Psychiatric Association. (1994). *Diagnostic and statistical manual of mental disorders* (4th ed.). Washington, DC: Author.

Apfel, R. J., & Simon, B. (2000). Mitigating discontents with children in war: An ongoing psychoanalytic inquiry. In A. C. G. M. Robben & M. M. Suarez-Orozco (Eds.), *Cultures under siege: Collective violence and trauma* (pp. 102-130). New York: Cambridge University Press.

Banyard, V. L., Williams, L. M., Siegel, J. A., & West, C. M. (2002). Childhood sexual abuse in the lives of Black women: Risk and resilience in a longitudinal study. *Women and Therapy, 25*(3/4), 45-58.

Bloom, S. L. (1998). By the crowd they have been broken, by the crowd they shall be healed: The social transformation of trauma. In R. G. Tedeschi, C. L. Park, & L. G. Calhoun (Eds.), *Posttraumatic growth: Positive changes in the aftermath of crisis* (pp. 179-213). Mahwah, NJ: Lawrence Erlbaum Associates, Inc.

Boorman, J. (Director). (1995). *Beyond Rangoon* [Motion picture]. United King-dom/United States: Castle Rock Entertainment & Columbia Pictures Corporation.

Bradley, R., & Davino, K. (2007). Interpersonal violence, recovery and resilience in in-carcerated women. *Journal of Aggression, Maltreatment, and Trauma, 14*(1/2), 123-146.

Braveheart-Jordan, M., & DeBruyn, L. (1995). So she may walk in balance: Integrating the impact of historical trauma in the treatment of Native American women. In J. Adelman & G.M. Enguidanos (Eds.), *Racism in the lives of women: Testimony, the-ory, and guides to antiracist practice* (pp. 345-368). Binghamton, NY: Haworth Press.

Brewin, C. R., Andrews, B., & Valentine, J. D. (2000). Meta-analysis of risk factors for post-traumatic stress disorder in trauma-exposed adults. *Journal of Consulting and Clinical Psychology, 68*(5), 748-766.

Burstow, B. (2003). Toward a radical understanding of trauma and trauma work. *Vio-lence Against Women, 9*(11), 1293-1317.

Cicchetti, D., & Garmezy, N. (1993). Prospects and promises in the study of resilience. *Development and Psychopathology, 5,* 497-502.

Cousineau, M., & Rondeau, G. (2004). Toward a transnational and cross-cultural anal-ysis of family violence. *Violence Against Women, 10*(8), 935-949.

Daigneault, I., Cyr, M., & Tourigny, M. (2007). Exploration of recovery trajectories in sexually abused adolescents. *Journal of Aggression, Maltreatment & Trauma, 14*(1/2), 165-184.

Daniel, J. H. (2000). The courage to hear: African American women's memories of ra-cial trauma. In L. C. Jackson & B. Greene (Eds.), *Psychotherapy with African American women: Innovations in psychodynamic perspectives and practice* (pp. 126-144). New York: The Guilford Press.

Danieli, Y. (1998). *International handbook of multigenerational legacies of trauma.* New York: Plenum Press.

De Girolamo, G., & McFarlane, A. C. (1996). The epidemiology of PTSD: A compre-hensive review of the international literature. In A. J. Marsella, M. J. Friedman, E. T. Gerrity, & R. M Scurfield (Eds.), *Ethnocultural aspects of posttraumatic stress disorder: Issues, research, and clinical applications* (pp. 33-85). Washington, DC: American Psychological Association

deVries, M. W. (1996). Trauma in cultural perspective. In B. A. van der Kolk, A. C. McFarlane, & L. Weisaeth, L. (Eds.), *Traumatic stress: The effects of overwhelm-ing experience on mind, body, and society* (pp. 398-413). New York: The Guilford Press.

Eisikovits, Z., Winstok, Z., & Fishman, G. (2004). The first Israeli national survey on domestic violence. *Violence Against Women, 10*(7), 729-748.

Eng, D. L., & Han, S. (2000). A dialogue on racial melancholia. *Psychoanalytic Dia-logues, 10*(4), 667-700.

Foster, R. P. (1996). Assessing the psychodynamic function of language in the bilin-gual patient. In R. P. Foster, M. Moskowitz, & R. A. Javier, *Reaching across bound-aries of culture and class* (pp. 243-263). Northvale, NJ: Jason Aronson, Inc.

Frueh, B. C., Hamner, M. B., Bernat, J. A., Turner, S. M., Keane, T. M., & Arana, G. W. (2002). Racial differences in psychotic symptoms among combat veterans with PTSD. *Depression and Anxiety, 16,* 157-161.

Gold, P. B., Engdahl, B. E., Eberly, R. E., Blake, R. J., Page, W. F., & Frueh, B. C. (2000). Trauma exposure, resilience, social support, and PTSD construct validity among former prisoners of war. *Psychiatric Epidemiology, 35,* 36-42.

Grossman, F. K., Cook, A. B., Kepkep, S. S., & Koenen, K. C. (1999). *With the phoenix rising: Lessons from ten resilient women who overcame the trauma of childhood sexual abuse.* San Francisco: Jossey-Bass Publishers.

Haeri, S. (2007). Resilience and post-traumatic recovery in cultural and political context: Two Pakistani women's strategies for survival. *Journal of Aggression, Maltreatment & Trauma, 14*(1/2), 287-304.

Hamby, S. L. (2000). The importance of community in a feminist analysis of domestic violence among America Indians. *American Journal of Community Psychology, 28*(5), 649-669.

Harris, M. (2003). Unto us a child: Abuse and deception in the Catholic Church. *Psychiatric Services, 54*(10), 1417-1418.

Harvey, M. R. (1996). An ecological view of psychological trauma and trauma recovery. *Journal of Traumatic Stress, 9*(1), 3-23.

Harvey, M. R. (2007). Towards an ecological understanding of resilience in trauma survivors: Implications for theory, research, and practice. *Journal of Aggression, Maltreatment & Trauma, 14*(1/2), 9-32.

Harvey, M., Liang, B., Harney, P., Koenan, K., Tummala-Narra, P., & Lebowitz, L. (2003). A multidimensional approach to the assessment of trauma impact, recovery and resiliency: Initial psychometric findings. *Journal of Aggression, Maltreatment & Trauma, 6*(2), 87-109.

Harvey, M. R., Mishler, E. G., Koenen, K., & Harney, P. A. (2000). In the aftermath of sexual abuse: Making and remaking meaning in narratives of trauma and recovery. *Narrative Inquiry, 10*(2), 291-311.

Helms, J. E., & Cook, D. A. (1999). *Using race and culture in counseling and psychotherapy: Theory and process.* Boston, MA: Allyn & Bacon.

Hernandez, P. (2002). Resilience in families and communities: Latin American contributions from the psychology of liberation. *The Family Journal: Counseling and Therapy for Couples and Families, 10*(3), 334-343.

Hobfoll, S. E., Jackson, A., Hobfoll, I., Pierce, C. A. & Young, S. (2002). The impact of communal-mastery versus self-mastery on emotional outcomes during stressful conditions: A prospective study of Native American women. *American Journal of Community Psychology, 30*(6), 853-871.

Hollingshead, A. B., & Redlich, F. C. (1958). *Social class and mental illness: A community study.* New York: Wiley.

Holtz, T. H. (1998). Refugee trauma versus torture trauma: A retrospective controlled cohort study of Tibetan refugees. *Journal of Nervous and Mental Disease, 186*(1), 24-34.

Jenkins, J. H. (1996). Culture, emotion, and PTSD. In A. J. Marsella, M. J. Friedman, E. T. Gerrity, & R. M Scurfield (Eds.), *Ethnocultural aspects of posttraumatic stress disorder: Issues, research, and clinical applications* (pp. 165-182). Washington, DC: American Psychological Association.

King, D. W., King, L. A., Foy, D. W., Keane, T. M., & Fairbank, J. A. (1999). Posttraumatic stress disorder in a national sample of female and male Vietnam veterans: Risk factors, war-zone stressors, and resilience-recovery variables. *Journal of Abnormal Psychology, 108*(1), 164-170.

Kogan, I. (1993). Curative factors in the psychoanalyses of Holocaust survivors' offspring before and after the Gulf War. *International Journal of Psychoanalysis, 74,* 803-814.

Koss, M. P., & Harvey, M. R. (1991). *The rape victim: Clinical and community interventions.* Thousand Oaks, CA: Sage Publications.

Kury, H., Obergfell-Fuchs, & Woessner, G. (2004). The extent of family violence in Europe: A comparison of national surveys. *Violence Against Women, 10*(7), 749-769.

Krug, E. G., Dahlberg, L. L., Mercy, J. A., Zwi, A. B., & Lozano, R. (2002). *World report on violence and health.* Geneva: World Health Organization.

Laney, M. D. (1996). Multiple personality disorder: Resilience and creativity in the preservation of the self. *Psychoanalysis and Psychotherapy, 13*(1), 35-49.

Loo, C. M. (1994). Race-related PTSD: The Asian American Vietnam veteran. *Journal of Traumatic Stress, 7*(4), 637-656.

Lyons, J. A. (1991). Strategies for assessing the potential for positive adjustment following trauma. *Journal of Traumatic Stress, 4*(1), 93-111.

Markus, H. R., & Kitayama, S. (1994). The cultural construction of self and emotion: Implications for social behavior. In, S. Kitayama & H. R. Markus (Eds.), *Emotion and culture: Empirical studies of mutual influence* (pp. 89-130). Washington, DC: American Psychological Association.

Marsella, A. J., Bornemann, T., Orley, J., & Ekblad, S. (Eds.). (1994). *Amidst peril and pain: The mental health and wellbeing of the world's refugees.* Washington, DC: American Psychological Association.

Masten, A. S., & Coatsworth, J. D. (1998). The development of competence in favorable and unfavorable environments: Lessons from research on successful children. *American Psychologist, 53*(2), 205-220.

Miller, D. B., & MacIntosh, R. (1999). Promoting resilience in urban African American adolescents: Racial socialization and identity as protective factors. *Social Work Research, 23*(3), 159-169.

Nair, M. (Director). (2001). *Monsoon wedding* [Motion picture]. India/United States: IFC Productions & Mirabai Films.

Peddle, N. (2007). Assessing trauma impact, recovery, and resiliency in refugees of war. *Journal of Aggression, Maltreatment & Trauma, 14*(1/2), 185-204.

Radan, A. (2007). Exposure to violence and expressions of resilience in Central American women survivors of war. *Journal of Aggression, Maltreatment & Trauma, 14*(1/2), 147-164.

Rinfret-Raynor, M., Riou, A., Cantin, S., Drouin, C., & Dube, M. (2004). A survey on violence against female partners in Quebec, Canada. *Violence Against Women, 10*(7), 709-728.

Roland, A. (1996). *Cultural pluralism and psychoanalysis: The Asian and North American experience.* New York: Routledge.

Schumacher, J. (Director). (1996). *A time to kill* [Motion picture]. United States: Regency Enterprises & Warner Bros.

Shepard, B. (2003). In search of a winning script: Moral panic vs. institutional denial. *Sexualities, 6*(1), 54-59.

Shirwadkar, S. (2004). Canadian domestic violence policy and Indian immigrant women. *Violence Against Women, 10*(8), 860-879.

Sorsoli, L. (2007). Where the whole thing fell apart: Race, resilience, and the complexity of trauma. *Journal of Aggression, Maltreatment & Trauma, 14*(1/2), 99-121.

Sue, D. W., Carter, R. T., Casas, J. M., Fouad, N. A., Ivey, A. E., Jensen, M., et al. (1998). *Multicultural counseling competencies: Individual and organizational development.* Thousand Oaks, CA: Sage.

Sue, D. W., & Sue, D. (1999). *Counseling the culturally different* (3rd ed.). New York: Wiley.

Tummala-Narra, P. (2005). Addressing racial and political terror in psychotherapy. *American Journal of Orthopsychiatry, 75*(1), 19-26.

Tummala-Narra, P. (2007). Trauma and resilience: A case of individual psychotherapy in a multicultural context. *Journal of Aggression, Maltreatment & Trauma, 14*(1/2), 205-225.

Walters, K. L., & Simoni, J. M. (2002). Reconceptualizing Native women's health: An "indigenist" stress-coping model. *American Journal of Public Health, 92*(4), 520-524.

Werner-Wilson, R. J., Zimmerman, T. S., & Whalen, D. (2000). Resilient response to battering. *Contemporary Family Therapy, 22*(2), 161-188.

doi:10.1300/J146v14n01_03

# SECTION TWO:
# ASSESSING RESILIENCE:
# MULTIPLE DIMENSIONS,
# MULTIPLE APPROACHES

# The Multidimensional Trauma Recovery and Resiliency Instrument: Preliminary Examination of an Abridged Version

Belle Liang
Pratyusha Tummala-Narra
Rebekah Bradley
Mary R. Harvey

**SUMMARY.** This paper describes two studies leading to the construction of and psychometric support for the MTRR-99, a shortened version

Address correspondence to: Belle Liang, PhD, Department of Counseling and Developmental Psychology, Lynch School of Education, Boston College, Campion 314, Chestnut Hill, MA 02461 (E-mail: liangbe@bc.edu).

[Haworth co-indexing entry note]: "The Multidimensional Trauma Recovery and Resiliency Instrument: Preliminary Examination of an Abridged Version." Liang. Belle et al. Co-published simultaneously in *Journal of Aggression, Maltreatment & Trauma* (The Haworth Maltreatment & Trauma Press. an imprint of The Haworth Press. Inc.) Vol. 14, No. 1/2, 2007. pp. 55-74; and: *Sources and Expressions of Resiliency in Trauma Survivors: Ecological Theory, Multicultural Practice* (ed: Mary R. Harvey. and Pratyusha Tummala-Narra) The Haworth Maltreatment & Trauma Press. an imprint of The Haworth Press. Inc.. 2007. pp. 55-74. Single or multiple copies of this article are available for a fee from The Haworth Document Delivery Service [1-800-HAWORTH, 9:00 a.m. - 5:00 p.m. (EST). E-mail address: docdelivery@haworthpress.com].

of the Multidimensional Trauma Recovery and Resiliency Scale (MTRR-135, formerly MTRR). In the first study, the original body of MTRR-135 data was reevaluated to remove psychometrically weak or theoretically unnecessary items. The remaining 99 items were then assessed for reliability, validity, and internal consistency. In the second study, the new MTRR-99 was applied to assess the recovery status of 164 incarcerated women prisoners with extensive abuse histories. Together, these two studies further document the utility of a multidimensional approach to assessing trauma impact, recovery, and resiliency; in addition, they provide preliminary evidence for the MTRR-99 as a viable measure for use with clinical and non-clinical populations. *doi:10.1300/J146v14n01_04 [Article copies available for a fee from The Haworth Document Delivery Service: 1-800-HAWORTH. E-mail address: <docdelivery@haworthpress.com> Website: <http://www.HaworthPress.com> © 2007 by The Haworth Press, Inc. All rights reserved.]*

**KEYWORDS.** Trauma, assessment, recovery, resiliency, MTRR-135, MTRR-99

After posttraumatic stress disorder (PTSD) was introduced into the third edition of the *Diagnostic and Statistical Manual of Mental Disorders* (DSM-III; American Psychiatric Association, 1980), a number of measures were developed to assess symptoms of PTSD. In this article we provide a preliminary report on the psychometric properties of a shortened version of the Multidimensional Trauma Recovery and Resiliency Measure (MTRR; Harvey, Liang, Harney, Koenen, Tummala- Narra, & Lebowitz, 2003) that goes beyond assessing PTSD symptoms to provide information about trauma recovery and resiliency.

The original Multidimensional Trauma Recovery and Resiliency measures, including a clinically directed interview (MTRR-I), a Q-sort (MTRR-Q), and a 135-item, observer-rated, Likert-type questionnaire and rating scale (MTRR-135; Harvey et al., 1994, 2003), were developed to address the limitations of previous trauma measures. The impetus for their development was threefold. First, they were designed to be applicable to more diverse samples, including female and treated and untreated trauma survivors. Second, they reflected unique patterns of harm across individuals, rather than uniform responses across survivors. Third, they focused on health and recovery, rather than on psychopathology. And finally, they utilize clinician reports, rather than self-reports.

Together, the various measures of the MTRR assess multifaceted and complex patterns of trauma response, and may potentially capture the variety of outcomes that patients in trauma-focused treatments can attain (Chambers & Belicki, 1998; Grossman, Cook, Kepkep, & Koenen, 1999; Lam & Grossman, 1997; Liem, James, O'Toole, & Boudewyn, 1997; Tedeschi, Park, & Calhoun, 1998).

## THE DEVELOPMENT
## OF THE ABRIDGED MULTIDIMENSIONAL
## TRAUMA RECOVERY AND RESILIENCY MEASURES

In response to the need for a shortened, more clinically accessible version of the MTRR-135, the current authors proposed an abridged, ninety-nine-item version, called the MTRR-99. The primary goals in the design of the MTRR-99 were the establishment of a measure that would reduce the number of items in the MTRR-135 while maintaining its content, psychometric acceptability, and methodology. Like the MTRR-135, the MTRR-99 relies on clinicians' observations and reports, rather than on self-report. Thus, it takes advantage of the clinical expertise of trained respondents, and does not rely on the self-reports of trauma survivors, who may suffer from significant impairments of memory and consciousness. Moreover, in the tradition of the original MTRR measures, the MTRR-99 assesses post-trauma functioning according to the domains outlined by Harvey's (1996) ecological framework: Authority Over the Remembering Process, Integration of Memory and Affect, Affect Tolerance and Regulation, Symptom Mastery, Self-Esteem, Self-Cohesion, Safe Attachment, and Meaning (see Table 1 for definitions). Finally, by reflecting, in a shortened format, the wide range of symptoms that apply to survivors of many types of traumatic histories (e.g., combat trauma, child sexual abuse, and domestic violence), the MTRR-99 provides an efficient new method for assessing trauma.

### Psychometric Studies Leading to the MTRR-99

The MTRR-135 (from which the MTRR-99 was derived) was developed and validated in a series of four studies (Harvey et al., 2003). The MTRR-135 demonstrated reasonable inter-rater reliability with both clinical and clinical research samples. Internal consistency was sound and, in the clinical sample, the measure drew significant distinctions be-

TABLE 1. Definitions of the Multidimensional Trauma Recovery and Resiliency Domains

---

Domain I. *Authority Over the Remembering Process*: the point in the recovery process at which the trauma survivor is able to choose to recall or not recall the experiences that once eluded meaningful appraisal and/or intruded unbidden into consciousness.

Domain II. *Integration of Memory and Affect*: the survivor's ability to feel what is remembered (i.e. to feel in the present some of the affects that attended the original experience) and to experience new feelings from remembering the past and reflecting upon it.

Domain III. *Affect tolerance and regulation:* the range of feelings trauma survivors are able to experience and the extent to which they can bear and manage difficult feelings.

Domain IV. *Symptom mastery:* the degree to which survivors can anticipate, manage, contain, or prevent the cognitive and emotional disruption that arises from posttraumatic arousal.

Domain V. *Self-esteem:* the experience of self-regard (i.e., regarding oneself as worthy of care) and the capacity for self-care (i.e., the behavioral expression of self-regard).

Domain VI. *Self-cohesion:* the extent to which survivors experience themselves as integrated or fragmented, in terms of thought, feeling, and action.

Domain VII. *Safe attachment:* the ability of the survivor to develop feelings of trust, safety, and enduring connection in relationships with others.

Domain VIII. *Meaning making:* the process by which a survivor struggles to understand and "metabolize" the impact and legacy of a traumatic past.

---

tween patients differing in clinician-estimated recovery status (Harvey et al., 2003). These findings supported the utility of the MTRR-135 in the detection and assessment of not only trauma symptoms, but also domain-specific expressions of trauma recovery and resiliency.

Findings also indicated that inter-rater reliabilities varied considerably among the 135 items comprising the MTRR-135, and each domain contained items with inter-rater reliabilities ranging from quite poor to quite good. These data, as well as the measure's long length, suggested a need to prune the MTRR-135 of less psychometrically sound items, shortening it for both ease of clinical administration and improved reliability. Another limitation of the MTRR-135 was that it was tested on fairly homogenous patients enrolled in trauma-focused treatments. It was clear that additional studies that included more diverse populations of trauma survivors would be required to establish the cross-cultural utility of the MTRR measures, as well as their applicability to untreated trauma survivors.

This paper presents two investigations designed to address the issues described above. Specifically, the first study provides a preliminary examination of a shortened and somewhat revised version of the MTRR-135, namely the MTRR-99. In doing so, the study also describes the process by which original MTRR-135 items were retained or eliminated to create the MTRR-99. In this same population, the interrater reliability and coefficient alphas for this new version are then presented. The second study presents the psychometric properties of this revised 99-item measure when used with a new and largely untreated population of trauma survivors. The purpose of these investigations was to examine the psychometric strength and practical utility of the MTRR-99 for research with diverse groups of trauma survivors.

## STUDY ONE:
## CONSTRUCTING AND EVALUATING THE MTRR-99

### Method

#### Participants

This study used data collected in the initial studies of the MTRR-135 (Harvey et al., 2003). Study participants were 181 adult trauma survivors (86% female and 14% male) who were in treatment for sexual abuse or physical abuse in childhood, adolescence, or adulthood. Eighty-two percent were Caucasian, 9% were African American, 8% were Latino, and 1% were Asian American. The mean age of participants was 37 years ($SD = 11$, range = 14-62).

Many participants reported multiple types of trauma: 64% had experienced child physical abuse, 62%, child sexual abuse, 45%, adult-incident rape, and 35%, a combination of war combat and childhood physical or sexual abuse. Participants were also categorized according to clinician-reported recovery status: 17% were rated as largely recovered, 54% as partially recovered, and 29% as largely unrecovered. The average time in current treatment as rated by clinicians was 30 months ($SD = 39$, range: less than one month to 240 months).

#### Measures

Like the original 135-item MTRR, the MTRR-99 instructs clinical observers (treating clinicians or clinical research interviewers) to rate the applicability of each item to the individual being rated. Ratings are made on a five-point, Likert-type scale ranging from *Not At All Descriptive* to *Highly Descriptive*. Sample items for each domain can be found in Table 2. The measure itself is included in this volume (see Ap-

TABLE 2. Sample Items from Abbreviated Multidimensional Trauma Recovery and Resilience Scale (MTRR-99)

| | |
|---|---|
| Domain I. Authority Over the Remembering Process | |
| 52. | Unwanted thoughts, memories or images intrude on consciousness. |
| 4. | Has difficulty recalling events from the very recent past. |
| Domain II. Integration of Memory and Affect | |
| 11. | When recalling painful or traumatic events s/he is able to remember feelings experienced at the time. |
| 94. | Can reflect upon painful events, including traumatic events, with varied and appropriate feeling. |
| Domain III. Affect Tolerance and Regulation | |
| 30. | Often feels emotionally numb. |
| 93. | Maintains a realistic view of situations even when emotions are strong. |
| Domain IV. Symptom Mastery and Positive Coping | |
| 13. | Is readily startled. |
| 44. | Practices and makes effective use of one or more stress management techniques (e.g., relaxation, meditation). |
| Domain V. Self Esteem (Self Care and Self Regard) | |
| 45. | Experiences impulses to behave in self-abusive ways, such as cutting, burning, whether or not s/he acts on these impulses. |
| 33. | Feels worthy of care and nurturance from others. |
| Domain VI. Self Cohesion | |
| 57. | Experiences dissociative states (e.g., feels like s/he leaves her/his body or that her/his feelings are somewhere else). |
| 79. | Feels like an integrated person whose actions and emotions fit together coherently. |
| Domain VII. Safe Attachment | |
| 31. | Is able to enter into and maintain safe and mutually satisfying relationships with intimate partners. |
| 36. | Is unusually sensitive to (or is preoccupied with) issues of power and control in relationships. |
| Domain VIII. Meaning | |
| 32. | Understanding of painful or traumatic past is marked by excessive and unreasonable self-blame. |
| 50. | Is able to feel a realistic sense of hope and optimism about the future. |

pendix A at the end of this volume). The MTRR-135 was designed with ample clinical input to enable clinicians and clinical researchers to rate patients and untreated research participants on each of the eight domains of functioning highlighted by Harvey's (1996) ecological framework. The process of creating the original 135 items has been described in an earlier paper (Harvey et al., 2003).

*Procedure*

Following the completion of the initial series of psychometric studies (Harvey et al., 2003) the MTRR-135 was subjected to further analysis in the current study. Original items were retained or eliminated from the measure based on several criteria: (a) inter-rater reliabilities for each of the 135 items, (b) the correlations between individual item and total domain scores for each of the eight subscales, (c) the number of items comprising a given domain of the MTRR-135, and (d) and the theoretical relevance of item content. The retained items and resultant subscales were then checked for internal consistency reliability (Chronbach's alpha) and inter-rater reliability (Pearson correlation's between pairs of raters).

More specifically, data from the original MTRR-135 study were reviewed item by item. For each item, inter-rater reliabilities from the original study were first considered. These reliabilities were based on the ratings of fifty-one patients (a subset of the total sample of 181 survivors) being seen in outpatient, trauma-focused psychotherapy, all with histories of child sexual abuse, child physical abuse, and/or adult incident rape, who had been independently rated on all 135 original items by pairs of clinicians, including: (a) thirty-one senior clinical staff members paired with clinical trainees (pre-doctoral psychology trainees, post-doctoral psychology fellows, psychiatric residents, or clinical social work interns) with whom they co-conducted initial evaluation interviews, (b) ten pairs of co-leaders rating patients in trauma-focused psychotherapy groups, and (c) ten pairs of clinicians having shared but not necessarily comparable knowledge of the patients (e.g., an individual therapist and a psychopharmacologist).

Those items that had relatively lower levels of inter-rater reliability and/or relatively low correlations with domain totals as well as those that would increase domain coefficient alphas if eliminated were subjected to careful content analysis. These items were typically eliminated. In a few cases, items were reworded when deemed theoretically important in preserving a domain construct. This process resulted in a shortened and slightly reworded 99-item measure. The construct validity of the revised MTRR-99 subscales was tested; and finally, validity, inter-rater reliability, and internal reliability were compared with those of the 135-item version.

## *Results*

Decisions regarding item retention were based on inter-rater reliabilities, number of items in the original subscale, examination of item-total correlations, and item content. Cutoff values were determined independently for each subscale, with the goals of: (a) producing shortened subscales with acceptable reliability and (b) preserving original subscale content.

*Reliability and Item Analysis*

Item analysis of the original 14 Authority over Memory items indicated that 13 items had an item-total correlation over .53. Two pairs of highly correlated items were combined, for a total of 11 items in the abbreviated subscale. The coefficient alpha for the shortened subscale was acceptable (.83) and comparable to that of the full Authority over Memory subscale (.85).

For the Integration of Memory and Affect subscale, item analysis indicated that four of the six original items had item-total correlations over .69. Of those remaining, one was deleted, but the other was retained due to vital item content. The coefficient alpha for the resulting five-item subscale was acceptable (.77) and similar to that of the full subscale (.75).

For the Affect Tolerance subscale, item analysis indicated that thirteen of the twenty-two items had item-total correlations over .50. Besides missing the item-total cut-off, most of the remaining items also had relatively low inter-rater reliability. Nevertheless, two of these were retained due to important item content. Internal consistency for the shortened subscale was good (.82) and comparable to the full Affect Tolerance subscale (.88).

Item analysis of the original seventeen Symptom Mastery items indicated that nine items had an item-total correlation over .50. Two of these items were considered theoretically unnecessary; and five of the items below this cut-off were seen as theoretically necessary. In sum, twelve items were retained for the abbreviated subscale. The coefficient alpha for the shortened subscale was acceptable (.76) and similar to that of the full subscale (.80).

As the original Self Esteem subscale included 30 items, a decision was made to reduce this subscale substantially. Item analysis indicated that seventeen of the thirty original items had item-total correlations over .55. Of the seventeen, seven were deleted as they had relatively low inter-rater reliability and expendable content. Six of those that missed the .55 cut-off, were retained due to important item content; two of these were combined as they were highly correlated. The coefficient alpha for the resulting fifteen-item subscale was good (.84) and comparable to that of the much longer subscale (.88).

For the Self Cohesion subscale, item analysis indicated that four of the twelve items had item-total correlations over .65. Two of these items were deleted as they had low inter-rater reliability and expendable content; four of the other items were retained due to important item content and good inter-rater reliability. Internal consistency for the short, eight-item subscale was acceptable (.72) and similar to that of the full subscale (.79).

Item analysis of the original twenty-one Safe Attachment items indicated that most of the safe attachment items were theoretically necessary, despite some relatively low item-total correlations and inter-rater reliabilities. Only four items were considered expendable. An additional item was created for the scale, and thus eighteen items were retained for the abbreviated subscale. The coefficient alpha for the shortened subscale was within acceptable range (.63) although lower than that of the full Safe Attachment subscale (.71).

As the original fifteen-item Meaning Making subscale was already relatively short and included theoretically important items, a decision was made not to reduce this subscale. All item-total correlations, most inter-rater reliabilities, and the internal consistency reliability for the subscale were fairly high ($\alpha = .85$).

The mean alpha for the eight subscales of the MTRR-99 was .78, which is considered within acceptable limits for widely used scales. Moreover, despite variability among clinician pairs in level of expertise and exposure to rated survivors, the inter-rater reliability was adequate for the composite MTRR-99 and all its domains (ranging from .78, $p < .001$ to .36, $p < .01$). When only the ten pairs of co-leaders of trauma groups (the type of pairs who would be expected to have the most comparable knowledge of patients) were assessed, inter-rater reliabilities for most domains increased. See Table 3 for a comparison of inter-rater reliabilities for the MTRR-135 (51 pairs of raters), the MTRR-99 (51 pairs of raters), and the MTRR-99 (10 pairs with comparable knowledge of patients).

## Construct Validity of the MTRR-99

Construct validity is demonstrated by establishing convergent validity (constructs that theoretically should be related to each are, in fact, observed to be related to each other) and discriminant validity (constructs that should not be related to each other are, in fact, observed to not be related to each other). Construct validity for the eight, MTRR do-

TABLE 3. Study One: Inter-Rater Reliability of MTRR-99 and MTRR-135 Scores

|  | MTRR-135 (N = 51 pairs) | MTRR-99 (N = 51 pairs) | MTRR-99 (N = 10 pairs of group co-leaders) |
|---|---|---|---|
| Composite | .71 *** | .66 *** | .80 ** |
| Authority over Memory | .49 *** | .49 *** | .43 * |
| Integration of Memory & Affect | .37 ** | .36 ** | .68 ** |
| Affect Tolerance | .50 *** | .48 *** | .76 ** |
| Symptom Mastery | .67 ** | .50 *** | .43 * |
| Self Esteem | .75 *** | .78 *** | .89 *** |
| Self Cohesion | .73 *** | .72 *** | .64 ** |
| Safe Attachment | .68 *** | .61 *** | .79 ** |
| Meaning-Making | .72 *** | .72 *** | .88 *** |

$^*p < .05,$ $^{**}p < .01,$ $^{***}p < .001$

mains was tested using the 181 clinician's ratings from the original study. The discriminant validity of the eight separate scales *versus* a composite score was assessed and supported when reliability coefficients for each of the subscales were higher than the inter-correlations between individual scales. The mean inter-correlation between MTRR scales was .61, with $r$'s ranging from .40 to .85 (see Table 4).

Convergent validity was further assessed by comparing the MTRR-99 scores with scores on a clinician rated index of recovery status because a putative measure of trauma resiliency and recovery would be expected to vary with other measures of recovery. Participants were categorized according to whether clinicians rated them as largely recovered, partially recovered, and largely unrecovered. A multiple analysis of variance using MTRR-99 domains as the dependent variables and recovery status as the independent variable revealed significant main effects for each of the eight scales at $p < .001$. $F$ values were: 18.56 for Authority over Memory; 25.54 for Integration of Memory and Affect; 43.34 for Affect Tolerance; 26.86 for Symptom Mastery; 48.49 for Self Esteem; 17.43 for Self Cohesion; 27.50 for Safe Attachment; 35.35 for Meaning Making. As expected, subjects rated by their clinicians as largely recovered indicated greater resiliency and fewer symptoms on each of the eight MTRR-99 scales (see Table 5).

Finally, when the MTRR-135 was compared to the MTRR-99, the latter appeared to be psychometrically and theoretically stronger in sev-

TABLE 4. Study One: Inter-Correlatons of Mean Scores Across MTRR-99 Domains (*N* = 181)

|  | 1 | 2 | 3 | 4 | 5 | 6 | 7 |
|---|---|---|---|---|---|---|---|
| 1. Authority over Memory |  |  |  |  |  |  |  |
| 2. Integration of Memory & Affect | .65 |  |  |  |  |  |  |
| 3. Affect Tolerance | .63 | .62 |  |  |  |  |  |
| 4. Symptom Mastery | .48 | .45 | .64 |  |  |  |  |
| 5. Self Esteem | .52 | .51 | .80 | .62 |  |  |  |
| 6. Self Cohesion | .56 | .48 | .62 | .60 | .63 |  |  |
| 7. Safe Attachment | .44 | .49 | .61 | .45 | .62 | .49 |  |
| 8. Meaning-Making | .49 | .62 | .68 | .60 | .64 | .50 | .56 |

For all correlations, *p* < .001.

TABLE 5. Study One: MANOVA Results for MTRR-99 Scores by Recovery Status (*df* = 2, *N* = 141)

|  | Recovery Status | *M* | *SD* | *F* |
|---|---|---|---|---|
| Composite | 1 | 3.80 | .34 | 60.58*** |
|  | 2 | 3.17 | .42 |  |
|  | 3 | 2.67 | .43 |  |
| Authority over Memory | 1 | 3.91 | .52 | 18.56*** |
|  | 2 | 3.35 | .60 |  |
|  | 3 | 2.94 | .74 |  |
| Integration of Memory & Affect | 1 | 3.77 | .66 | 25.54*** |
|  | 2 | 3.23 | .73 |  |
|  | 3 | 2.56 | .63 |  |
| Affect Tolerance | 1 | 3.59 | .47 | 43.34*** |
|  | 2 | 2.90 | .56 |  |
|  | 3 | 2.35 | .51 |  |
| Symptom Mastery | 1 | 3.77 | .40 | 26.86*** |
|  | 2 | 3.23 | .59 |  |
|  | 3 | 2.72 | .62 |  |
| Self Esteem | 1 | 4.13 | .45 | 48.49*** |
|  | 2 | 3.44 | .57 |  |
|  | 3 | 2.75 | .61 |  |
| Self Cohesion | 1 | 4.07 | .60 | 17.43*** |
|  | 2 | 3.42 | .72 |  |
|  | 3 | 3.00 | .77 |  |
| Safe Attachment | 1 | 3.89 | .73 | 27.50*** |
|  | 2 | 3.29 | .46 |  |
|  | 3 | 2.92 | .45 |  |
| Meaning | 1 | 3.42 | .47 | 35.35*** |
|  | 2 | 2.76 | .57 |  |
|  | 3 | 2.28 | .51 |  |

***p* < .001
Recovery status: 1 = largely to fully recovered; 2 = partially recovered; 3 = largely unrecovered.

eral respects. First, it maintained similar levels of internal reliability consistency per domain, despite the fact that large numbers of items typically contribute towards boosting alphas. Second, inter-rater reliability for each domain was greater for the MTRR-99 based on trauma group leaders' ratings. Third, whereas several domains in the MTRR-135 were not significantly related to trauma recovery ratings, all of the domains in the MTRR-99 were significantly related to trauma recovery ratings.

## STUDY TWO:
## PSYCHOMETRICS OF THE MTRR-99 IN A SECOND SAMPLE

The goal of this study was to examine data bearing on the reliability and validity of the MTRR-99 in a second sample. Following Study One, four new items were created for the measure, three pairs of items that were highly correlated and related in content were consolidated to three single items, several items with relatively low inter-rater reliability were slightly reworded to clarify, but not change, their meanings. Study Two was conducted to assess the validity and reliability of the scales following these minimal revisions. Four domains of reliability and validity were assessed: (a) the coefficient alpha for each scale; (b) the inter-rater reliability using a sub-sample of 20 MTRR-99 protocols; (c) the disciminant validity of eight separate scales versus the use of a composite score by comparing correlations among MTRR scales and subscale alphas; and (d) construct validity by comparing MTRR subscale scores with scores on another trauma measure that assesses criteria for Disorders of Extreme Stress not Otherwise Specified (DESNOS) or "complex" PTSD.

### Method

*Participants*

Of the approximately 200 women recruited for the study, 175 agreed to participate in an interview. Of the 175 interviews, 164 yielded complete, valid protocols. The sample included 61% African American, 38% Caucasian, and 1% Latina women, most of whom had a high school education or less (72%). They reported relatively low household incomes (35% less than $12,000/year; 74% less than $36,000 /year). Most had children (86%) and were currently not married (81%). Sixteen percent of the participants reported that they were HIV positive, the most prevalent medical condition in the sample. The majority of the women reported surviving multiple types of abuse across four categories: childhood sexual abuse, child physical abuse, adult sexual assault, and adult physical assault. Forty-two percent reported having experienced all four types of abuse; only 5% of the participants had experienced none of these abuses.

## Procedure

One hundred and sixty-four women incarcerated in a medium security women's prison in South Carolina were interviewed as part of a study of "women's life experiences." The prison facility served as the "special needs" prison for women in the state, meaning that all female prisoners in need of chronic medical or psychological care were housed there. Participants were recruited in three ways: (a) individuals referred by prison mental health staff; (b) individuals selected at random from a list of the inmates and asked to participate in an interview; and (c) individuals who had heard of the study from other participants and requested participation. The interviews normally lasted 2-3 hours and involved administration of: (a) the MTRR-I, (b) interviews regarding history of physical and sexual assault in childhood and adulthood, and (c) a set of self-report measures. More details of the study are described elsewhere (Bradley & Davino, this volume; Davino, 2000).

Interviewers included a doctoral candidate in clinical psychology, six other graduate students in clinical psychology, and one advanced undergraduate student. The principal investigator completed 87 interviews, the undergraduate interviewer completed 40 interviews, and the group of graduate interviewers completed 48 interviews. All interviewers received training in the impact of trauma on mental health, and in the administration of the interview protocols, including the MTRR-I. Four taped MTRR interviews were conducted by the principal investigator at a battered women's shelter, then listened to and scored by each interviewer. Scoring for these training tapes was reviewed and discussed with the principal investigator until consistency of scoring between interviewers was achieved. These four interviews were not included in the data set for this study.

After training was completed, twenty interviews were conducted and scored twice for inter-rater reliability analysis. To do this, interviewers observed the principal investigator conduct an MTRR interview with one of the participants in this study. Then both the principal investigator and observer scored the participant on the MTRR items. In addition, the principal investigator observed each interviewer conduct an MTRR interview with one of the participants. Then both the principal investigator and the observer scored the participant on the MTRR items.

*Measures*

The data presented in Study Two (which represent a subset of data collected in a larger study) include demographics, the MTRR-99 (rated based on the MTRR-I which is designed to collect MTRR-99 data), physical and sexual assault histories collected via a structured interview (see Bradley & Davino, this volume; Davino, 2000), and the Structured Interview for Disorders of Extreme Stress (SIDES; Pelcovitz, van der Kolk, Roth, Mandel, Kaplan, & Resick, 1997; Zlotnick & Pearlstein, 1997). Only the SIDES will be described in detail here because the other measures have already been discussed in Study One or in other articles presented in this volume.

The SIDES is a structured interview and diagnostic criteria set for symptoms across seven functional domains: regulation of affect and impulses, regulation of attention and consciousness, self-perception, perception of the perpetrator, relationships with others, somatization, and systems of meaning. These domains are based on the diagnosis of "complex" PTSD or Disorders of Extreme Stress Not Otherwise Specified, a diagnostic category within the PTSD spectrum (Herman, 1992; Pelcovitz et al., 1997). Typically a diagnosis of DESNOS is made if interviewees report clinically significant symptoms in 6 of the 7 domains–symptoms in the domain regarding perception of the perpetrator are not required. However, the somatization subscale was not administered, as it was not a focus of this study. Thus, in this study, participants needed to meet 5 of 6 criteria for a diagnosis of DESNOS. The SIDES has previously demonstrated reliability and validity (Pelcovitz et al., 1997; Zlotnick & Pearlstein, 1997), including an inter-rater reliability of .81 and coefficient alphas ranging from .53-.96. The SIDES also had good internal reliability in the current study (alphas ranging from .51-.82).

### Results

*Reliability*

As with Study One, the data supported the internal reliability of the MTRR-99 subscales with an average coefficient alpha of .85, and subscale alphas ranging from .76 to .89 (see Table 6). Moreover, based on 20 pairs of raters, inter-rater reliabilities for each subscale were adequate with a mean of .67 (see Table 6).

### Preliminary Psychometric Properties

Reliability coefficients for each of the subscales were higher than the inter-correlations between individual scales supporting the use of eight separate scales *in addition to* a composite score. The mean inter-correlation between MTRR scales was .59, with $r$'s ranging from .38 to .72 (see Table 7).

We conducted a preliminary analysis of construct validity by testing whether MTRR domain scores predict current DESNOS diagnostic status. A 2 × 2 between-subjects multivariate analysis of variance was conducted for each of the MTRR scales and the MTRR composite score as dependent variables and DESNOS diagnostic criteria (scored as yes/no) as the independent variable. The data yielded a significant overall MANOVA using the Wilks Criterion, $F(8,154) = 8.19, p < .001$). In follow up univariate ANOVAs, we found lower scores on each of the MTRR-99 subscales for the women meeting SIDES criteria for DESNOS ($n = 102$), as compared to those not meeting the criteria ($n = 61$; see Table 6). That is, those who met the SIDES criteria for DESNOS also showed lower levels of trauma recovery and resiliency as assessed by the MTRR-99.

## DISCUSSION

The shortened MTRR-99 is a 99-item theory based, paper and pencil instrument that measures eight dimensions of trauma recovery and resiliency. The instrument is easy to complete, and it can generate both a graphic profile of an individual's areas of relative resiliency and deficit, a textual description of strengths and weaknesses within those domains, and treatment outcome goals linked to specific domains and to specific items within these domains.

Most other indices of "trauma recovery and resiliency" are criterion-referenced, in that they measure how closely the respondent matches a set of characteristics or behaviors thought to be associated with trauma recovery and resiliency. It is difficult to establish reliability and validity for such indices. As a theory-based measure, the MTRR-99 can meet

TABLE 6. Study Two: Descriptive Statistics of Multidimensional Trauma Recovery and Resiliency

| Domain | Full Sample M (SD) (N = 164) | Alpha | Inter-Rater correlation | DESNOS + M (SD) (N = 102) | DESNOS – M (SD) (N = 61) | F(1,161)[a] |
|---|---|---|---|---|---|---|
| Authority over the remembering process | 3.60(.87) | .84 | .71** | 3.85 (.84) | 3.16 (.73) | 27.47*** |
| Integration of memory and affect | 3.57 (.96) | .78 | .54* | 3.82 (.88) | 3.12 (.96) | 20.75*** |
| Affect tolerance/regulation of trauma affect | 3.18 (.93) | .89 | .68** | 3.54 (.83) | 2.56 (.74) | 57.68*** |
| Symptom mastery and positive coping | 3.44 (.74) | .76 | .61** | 3.71 (.69) | 2.97 (.57) | 49.29*** |
| Self-esteem (self-care and self-regard) | 3.78 (.83) | .88 | .77** | 4.1 (.73) | 3.3 (.78) | 39.26*** |
| Self-cohesion | 4.13 (.87) | .86 | .82** | 4.40 (.73) | 3.70 (.94) | 28.88*** |
| Safe attachment | 3.28 (.80) | .87 | .49* | 3.5 (.79) | 2.8 (.64) | 31.73*** |
| Meaning | 2.90(.83) | .88 | .70** | 3.47 (.79) | 2.45 (.68) | 35.49*** |

*$p < .05$, **$p < .01$, ***$p < .001$
[a] $F$ statistic for the univariate ANOVA comparing women in DESNOS+ group and DESNOS– group on each MTRR subscale

TABLE 7. Study Two: Inter-Correlations of Mean Scores Across MTRR-99 Domains (N = 164)

|                                    | 1   | 2   | 3   | 4   | 5   | 6   | 7   |
|------------------------------------|-----|-----|-----|-----|-----|-----|-----|
| 1. Authority over Memory           |     |     |     |     |     |     |     |
| 2. Integration of Memory & Affect  | .68 |     |     |     |     |     |     |
| 3. Affect Tolerance                | .63 | .50 |     |     |     |     |     |
| 4. Symptom Mastery                 | .59 | .46 | .72 |     |     |     |     |
| 5. Self Esteem                     | .58 | .38 | .76 | .72 |     |     |     |
| 6. Self Cohesion                   | .63 | .44 | .66 | .54 | .64 |     |     |
| 7. Safe Attachment                 | .52 | .42 | .68 | .69 | .58 | .50 |     |
| 8. Meaning-Making                  | .62 | .49 | .68 | .69 | .67 | .46 | .58 |

For all correlations, $p < .001$.

the standard scientific criteria for a valid psychometric instrument. Further, the MTRR-99 emphasizes behavior and specific experiences rather than general states of well-being and attitudes. Thus, the instrument is less susceptible to differences in interpretation by raters and it is more generalizable than other tests commonly in use.

The scales of the MTRR-99 demonstrated reasonable reliability and validity in clinical and non-clinical samples, supporting the utility of the MTRR-99 in the detection and assessment of not only trauma symptoms, but also resiliency and recovery status. Moreover, the domains of the MTRR-99 improve upon those of MTRR-135 in that they are shorter and are more highly related to recovery and resiliency status. That is, several domains of the MTRR-135 (i.e., Authority over Memory, Self-Cohesion, and Self-Esteem) were not significantly related to recovery status at the $p < .05$ level (Harvey et al., 2003); in contrast, all the domains of the MTRR-99 were significantly related to recovery status with higher $p$ levels and $F$ scores. Moreover, the MTRR-99 demonstrates increased inter-rater and internal reliability in a sample of incarcerated women.

Items on the MTRR-135 and MTRR-99 reflect actual experiences described in interviews of a directed sample of trauma survivors representing cross-cultural and situational diversity (i.e., multicultural survivors of domestic violence, child abuse, and war trauma) as well as symptoms and experiences observed by trauma experts. In the current study, each of the 135 resulting descriptions of trauma recovery and resiliency were used to rate 51 trauma survivors by pairs of clinicians. Experts then reviewed the 135-item pool and items were deleted or reworded which had relatively poor inter-rater reliability or low item-total correlations. The eight new subscales, based on 99 items were then tested for inter-rater reliability and internal consistency reliability. In Study One, they had adequate inter-rater reliabilities and coefficient alpha levels of .72 or better (except for Safe Attachment's Alpha of .63). In Study Two, they had significantly higher inter-rater reliability and internal consistency–most alphas, including Safe Attachment, were above .84, meeting or exceeding the standard reliability criterion for individual and group psychometric diagnosis (DeVellis, 1991; Nunnally, 1978).

The validity of the MTRR-99 was confirmed in a variety of ways. In Study One, content validity was established by using actual experiences and statements drawn from interviews, along with the reliable confirmation and categorization of these by both raters and experts. Both studies provided preliminary evidence for construct validity–the MTRR-99 subscales' successfully predicted a clinician rated index of Trauma Recovery Status in Study One (Harvey et al., 2003), and DESNOS status in Study Two. As expected, greater resiliency and fewer symptoms as indicated by the MTRR-99 Scales are positively associated with clinician rated trauma recovery and negatively associated with DESNOS status.

Finally, content and discriminant analysis established that the items constituted eight distinct dimensions of trauma recovery and resiliency (Authority over Memory, Integration of Memory and Affect, Affect Tolerance, Symptom Management, Self-Esteem, Self Cohesion, Safe Attachment, and Meaning Making). The assumption that the domains are separate but related to trauma recovery and resiliency is supported in the construct validity tests and by the correlations between MTRR-99 subscales for both studies. Correlations between scales are significant but modest indicating that the scales are related but separate and provide unique information.

Based on this process of developing and testing the MTRR-99 for reliability and validity, it is fair to conclude that the instrument is measuring the affective, cognitive, and behavioral characteristics described by Harvey's (1996) stage by dimension theory and that these characteristics can be reliably rated by clinicians treating trauma survivors, and researchers interviewing participants in a non-clinical setting.

## Limitations and Future Directions

The low number of study participants in certain subgroups, including male gender, trauma-type, and cross-cultural populations may limit the generalizability of these findings. Study Two supported the reliability, validity, and utility of the English-language MTRR-99 in a sample of ethnic minority trauma survivors, however, and other studies presented in this volume (e.g., Daigneault, Cyr, & Tourigny, this volume; Radan, this volume) using non-English language versions of the measure are promising with respect to the MTRR-99's potential for cross-cultural studies. More such studies are needed and are in progress.

Another limitation is that for Study One clinician's assessments of recovery status and their responses on the MTRR-99 shared method variance (i.e., they both relied on clinician-reports to structured questionnaire items), and this may have increased the relationship between the two. The same is true for Study Two in that clinicians' provided ratings for the MTRR-99 and the SIDES (measure of DESNOS status). Concurrent and construct validity may be further confirmed by examining the MTRR-99's relation to multi-method indicators of trauma outcome.

In summary, the relatively wide variety of symptoms and strengths addressed by this measure may support its use, not only as a clinical measure, but also as a research measure, to be used in testing hypotheses about trauma recovery and resiliency. In examining trauma survivors' profiles, both the patterns that reveal universal human capacities and unique protective factors for each individual or subgroup that contribute to recovery and resiliency are important findings that may inform the design of specific interventions across cultures and diverse populations.

## REFERENCES

American Psychiatric Association (1980). *Diagnostic and statistical manual of mental disorders* (DSM III) (3rd ed.). Washington, DC: Author.

Bradley, R. G., & Davino, K. M. (2007). Interpersonal violence, recovery and resilience in incarcerated women. *Journal of Aggression, Maltreatment & Trauma, 14*(1/2), 123-146.

Chambers, E., & Belicki, K. (1998). Using sleep dysfunction to explore the nature of resilience in adult survivors of childhood abuse or trauma. *Child Abuse & Neglect, 22,* 753-758.

Daigneault, I., Cyr, M., & Tourigny, M. (2007). Exploration of recovery trajectories in sexually abused adolescents. *Journal of Aggression, Maltreatment & Trauma, 14*(1/2), 165-184.

Davino, K. (2000). *Exploring a feminist-relational model of the mental health effects of interpersonal violence among incarcerated women.* Unpublished doctoral dissertation, University of South Carolina, Columbia, SC.

DeVellis, R. F. (1991). *Scale development:Theory and applications*. Newbury Park, CA: Sage.

Grossman, F. K., Cook, A. B., Kepkep, S. S., & Koenen, K. C. (1999). *With the phoenix rising: Lessons from ten resilient women who overcame the trauma of childhood sexual abuse*. San Francisco: Jossey-Bass.

Harvey, M. R. (1996). An ecological view of psychological trauma and trauma recovery. *Journal of Traumatic Stress, 9*(1), 3-23.

Harvey, M. R., Liang, B., Harney, P., Koenan, K., & Tummala-Narra, P., & Lebowitz, L. (2003). A multidimensional approach to the assessment of trauma impact, recovery and resiliency: Five psychometric studies. *Journal of Aggression, Maltreatment & Trauma, 6*(2), 87-109.

Harvey, M. R., Westen, D., Lebowitz, L., Saunders, E., Avi-Yonah, O., & Harney, P.A. (1994). *Multidimensional trauma recovery and resilience scale* (MTRR-135). Unpublished manuscript.

Herman, J. L. (1992). *Trauma and recovery*. New York: Basic Books.

Lam, J. K., & Grossman, F. K. (1997). Resiliency and adult adaptation in women with and without self-reported histories of childhood sexual abuse. *Journal of Traumatic Stress. 10*, 175-196.

Liem, J. H., James, J. B., O'Toole, B. A., & Boudewyn, A. C. (1997). Assessing resilience in adults with histories of childhood sexual abuse. *American Journal of Orthopsychiatry, 67*, 594-606.

Nunnally, J. C. (1978). *Psychometric theory* (2nd ed.). New York: McGraw-Hill.

Pelcovitz, D., van der Kolk, B., Roth, S., Mandel, F., Kaplan, S., & Resick, P. (1997). Development of a criteria set and a structured interview for disorders of extreme stress. *Journal of Traumatic Stress, 10*, 3-16

Radan, A. (2007). Exposure to violence and expressions of resilience in Central American women survivors of war. *Journal of Aggression, Maltreatment & Trauma, 14*(1/2), 147-164.

Tedeschi, R. G., Park, C. L., & Calhoun, L. G. (1998). *Posttraumatic growth: Positive changes in the aftermath of crisis* (Volume VII: The LEA Series in Personality and Clinical Psychology). Mahwah, N.J.: Lawrence Erlbaum Associates, Inc.

Zlotnick, C., & Pearlstein, T. (1997). Validation of the Structured Interview for Disorders of Extreme Stress. *Comprehensive Psychiatry, Vol 38*(4), 243-247.

doi:10.1300/J146v14n01_04

# The Story of My Strength:
# An Exploration of Resilience
# in the Narratives of Trauma Survivors
# Early in Recovery

Shannon M. Lynch
Amy L. Keasler
Rhiannon C. Reaves
Elizabeth G. Channer
Lisa T. Bukowski

**SUMMARY.** The purpose of this study was to explore the narratives of 18 survivors of trauma for elements of resilience present in their stories at a time when they were seeking treatment for their psychological dis-

---

Address correspondence to: Shannon M. Lynch, Department of Psychology, Idaho State University, Garrison Hall, Room 427, Campus Box 8112, Pocatello, ID 83209 (E-mail: lyncshan@isu.edu).

First and foremost, the authors thank the participants who chose to share their life stories. Next, they want to thank the University Research Council at Western Illinois University for their support of this work. The authors also thank Mary Harvey for her support of research aimed at understanding individuals' recovery as well as their pathology. They also express our appreciation to Rachel Wolfe for her work as an interviewer on this project. Finally, the authors thank our colleagues, Virginia Diehl, Alice Michael, and Lynn Sorsoli, who provided us with feedback and suggestions about this manuscript.

[Haworth co-indexing entry note]: "The Story of My Strength: An Exploration of Resilience in the Narratives of Trauma Survivors Early in Recovery." Lynch, Shannon, M. et al. Co-published simultaneously in *Journal of Aggression, Maltreatment & Trauma* (The Haworth Maltreatment & Trauma Press, an imprint of The Haworth Press, Inc.) Vol. 14, No. 1/2, 2007, pp. 75-97; and: *Sources and Expressions of Resiliency in Trauma Survivors: Ecological Theory, Multicultural Practice* (ed: Mary R. Harvey, and Pratyusha Tummala-Narra) The Haworth Maltreatment & Trauma Press, an imprint of The Haworth Press, Inc., 2007. pp. 75-97. Single or multiple copies of this article are available for a fee from The Haworth Document Delivery Service [1-800-HAWORTH. 9:00 a.m. - 5:00 p.m. (EST). E-mail address: docdelivery@haworthpress.com].

Available online at http://jamt.haworthpress.com
doi:10.1300/J146v14n01_05

tress. While these participants appeared to be struggling in some or even several aspects of their lives, analyses suggested that they had personal characteristics and experiences of supportive relationships similar to those of individuals often labeled as resilient. In particular, their narratives conveyed motivation to cope and recover, recognition of how traumatic events had influenced them, and faith in the possibility of a better life. The participants also seemed to be in a process of noticing their capacity to make active choices to take care of themselves and developing a sense of themselves as worthy of care. doi:10.1300/J146v14n01_05 *[Article copies available for a fee from The Haworth Document Delivery Service: 1-800-HAWORTH. E-mail address: <docdelivery@haworthpress.com> Website: <http://www.HaworthPress.com> © 2007 by The Haworth Press, Inc. All rights reserved.]*

**KEYWORDS.** Resilience, trauma, child abuse survivors, coping, narrative study

Researchers in the field of interpersonal violence have investigated many potential adverse effects of childhood abuse, partner violence, and sexual assault. Most of the empirical work in this field has focused on the multitude of negative outcomes that can follow experiences of traumatic events (Bybee & Sullivan, 2002; Hall, 2003; Heller, Larrieu, D'Imperio, & Boris, 1999; McGloin & Widom, 2001; Spaccarelli & Kim, 1995). However, many individuals do recover from experiences of interpersonal violence and, yet, remarkably little empirical research exists that examines the process of recovery (Harvey, Liang, Harney, Koenen, Tummala-Narra, & Lebowitz, 2003). Greater understanding of what factors or processes aid individuals in recovering from traumatic events clearly offers the potential to improve current prevention programs and intervention strategies for treating survivors of violence. Thus, it is not surprising that there is increasing interest among researchers and practitioners in identifying individuals' strengths in the aftermath of a traumatic event as well as in assessing the extent of an individual's psychological distress (Bybee & Sullivan, 2002; Davis, 2002; Harvey et al., 2003, Heller et al., 1999; Richardson, 2002). In fact, a number of researchers have noted the resilient nature of some individuals' responses to adversity; identifying innate qualities, interpersonal skills, and positive coping strategies that survivors of traumatic events have utilized to overcome the difficult events in their lives (see Harvey, 1996, this volume; Richardson, 2002).

Thus, there is a growing body of research on individuals' resilience in response to traumatic events. Theorists appear to concur on a definition of resilience as a state of competent functioning despite serious threats to development (Masten, 2001; McGloin & Widom, 2001). However, there remains substantial variation in the operationalization of resilience in studies (Luthar, Cicchetti, & Becker, 2000; Olsson, Bond, Burns, Vella-Brodrick, & Sawyer, 2003). In research examining positive outcomes for trauma survivors, for example, a typical method of representing resilience as an outcome variable relies on measuring the absence of clinically significant symptoms with self report scales (e.g., Feinauer & Stuart, 1996; Liem, James, O'Toole, & Boudewyn, 1997). In contrast, researchers and practitioners have increasingly argued that assessing symptom absence alone does not fully capture an individual's level of functioning (Harvey et al., 2003; Heller et al., 1999; McGloin & Widom, 2001). Furthermore, little is known regarding the extent to which strengths and strategies associated with resilience are present in the lives of individuals who are both symptomatic and in the process of recovering from past traumatic events (Hall, 2003). Thus, the purpose of this study was to explore the narratives of individuals seeking trauma focused treatment who typically would not be described as resilient for their potential strengths and utilization of positive strategies in their lives.

Given the aims of this study, it is important to note that some researchers have developed a more complex measure of resilience (i.e., as something more than the absence of symptoms). In a study of resilience among individuals who were abused or neglected as children ($N = 676$) and a group of matched controls ($N = 520$), McGloin and Widom (2001) identified several domains that they asserted more closely represented overall competent functioning. To be designated resilient in this study, individuals could not have a current or past psychiatric diagnosis, a history of substance abuse, employment problems or several jobs within five years, less than a high school degree, a history of homelessness, or a history of criminal behavior. In addition, they were required to have been engaged in regular social interaction with other individuals or in an organized activity during the past year. McGloin and Widom determined that individuals who functioned competently in six or more of these domains should be considered resilient. Twenty-two percent of the sample who had experienced abuse and/or neglect met these stringent criteria. While this definition of resilience seems to more accurately represent the complexity of competent functioning than symptom absence and although the percentage of individuals who met criteria is encouraging, the categorical nature of this form of assessment did not provide information about partial recovery or the path of recovery for individuals labeled non-resilient. Participants either had received a diagnosis, had problems in work and interpersonal relationships, or they had not. One goal of the current study was to use methodology to assess individuals' perceptions of the shifts in their functioning over time.

The representation of resilience as a complex construct in research also has been facilitated by increased efforts to examine not only the qualities of individuals who appear resilient, but also the process of becoming resilient (Olsson et al. 2003; Richardson, 2002). These research endeavors highlight potential protective and risk factors, the adaptive or maladaptive choices individuals make in response to threats to their development, and examines how these interrelated factors are associated with positive and negative outcomes. Consistent with an ecological perspective (Harvey, 1996), this research incorporates person, event, and environmental level variables into models developed to test predictors of resilience or pathology.

For example, several researchers have examined the association of such variables as self-esteem, locus of control, blame attribution, and support from caregivers and peers with positive outcomes after experiences of abuse (Feinauer & Stuart, 1996; Herrenkohl, Herrenkohl, & Egolf, 1994; Hobfoll et al., 2002; Spaccarelli & Kim, 1995). Thus, we can identify specific characteristics of individuals and resources in their environments that appear related to recovery. However, the nature of these quantitative data constrict the extent to which we can explore how these factors interrelate, where these individuals may be in the process of adaptation to adversity, and what their perceptions are of their recovery process. It also remains unclear whether there are aspects of resilience not captured by the objective, standardized measures commonly used in these studies.

Higgins (1994) explored resilience qualitatively and retrospectively by interviewing 40 adults who had overcome self-defined traumatic experiences and who subsequently were successful in multiple life domains. The author described this sample as having above average intelligence, exceptional talents, long-standing reciprocal relationships, high job satisfaction, and involvement in political or social activism. Higgins identified characteristics of her participants that she felt facilitated their resilience: a commitment to reflection and flexible problem solving, high tolerance for negative affect, the ability to find positive meaning in negative events, and perhaps most importantly, the capacity to build mutual, caring relationships with others. She also noted their general tenacity across life experiences, a strong desire to avoid repeating their parents' mistakes, and faith in the possibility of a better, different world. Higgins asserted that these qualities of resilience are amplified in the participants in her study, but present in everyone. However, there are few studies of the extent to which survivors of trauma who are suffering from psychological distress demonstrate such qualities.

To begin to address this gap in the trauma literature, Harvey and her colleagues (Harvey et al., 2003; Liang, Tummala-Narra, Bradley, & Harvey, this volume) developed a scale and interview designed to assess survivors' strengths as well as their distress and symptoms. This set of instruments, the Multi-Dimensional Trauma Recovery and Resiliency Scale (MTRR-99; see Appendix A at the end of this volume) and Interview (MTRR-I; see Appendix B at the end of this volume), allows clinicians to measure individual variation across a variety of domains and to recognize when individuals have greater as well as lesser capacity in these different aspects of functioning (Harvey et al., 2003). These domains are assessed though an open-ended interview (the MTRR-I) that invites the individual to share the story of her/his life, which the interviewer can rate using the MTRR-99. However, the focus of this study is on the participants' narratives.

The current study presents an analysis of the narratives of 18 survivors of interpersonal violence who completed the MTRR-I. A majority of the participants were survivors of chronic childhood abuse and most had experienced multiple forms of abuse over the course of their lives. They typically would not be the focus of a study of resilience given their current levels of distress and symptomology. Our purpose was to explore the extent to which the qualities and strategies generally associated with resilience were present in the lives of these highly symptomatic individuals; essentially, to apply the concept of resilience more broadly in order to learn about similarities between trauma survivors seeking treatment for their distress and survivors functioning well in many life domains. We were interested in exploring what elements of resilience the participants exhibited in different periods and/or aspects of their lives. We did not require these strengths to be stable over time or across multiple domains; instead, we defined elements of resilience as the adaptive choices individuals made or seemed to be in the process of making subsequent to a traumatic event in any life domain or in any period of their adult life.

## METHOD

### Participants

The demographic characteristics of the 18 clients who chose to participate in the interview were similar to the majority of individuals presenting for treatment at a center for trauma-focused treatment. Most were Caucasian, female, from the surrounding urban area, eligible to receive free psychological services, and met diagnostic criteria for Post Traumatic Stress Disorder and/or Major Depressive Disorder. Two of the 18 participants were Caucasian males. Two of the women identified as Hispanic-American and one woman as Asian-American. The majority of the participants had completed high school; several had attended college, and four had completed graduate school. They ranged in age from 21 to 52 years of age, with an average age of 35 years. None were currently married; a few indicated they had current, long-term partners. Six identified as lesbian. The participants reported experiencing the following forms of interpersonal violence: eight reported histories of childhood sexual abuse, thirteen stated they had experienced physical abuse during their childhoods, eight indicated they had been sexually assaulted as adults, and nine described having had abusive partners in their adulthoods. Twelve described experiences of multiple forms of violence. Three of the participants reported experiencing interpersonal violence as adults but not as children.

### Procedure

An invitation to participate in this study was offered to all new clients who presented for individual, trauma focused treatment at an urban outpatient clinic when they completed an initial packet of self-report questionnaires between 1999 and 2001. Many clients seeking treatment at this facility had sought treatment previously at other sites but remained highly symptomatic. Most were referred after an inpatient hospitalization or were currently in a state of crisis. In addition, because of their limited economic resources and lack of health benefits, clients at the center typically qualified for free or reduced fee care. Participation was completely voluntary and all clients were informed that participation would have no effect on the services they received. Individuals who expressed interest in the study were called and scheduled for an appointment. Several individuals cancelled multiple appointments or did not return for therapy after an initial visit and thus were not interviewed.

Informed consent was discussed at the beginning of each interview. Participants received twenty dollars for the interview regardless of whether or not it was completed. They were invited to stop the interview at any time, could decline to answer questions they did not wish to answer, decline audio-taping of the interview, and take breaks if/when needed. One participant stopped the interview and another later requested that we not use her interview for personal reasons. In the former case, safety was assessed and resources offered prior to ending the meeting. Another interview was not included in these analyses because the participant appeared to be delusional and manic at the time of the interview and we felt we were unable to adequately represent or interpret her experiences.

## *Interview and Method of Analysis*

Many authors have noted the opportunity to understand human experience provided by the study of narratives (e.g., Mishler, 1986). The MTRR-99 and MTRR-I were designed to assess an individual's areas of strength and weakness across multiple domains of functioning.

The MTRR-I begins with an expression of appreciation to the participant for being willing to share his/her experiences. Next, the interviewer explains our interest in various aspects of the participant's life history and invites the participant to tell his/her story. Subsequently, if these concepts were not addressed in the participant's free-flowing narrative, the interviewers use semi-structured prompts to ask more about these subjects. For example, if a participant did not convey the quality of significant relationships with others in his/her narrative, the interviewer asked "Are there ways that you take care of other people and that other people take care of you?" In this study, the average length of the interview was 90 minutes. The interviewers were three female, Caucasian, clinical psychologists at the treatment center. While the majority of the participants were also female and Caucasian, it is important to acknowledge that the gender and/or the ethnicity of the interviewers may have influenced the participants' comfort and willingness to disclose during the interview. Therapists never interviewed their own clients.

The first three authors transcribed the taped interviews and then all authors met regularly for approximately ten months to conduct thematic analyses of the transcribed interviews. We employed a strategy of open coding in our analyses. This coding technique is derived from the grounded theory approach (Charmaz, 2000) and is used to focus the analysts on the participants' experiences and to extract meaning based as closely as possible on their words and experiences. We conducted this type of analysis with the stated purpose of generating theory rather than confirming preconceived hypotheses (Charmaz, 2000). Thus, our goal for this project was not to confirm the existing MTRR domains but rather to conduct an open ended exploration of the elements of resilience that the participants included in their narratives.

We began by coding five of the interviews line-by-line. In other words, we worked to represent every emotion, event, or action described in each line of text. During this stage of our coding process, several concepts were linked with a single sentence. For example, we identified independence, work, school, quitting, and motivation in the following segment of text: "I left school but I ended up going back after working for a while." Next, we reviewed the initial codes derived from our line-by-line analysis, and by comparing them within and across the five interviews, we generated a list of 54 codes. We then grouped these 54 codes into several general conceptual categories: self, connections with others, actions/coping, affect, type of violence, health, structure, and quality of the narrative. The generated codes both represented the participants' variety of experiences and allowed us to combine similar concepts or experiences into one term. The following are examples of the codes we generated: creativity, insight, anger, setting boundaries, positive connections, seeking help, paid work, psychological distress, control, identity, vulnerability, humor, and taking responsibility. We then read and independently applied these codes to eight additional interviews. For each of these eight narratives, we continued to meet and discuss how we had coded the transcripts. When individuals' experiences did not seem to be captured by the list, we generated additional codes, ultimately adding four to our initial list for a total of 58 terms. As we discussed our coding of each interview, we noticed that we typically agreed in our use of the codes. When we disagreed, we discussed our reasoning, and through this dialogue, reached agreement. Based on these discussions, we independently coded the remaining six interviews.

All the codes that we agreed on for the 18 interviews were attached to relevant lines of text using the qualitative software program WinMax (Kuckartz, 1998). The software was used to sort groups of quotations by each code so that we could further examine commonalities and differences across the different narratives within each code category and identify common themes. Although we entered all of the codes into the software program, for this project we chose to focus on only those codes that seemed to represent participants' strengths or adaptive choices subsequent to threats such as traumatic events or subsequent trauma-related distress. We read over the quotations organized by these codes that seemed to convey positive experiences and choices, such as accomplishment or self care, and worked to identify the common themes from across the narratives in each of these codes. We also compared quotations from similar code categories such as assertiveness and boundaries within and across the narratives. In this way, we identified critical themes drawn from the code categories that we believed illustrated resilience (see Table 1). Once the themes were identified, we aimed to include both illustrative quotations from participants and examples that seemed most representative of their experiences. This is the data that comprises the results section.

We also invited a colleague to read the narratives as well as the identified themes and supporting quotations that we had selected. We explained we were interested in her opinion about whether our selections seemed representative of the strengths in all of the narratives. Our colleague responded that the themes and selected quotations appeared representative of the participants' narratives. Our effort to make our focus on resilience explicit, to include themes that represented the participants' experiences as accurately and as closely as possible with their own words, to use a process of coding and interpretation that was collaborative and highly visible, and our invitation to a colleague to check the accuracy of our work demonstrates our attention to rigorous, feminist methods of inquiry (Hall, 1991).

## RESULTS

Below, we describe the different themes that emerged from our exploration of strengths in the participants' narratives. Some were relevant to their past, whereas others were strengths they displayed at the time of the interview. While it is important to acknowledge that the respondents were suffering from substantial psychological distress, we found numerous examples of their capacity for recovery within their stories. First, we noted their ability to make and sustain positive connections with other individuals and as members of a group, in essence to trust others even after experiencing interpersonal violence. Next, they clearly demonstrated the capacity to utilize opportunities to be successful and in that action, to recognize their skills and competencies even though many struggled with negative feelings about themselves. Finally, they all seemed to describe a process of self change that included

TABLE 1. Codes Illustrating Strengths and Associated Times

| Code Types | Codes Illustrating Strengths | Themes |
|---|---|---|
| Self Codes | Accomplishment<br>Determination/goal setting<br>Identity<br>Positive Self [evaluation] | Taking Opportunities<br>Taking Opportunities<br>Processes of Self Change<br>Processes of Self Change &<br>Taking Opportunities |
| Connection Codes | Boundaries<br>Breaking connections<br>Positive connection<br>Supportive Others | Assertiveness/Limits<br>Assertiveness/Limits<br>Inspiration thru Connection<br>Inspiration thru Connection |
| Action Codes | Assertiveness<br>Avoidance<br>Creativity<br>Insight<br>Self care | Assertiveness/Limits<br>Self Care and Coping<br>Self Care and Coping<br>Processes of Self Change<br>Self Care and Coping |
| Affect Codes | Anger<br>Blame<br>Hope | Responsibility<br>Responsibility<br>Processes of Self Change |

developing and maintaining multiple, active coping strategies, a shift in the attribution of responsibility for the violence, a current focus on making different life choices, and holding onto hope through difficult times.

## *Inspiration through Connection*

The majority of the participants described positive connections with important others. Their closest connections seemed to be with others who could be relied on consistently, through good and bad times. For some, it also seemed critical that those around them understand their experiences, either through having a similar history or simply by being a good listener.

> If it hadn't, if it wasn't for my mother, I don't know where I would be right now, because she was always there for me, she always helped me out, if I needed to talk to her I'd have someone to talk to.

> She's the one person that actually in my life has sort of a similar background in terms of dysfunctional families and dealing with the whole thing about you know getting a higher education than where you came from and then not being able to go home . . . she's the really one person that I have that I feel like I have some major things in common with.

Two women that I met at work are sort of like my cool mom, who I can talk to about anything.

A number of participants also specifically identified important others who served as mentors to them. They found individuals outside of their families–generally teachers, therapists, or work supervisors–to provide them with recognition and praise for abilities that otherwise often went unappreciated. In addition, these important others seemed to provide tools for learning and strategies that facilitated the participants' success. At times, they also gave direct assistance. For example, one woman explained that her art teacher paid an application fee and drove her to a contest for an art scholarship, a scholarship that she won and used to attend school.

I had a teacher who was really good for me. She was my English teacher and thought I was an incredible writer and she wrote me a letter about how talented I was and how special I was to her and she was really a positive force. I did well in her classes and completed things. She taught me how to study, how to take notes in class, how to do things like that. That was extremely helpful.

Well I think one person that meant a lot to me was my biology teacher when I was a freshman in high school . . . she was also my counselor and she was the first person I went to for . . . just to talk. You know, just to talk about problems and issues in my life at that time, things that I was struggling with. So she was very important to me, and I loved her because she was there for me.

Finally, a few participants indicated that positive connections with others had offered them protection from the violence. Again, participants actively engaged individuals outside of their families, adults who indicated that they did not agree with how the participant was being treated and who in some way offered concrete assistance to them.

I would always run to my neighbors' house . . . they were always like very nice to me but back then you know the thing is that people didn't really want to believe that something like any form of child abuse existed, or that if it did, they should remain outside of it, but although she did voice her opinion many times, you know to my mother, you know it just never . . . I was grateful that I had someplace to run to.

I went to a center for women when I was still married and I knew
something was wrong. I knew that I was in danger . . . there was an
advocate and she walked me through the initial steps of having my
husband removed from the house and I think if it wasn't for her I'd
still be with my husband today.

The majority of participants also indicated that much of their strength
and determination came from the reciprocal nature of their relationships
with group members. Their descriptions suggested that membership in
groups through paid work, volunteering, spirituality, and "self-help" organizations energized them and confirmed a sense of themselves as valued and capable contributors to the community. In particular, others in
the groups seemed to serve as role models, to provide confirmation of
shared values, and to offer an opportunity and motivation to heal oneself through connections with others.

I think the job kind of solidified things–I mean we worked with all
these women from different conflict areas, most of them have experienced major, major trauma and uh, there was something about
listening to these stories . . . it was very hard to listen to them speak
about their pain and their experiences. But another part was seeing
these women who had gone through, you know, you see–awful,
awful experiences and had come out stronger and you know just
these amazing women and I think the combination of that and just
the support I felt from the other, the other women I worked with
and you know none of them had any idea what I was going through
but they were still a support there and I think that really kind of
made a difference for me, kind of gave me a focus and put things in
perspective . . .

So like, it felt like a community with the organization that I
volunteered with you know, everybody really liked what they
were doing, they felt that it was necessary. Nobody that I met
that volunteered felt that being a volunteer there would get us into
heaven–we just did it cause we liked doing it and felt it was important so I felt like a community with them.

It's a group of mostly men and women of color who come together
and, the thing about it is that we're not just talking about it, we're
actually planning things, we're, you know, writing letters, campaigns, you know, protests, that's what makes, that's what excites

me is to be doing something as opposed to just talking about it . . . So, that's been an incredible experience.

I'm doing the 12 steps in the program of AA . . . People recognize things in me . . . I don't know–they just help me ground myself and they give me advice . . . they tell me when I'm, they call me on my shit ya know (laugh).

## *Taking Opportunities to be Successful*

In addition to demonstrating the capacity to develop trusting, reciprocal relationships with others, most of the respondents shared a history of achievement in their schooling and success at work for some period of time in their lives. Some who described themselves as smart indicated that they struggled to focus in school and did not necessarily demonstrate their ability through their academic records, but still were successful in graduating and pursuing occupational or academic goals. Incredibly, although all of the participants encountered obstacles in their pursuit of a college education, most returned to school later in their lives and balanced work and school, and sometimes parenthood, while obtaining a degree. A few indicated that the effort of meeting the demands of work or school assisted them in keeping psychological distress at bay. Perhaps not surprisingly, about a fourth of the sample described choosing to work in jobs aimed at providing help to others and indicated pleasure and satisfaction in assisting others to change their lives. Finally, as readers of the narratives, we noticed that participants' descriptions of their work conveyed the clearest and most consistent sense of accomplishment and suggestion of positive self worth across the narratives.

The best times were when, and I worked in the divorces mostly, but, domestic violence and, there would be those moments with those women where you could hear in their voice that they–probably wouldn't last–but that they realized they deserved better and that talking with you helped them to see that and those were incredible, that I could do that.

I ended being really successful . . . The center ended up hiring me fulltime and I ended up getting promoted. I loved my job–I was the director of the women's center and I also was the supervisor of the lesbian/gay/bisexual center.

> I was getting all the kudos and I kept progressing at work and get-
> ting promotions and pretty soon I had my own crew and I was, I
> was a supervisor within I guess six months of working there.

Whereas the majority of participants' stories suggested that they experienced a sense of accomplishment at work, a few indicated that they
felt most accomplished when they expressed themselves creatively or
through physical activity. In these cases, the participants seemed not
only to feel successful but their descriptions also depicted that these activities were mechanisms for coping with their experiences of violence.

> I think the way I healed was just by overstepping my own bound-
> aries and I was able to put a lot of work together and have an ex-
> hibit right away and so um, in that sense you know I was able to
> actually just turn around all that and be able to surpass it and that
> was I would say that was tremendously successful.

> When I was playing sports I pretty much could forget about every-
> thing and I didn't, you know I was, I had some talent so I was
> pretty good and it was fun and um you know I pretty much did a lot
> of that, I mean I was on the cross country team and I would come
> home from practice and eat dinner and go out and run again
> {laughs} for two hours and um you know I, I, that's, that's pretty
> much how I coped. I mean I was so physically active and for me it
> was fun, I really enjoyed playing, for me those are my, my best
> memories are definitely playing sports and being involved in
> sports.

### Processes of Self-Change

Participants' descriptions of their accomplishments were often located in their recent past. At the time of the interview, most were focused on coping with substantial psychological distress, particularly
intense, unwanted affect. However, even at this critical time, it was
clear that they were working on how they might increase their capacity
to deal with their distress. All of the participants' narratives suggested
they were engaged in a process of recovery represented by their determination to confront their unwanted memories and to manage overwhelming affect. Similarly, they indicated they were increasingly
prepared to take care of themselves through asserting their right to meet

their own needs and setting limits in relationships with others. They also seemed to demonstrate growing recognition of how their experiences had affected them, attributing responsibility for the violence to their perpetrators while acknowledging that the choice to make their lives different now is their own. Finally, they demonstrated the belief that they could live their lives differently as a result of their own actions and faith. The participants' descriptions of these effortful changes in strategies of coping and relating, of attributing responsibility, and in holding onto their hope, conveyed their insight into the challenges they faced and a sense of power to make the changes. In each case, they seemed to be recognizing how past events might affect them now and to be exploring their capacity to be the actor, in control of one's self in the present.

*Self-care and coping.* All of the participants described multiple forms of coping and the majority seemed committed to working on taking care of themselves physically as well as mentally. The predominant underlying theme across these descriptions seemed to us to be persistent, ongoing determination to cope. This involved dealing with overwhelming affect in healthy ways, specifically, enhancing their abilities to stay present, to tolerate affect and memories, and to self soothe. For example, they described writing, cooking, listening to music, walking, and exercising; painting pictures and a multitude of ways that they worked to release tension and cope with negative affect.

> I think throughout my life I've used um music and films as, and art as ways, not that I'm an artist but I love art and you know any kind of creativity. I used to keep a journal more, more diligently than I have been but any form of creativity, I try to escape that way as opposed to doing something self-destructive.

> (Any changes in way you cope with stress?) Yeah. There's more . . . there's more process, there's more, instead of just stuffing it in and trying to keep it out of sight, I'm trying more to look at it, let it out, um, understand it better, and uh . . . feel it, so yeah.

> I try to just break down each moment into the space of a breath and that I will feel whatever I'm feeling and just tell myself that it's OK, whatever I feel, not judge the feeling, is this good or bad, do I want to feel this way, none of this and know that it will pass. It will pass as long as I keep breathing and keep focusing and start to do things . . .

I let time go by and it's not as stressful to me. I don't know if that makes sense . . . and then I tackle it one at a time.

A mental thing that I do just to be okay is . . . this is now and you're just telling this person um here what went on–that goes on, that's my . . . I call it head talk . . . If things get really bad . . . I get ice–which generally is really helpful to me. . . . It's a form of action, the ice or some other grounding, I've used a watch when I can't get to ice . . . I take my watch and I take the stem and I push the stem into my wrist, not hard enough to do some damage, it's just like a little pinch that tells you ok, you are real, this is, this is a real place, this is something you're remembering, it's not actually happening, just enough of a little pinch to get, bring me back to where I need to be.

*Assertiveness and limits.* One way that many of the participants conveyed an increased investment in taking care of themselves was in their descriptions of times they asserted their right to be respected and to have their own needs met. For many, this was an ongoing process of realizing they could assert these rights and they were trying out new and varied strategies. They also described a process of learning to set limits in relationships and, at times, considered ending relationships when they recognized their needs were not being met or simply to protect themselves.

Her check wouldn't go through and I remember asking her very nicely if it was from out of state and she was very, very snotty with me and like put her face in mine . . . and I remember like telling her hold it right there, I asked you a question very nicely and I want you to answer my question very nicely as well and you know she was taken aback by that in the sense of you know not expecting me to have to say to her well you know I'm speaking to you nicely and I'm asking you a question for a reason, so she ended up apologizing.

I was always very much the caretaker and taking care of other people's needs and I am beginning to realize you know that I deserve the same nurturance or sustenance or support that I was giving to others.

I'm learning how to make boundaries with people so I have to learn how to say no, like I can't do this or I can't do that. I'm getting better at it.

I'm more willing to remove myself from a relationship than I used to be. A lot more willing to remove myself from my relationship. (You mean end the relationship?) End it or take a break, whatever it takes, to complete . . . [long pause] . . . I'm more comfortable with the idea of being alone . . . I want to work things out. But I'm learning to accept the fact that what one person wants doesn't determine the outcome of the relationship.

*Responsibility.* The narrators described shifts in their perceptions of past relationships as well as changes in their expectations in current relationships. In particular, they seemed to be developing a more complex understanding of the traumatic events in their lives. Although several participants still felt shame and anger directed at themselves, they also expressed a growing cognitive awareness that it was the perpetrators of the violence who were at fault, clearly distinguishing between the role of a child and a caregiver/adult. In addition, while most did not describe themselves as having forgiven their perpetrators for their actions, they indicated some acceptance or understanding that the perpetrators were likely influenced by experiences in their own lives and consequently made the choices to act as they did. Finally, the participants seemed aware of how traumatic events may have influenced some of their previous, unhealthy, choices, but noted that in the present time, they are the ones who have control over their actions.

Had I had a better childhood I would have liked myself a lot better than to get involved with the people that I got involved with but I don't feel like, I don't ever feel like look at what the world has done to me. I mean I know that you know you have to learn you know why you got into certain situations and how not to have them you know come back into your life.

I understand it's the choices people in my life have made and its affected me and . . . potentially affected the choices that I make in my life. But I also realize the, both internal and external forces upon those choices and . . . so it's a very sort of complex understanding.

I think that my parents came from where they came from and came up in a time where it wasn't acceptable to seek help. They brought what they brought to the relationship. I believe they loved me, I believe they did the best they could with what they had. . . . I'm learning there is no way, there's no way it's all my fault . . . you're still responsible for your own reaction to what happens to you, more so, more so if the person to whom you're reacting is a child and you're an adult. More so still if the person to whom you're reacting is a child and you're that child's parent, or caretaker.

*Hope.* Although their experiences of interpersonal violence clearly challenged the basic assumption of a benevolent world, all the participants conveyed some hope that their life would change for the better as a result of their efforts. Some seemed uncertain of whether they would attain the wishes they had for themselves, but all described beliefs that their efforts could lead to meaningful lives through their work, helping others, spirituality, or through healing themselves. Underlying this faith seemed to be a sense that life can be meaningful if one is determined enough and recognizes the power to make choices as adults. Several participants clearly communicated their understanding that their future is in their own hands.

> It [spirituality] gives me a lot of strength . . . and even when I can't get to the point where I can get strength from it, I get hope from it and then once I get hope I get strength.

> I hope, my hope is to again to, I would love to be able to really find work that uh I can honestly . . . feel like I'm doing something I believe in I guess, give me a sense of purpose, a sense of feeling connected to the world and people.

> I mean it's a really uncomfortable process and I guess I was aware and prepared that there would be times that I was going to feel it even worse before I really started to feel consistently better . . . but . . . there's a difference between knowing that ahead of time and then actually being in the moment and having all this stuff dredged up, having to think about it and process it, and having it be painful or realizing your, you know this pain is really old, this pain is really old, and it stings and it hurts and god this sucks why am I even doing this I should quit [soft laughter], but knowing that it's like having a bad tooth [laughs] . . . It's got to be taken care of and I'll feel a lot better once it is.

> On the other hand I don't think anything is so bad that I can't pull my life together. There is always that element that I think I can do it.

## *DISCUSSION*

The individuals who took part in this study were highly symptomatic at the time of the interview and reported experiencing periods of substantial psychological distress over the course of their lives. However, they also displayed many qualities that have been identified as contributing to resilience. The majority of the participants described themselves as smart and most displayed a sense of humor as they told their stories. All indicated that they had positive relationships with at least one important other, and most had engaged the interest of individuals outside their families of origin who provided them with encouragement, praise, and support. Some also indicated that their positive connections with others, particularly in groups, provided them with a sense of shared values and the knowledge that they were not alone as well as with examples of how to overcome the adversity in their lives. These characteristics and experiences of supportive relationships clearly mirror those of resilient children and adults described in reviews of the resilience literature (Olsson et al., 2003; Richardson, 2002). In addition, the underlying themes of determination, insight, and hope reflect those identified in qualitative analyses of resilient adults (Higgins, 1994). Thus, while these participants appeared to be struggling in some or even several domains of functioning in their lives, they also exhibited a powerful motivation, an ability to connect with others, and faith in the possibility of a better life. Together, these characteristics suggest that although they do not meet the stringent criteria defining an adult as resilient or not resilient (e.g., McGloin & Widom, 2001), they are engaged in a process of adaptation or recovery from trauma and they bring these strengths with them to that process when they seek out treatment.

Many of the participants described a sense of accomplishment based on their experiences at work. Higgins (1994) identified success and satisfaction at work as a central characteristic of the resilient adults that she interviewed. Although some of the participants of this study were not working at the time of the interview, we felt that their depictions of their competency at work for a period of time during their life seemed similar in nature to Higgins' (1994) portrayal of her sample. Specifically, the participants in this study conveyed a capacity to contribute, even to excel, at work that they rarely described in other contexts. Even when they were severely distressed, work was a domain in which a majority of the respondents had experienced success. In addition, many participants made positive connections with co-workers or supervisors that offered them support and encouragement. Across the narratives, the workplace appeared to offer unique opportunities to be successful and to feel positively about themselves in these individuals' lives. This finding is similar to the quantitative results of a study focused on associations among partner violence, paid work, and sense of self (Lynch & Graham-Bermann, 2004). In that study, women's experiences at work ($N = 100$) were significantly and positively associated with women's sense of self, suggesting that paid work may serve as a source of positive feedback in the context of partner violence. However, unless problems at work are part of a presenting complaint, the quality of individuals' experiences at work is not typically included in initial assessments of functioning. Generally, we investigate the length of time of employment, reasons for leaving jobs, and number of jobs held. Although further studies would be necessary to generalize the results from this study, our analyses suggest that attending to a trauma survivor's past and current positive work experiences, rather than focusing solely on how symptoms and distress impair their functioning at work, may be one avenue to discovering what potential strengths they bring to treatment.

All of the narratives illustrated ongoing efforts to develop and maintain coping strategies aimed at dealing with overwhelming affect and memories. Many participants also indicated they were coming to an understanding about the traumatic events they experienced, including shifting blame from themselves to the perpetrators of the violence while simultaneously comprehending that the perpetrators' actions and decisions were often influenced by events in their own lives. In essence, the participants seemed to be in a process of noticing the ways in which they were influenced by events in their lives but also recognizing their capacity to make different choices to protect and nurture themselves as well as their loved ones at this point in their lives. These shifts were accompanied by an increased willingness to assert boundaries in their relationships with others and to take care of themselves by meeting their own needs, replicating some of the positive self transitions identified by Hall (2003) in her work with women who were survivors of child abuse. While the nature of this research does not allow for conclusions about causality, it seems probable that these self processes are interrelated and indicative of an increased sense of power to act for oneself and a developing internal belief that one is worthy of protection and self care. Again, it seem critical to note that these participants recently had initiated or reinitiated treatment at the time of the interview and thus, appear to be bringing these active, engaged self processes to treatment.

The purpose of using a qualitative approach grounded as closely as possible in the participants' actual experiences and voices is to gain access to information not well captured by standardized measures and to inform developing theory (Charmaz, 2000). Thus, while it is important to note that the sample size and nature of the study prevent generalizing these results to all survivors of multiple traumas, this qualitative analysis provides insight into potential strengths that is not typically obtained with current commonly used self report measures. For example, listening closely to the participants' actual words conveys several reasons why a mentor is useful: as a source of praise and feedback as well as information about tools and strategies, and as a person who offers direct, concrete assistance. Similarly, we can notice shifts in perspectives and changes in behaviors, such as the different self processes identified in the analyses that are not easily assessed with measures of self-esteem or efficacy. Clearly, these analyses of processes of change are limited by the retrospective nature of this data, given that we only interviewed the participants one time. However, the analyses are based on the participants' knowledge of their life experiences and on the perceptions they shared regarding how they have changed over time. The current analyses also suggest avenues for future studies. For example, a study that initially included an assessment of strengths as well as pathology and then followed participants over time would allow us to make stronger conclusions about ways in which potential strengths are used in the process of recovery and provide evidence of the utility of incorporating an explicit assessment of strengths early in the therapeutic process.

Finally, typical assessments of individuals who present for treatment related to traumatic experiences are focused on ascertaining the scope of the presenting problem, severity and duration of symptoms, treatment history, orientation to reality, a brief psychosocial history, and possibly sources of social support. This comparably narrow focus is due to a combination of time constraints for assessment, a limited number of total sessions, and the demand for an immediate diagnosis. Yet even when there are a finite number of sessions, the narratives of these participants suggest the potential utility of conducting an initial interview that explicitly explores characteristics associated with resilience, regarding both the person and his/her environmental context. This study suggests that potential aspects of an individual's life to assess are the presence of reciprocal, consistent relationships with others, meaningful involvement in a group, quality of work experiences, and the extent to which individuals seem to be developing an understanding of their experiences that conveys their right to assert and meet their needs, and the ability to make choices that will impact their life at this time. Masten (2001) suggested that it is the ability to use ordinary, basic human skills, connections, and experiences to aid in one's recovery that is of the greatest interest to scientists and practitioners. It is our hope that this study contributes insight into what those ordinary strengths, experiences, and skills might be in the process of adapting to adversity for survivors of trauma.

> Bad things happened. I can't change what happened but I can try to like put my life back together and move on and hopefully help other people who had the same experience get better.

## REFERENCES

Bybee. D. I., & Sullivan, C. M. (2002). The process through which an advocacy intervention resulted in positive change for battered women over time. *American Journal of Community Psychology, 30,* 103-133.

Charmaz, K. (2000). Grounded theory: Objectivist and constructivist methods. In N. K. Denzin & Y. S. Lincoln, Y.S. (Eds), *Handbook of qualitative research* (2nd ed., pp. 509-535). Thousand Oaks: Sage.

Davis, R. E. (2002). The strongest women: Exploration of the inner resources of abused women. *Qualitative Health Research, 12,* 1248-1263.

Feinauer, L. L., & Stuart, D. A. (1996). Blame and resilience in women sexually abused as children. *American Journal of Family Therapy, 24*(1), 31-40.

Hall. J. (1991). Rigor in feminist research. *Advances in Nursing Science, 13*(3), 16-29.

Hall. J. (2003). Positive self transitions in women child abuse survivors. *Issues in Mental Health Nursing, 24,* 647-666.

Harvey, M. R. (1996). An ecological view of psychological trauma and trauma recovery. *Journal of Traumatic Stress, 9*(1), 3-23.

Harvey, M. R. (2007). Towards an ecological understanding of resilience in trauma survivors: Implications for theory, research, and practice. *Journal of Aggression, Maltreatment & Trauma, 14*(1/2), 9-32.

Harvey, M. R., Liang, B., Harney, P. A., Koenen, K., Tummala-Narra, P., & Lebowitz, L. (2003). A multidimensional approach to the assessment of trauma impact, recovery and resiliency: Five psychometric studies. *Journal of Aggression, Maltreatment & Trauma, 6*(2), 87-109.

Heller. S. S., Larrieu, J. A., D'Imperio, R., & Boris, N. W. (1999). Research on resilience to child maltreatment: Empirical considerations. *Child Abuse and Neglect, 23*(4), 321-338.

Herrenkohl, E. C., Herrenkohl, R. C. & Egolf, B. (1994). Resilient early school-age children from maltreating homes: Outcomes in late adolescence. *American Journal of Orthopsychiatry, 64*(2), 301-309.

Higgins, G. O. (1994) *Resilient adults: Overcoming a cruel past.* San Francisco: Josey-Bass.

Hobfoll, S. E., Bansal, A., Schurg, R., Young, S., Pierce, C. A., Hobfoll, I. et al. (2002). The impact of perceived child physical and sexual abuse history on Native American women's psychological well-being and AIDS risk. *Journal of Consulting and Clinical Psychology, 70*(1), 252-257.

Kuckartz, U. (1998). *WinMAX 98 Pro* [computer software]. Thousand Oaks, CA: Sage.

Liang, B., Tummala-Narra, U., Bradley, R., & Harvey, M. R. (2007). The Multidimensional Trauma and Resilience Instrument: Preliminary examination of an abridged version. *Journal of Aggression, Maltreatment, and Trauma, 14*(1/2). 55-74.

Liem, J. H., James, J. B., O'Toole, J. G., & Boudewyn, A. (1997). Assessing resilience in adults with histories of childhood sexual abuse. *American Journal of Orthopsychiatry, 67*(4), 594-606.

Lynch, S. M., & Graham-Bermann, S. A. (2004). Exploring the relationship between positive work experiences and women's sense of self in the context of partner abuse. *Psychology of Women Quarterly, 8*(2), 159-167.

Luthar, S. S., Cicchetti, D., & Becker, B. (2000). The construct of resilience: A critical evaluation and guidelines for future work. *Child Development, 71*(3), 543-562.

Masten, A. S. (2001). Ordinary magic: Resilience processes in development. *American Psychologist, 56*, 227-238.

McGloin, J. M., & Widom, C. S. (2001). Resilience among abused and neglected children grown up. *Development and Psychopathology, 13*, 1021-1038.

Mishler, E. G. (1986). *Research interviewing: context and narrative*. Cambridge, MA: Harvard University Press.

Olsson, C. A., Bond, L., Burns, J. M., Vella-Brodrick, D. A., & Sawyer, S. M. (2003). Adolescent resilience: A concept analysis. *Journal of Adolescence, 26*, 1-11.

Richardson, G. E. (2002). The meta-theory of resilience and resiliency. *Journal of Clinical Psychology, 58*, 307-321.

Spaccarelli, S., & Kim, S. (1995). Spotlight on practice: Resilience criteria and factors associated with resilience in sexually abused girls. *Child Abuse and Neglect, 19*, 1171-1182.

doi:10.1300/J146v14n01_05

# Where the Whole Thing Fell Apart:
# Race, Resilience, and the Complexity
# of Trauma

Lynn Sorsoli

**SUMMARY.** This article examines the intersection of societal prejudice and psychological trauma. In an instrumental case study created
through a layered narrative analysis, the author highlights the potentially
traumatic effects of racism and discrimination, while also exploring the
phenomenon of resilience in a complex ecological system. The findings
suggest that the enduring and continual strain of racial prejudice may
cause significant psychological distress, particularly when those experiences reinforce early negative experiences within a family; and that assessments of resilience need to consider the contribution of ecological
context to psychological outcomes as well as to an individual's ability to
mobilize personal resources when such a context finally shifts.
doi:10.1300/J146v14n01_06 *[Article copies available for a fee from The
Haworth Document Delivery Service: 1-800-HAWORTH. E-mail address:
<docdelivery@haworthpress.com> Website: <http://www.HaworthPress.com>
© 2007 by The Haworth Press, Inc. All rights reserved.]*

**KEYWORDS.** Trauma, race, resilience, case study, narrative analysis

Address correspondence to: Dr. Lynn Sorsoli, Center for Research on Gender and
Sexuality, 2017 Mission Street, Suite 300, San Francisco, CA 94110.

[Haworth co-indexing entry note]: "Where the Whole Thing Fell Apart: Race, Resilience, and the Com-
plexity of Trauma." Sorsolii, Lynn. Co-published simultaneously in *Journal of Aggression, Maltreatment &
Trauma* (The Haworth Maltreatment & Trauma Press, an imprint of The Haworth Press, Inc.) Vol. 14, No.
1/2, 2007, pp. 99-121; and: *Sources and Expressions of Resiliency in Trauma Survivors: Ecological Theory,
Multicultural Practice* (ed: Mary R. Harvey, and Pratyusha Tummala-Narra) The Haworth Maltreatment &
Trauma Press, an imprint of The Haworth Press, Inc., 2007, pp. 99-121. Single or multiple copies of this article are available for a fee from The Haworth Document Delivery Service [1-800-HAWORTH, 9:00 a.m. -
5:00 p.m. (EST). E-mail address: docdelivery@haworthpress.com].

Available online at http://jamt.haworthpress.com
© 2007 by The Haworth Press, Inc. All rights reserved.
doi:10.1300/J146v14n01_06

The only community I ever thought I would be a part of is an academic community and I felt like I was *robbed* of that because people were relating to my race. What the hell does Blackness have to do with 15th century art? Nothing.

We weren't taught that we were special in and of ourselves and that's where the whole thing fell apart once we got out into the world.

According to the Diagnostic and Statistical Manual of Mental Disorders (American Psychiatric Association [APA], 1994), the criteria for a "traumatic" stressor stipulate that the event or events "involved actual or threatened death or serious injury" (p. 463) and that the emotional responses to these events entailed fear, helplessness, or horror. Although the specificity of these criteria has led to powerful and important understandings of a particular form of traumatic stress, many clinicians and researchers embrace a broader definition of "trauma" in their work, acknowledging that psychological harm can arise from a wide array of experiences, many of which may greatly impact developmental processes (Garbarino, Guttmann, & Seely, 1986; Hart, Binggeli, & Brassard, 1998). Recognizing the complexity of psychological trauma, these broader definitions tend to incorporate a greater range of experiences, including complicated social and emotional experiences not specifically related to physical integrity. Other researchers have in addition taken an "ecological view" of trauma and recovery (Harvey, 1996), arguing that rather than happening in a vacuum, potentially traumatic events occur within an ecological system and that individual differences in trauma responses and recovery are the result of complicated interactions between event, person, and environment. As Shalev (2002) argues, "Events are never 'traumatic' just because they meet a threshold criterion. Extreme events become traumatic . . . when the individual exposed is, for some reason, vulnerable to their effect" (p. 161).

This important shift away from an event/criterion-based definition of trauma allows for the existence of individual vulnerabilities, which from an ecological perspective can occur anywhere in the person-event ecosystem, such as when events and environment conspire to corrupt potential sources of resiliency; and encourages us to consider experiences that are not distinct or discrete but rather enduring or continual. For example, although racism obviously can lead to serious violence, it is often more subtle and insidious. Yet, it is clear that discrimination and hostility based on race and class, both pervasive elements of the social system, can have effects that are harmful both economically and psychologically (e.g., Eyerman, 2001) and can interrupt sources of personal strength and resiliency (e.g., Allen, 2001), even when the experiences are not life-threatening. In fact, years of systematic discrimination and segregation may have left Black children in a particularly vulnerable position in this society (Edelman, 1985). Though perhaps never quite meeting the diagnostic threshold of a traumatic stressor, it seems possible that, for some children, exposure to discrimination could produce a set of psychological symptoms mirroring the effects of trauma.

Redefining the experience of racism as potentially traumatic (Burstow, 2003; Daniel, 2000; Harvey, 1996; Sanchez-Hucles, 1999) encourages us to listen closely for signs of complex trauma (Herman, 1992a), a particular collection of symptoms normally following early and prolonged exposure to interpersonal violence that may be heard in personal narratives, including a lack of predictable sense of self, a poor sense of separateness, and a disturbed body image; poorly modulated affect and impulse control; and an uncertainty about the reliability and predictability of others (van der Kolk, 2002). A person of color may encounter instance after instance of racism throughout his or her lifetime; such exposure–though not necessarily life-threatening–would understandably tear at self-esteem, shape one's relationship with the larger world, and, potentially, have a complexly traumatic impact on the developing individual. At the same time, because racial hegemony has been woven into the fabric of American society, the context in which these events are experienced also colors the experiences, as well as expressions of resilience and subsequent pathways to recovery.

The subject of this case study, Patti,[1] is a Black woman (she preferred the term Black over African American, saying emphatically "Just please call me Black 'cause I'm Black") in her late thirties. One of the youngest in a large family, she had been raised in a large northeastern city. After attending a well-known college, she completed a graduate degree and is now actively pursuing a career as an artist. In some senses, the experiences Patti narrated were more like normal, everyday experiences than the horrific childhood experiences of violence and abuse that one might hear in interviews open to these stories; however, there was no question that she had been deeply affected by her childhood and in ways reminiscent of trauma survivors. Like past studies in which narrative methods have been used to understand the lived experiences of trauma survivors (Harvey, Mishler, Koenen, & Harney, 2000; Rogers, 1999; Sorsoli, 2004), this case study relies on narrative analysis to provide insight into the intriguing intersection between trauma and race. A rigorous exploration of Patti's experiences and childhood environment yields a portrait of the potentially traumatic impact of experiences with racism and discrimination. Moreover, paying close attention to the ways this particular Black woman narrated her life experiences, including distressing experiences involving racism and discrimination, provides a deep understanding of the ways the relationships between an individual, her experiences, and her environment can contribute to her resiliency or hamper her recovery.

## METHOD

Although in quantitative research a larger sample can offer greater statistical power, the object of qualitative research is often not to generalize to a larger population but to optimize the understanding of the topic, or case, at hand (Stake, 1998) as well as to generate theory (Strauss & Corbin, 1998) or hypotheses for subsequent quantitative research. The complexity of the phenomenon of resilience suggests that case study analysis would be an appropriate and useful research method for this topic (Yin, 1994). In this article, an instrumental case study (Stake, 1998) offers insight both into the intersection of racism and trauma and the complexity of resilience in a person-event ecosystem, while also providing a thorough and systematic exploration of the reasons Patti, a woman who had not experienced significant direct exposure to maltreatment or violence, was narrating many symptoms of trauma; and in addition, why she should be considered particularly resilient.

As a part of a larger study focusing on the experience of disclosing painful or traumatic events (Sorsoli, 2003), I conducted two interviews with Patti. The first interview (the Multidimensional Trauma Recovery and Resiliency Interview; Harvey, Liang, Harney, Koenan, Tumamal-Narra, & Lebowitz, 2003) was semi-structured, and sought information about life history, including early experiences and relationships, work history and current relationships, coping with stress and emotions, expectations of the future, and the meaning-making process. The second interview was more open-ended, though focused on the process of disclosing painful or traumatic events in relationships across the lifespan. Together these interviews served as vehicles for understanding the intricacies and nuances of Patti's relationships with culture, context, and experience and the ways in which these factors shaped her identity and her encounters with trauma. Patti's two interviews were relatively long, lasting between two and three hours each.

The audio-taped interviews were transcribed verbatim, including pauses, voice drops (both volume and pitch), laughter, stammers, and repetitions. When available and appropriate, information from post-interview notes about body language, gestures, and gaze was also included. The full annotated transcripts were first coded line by line to capture the thematic content of repetitive or commonly made statements utilizing an open-coding technique (Miles & Huberman, 1994; Strauss & Corbin, 1998). As a second layer of analysis, again coding inductively, a clean transcript was reviewed to identify and thematically code personal narratives (stories with a beginning, middle, and end); finally, certain segments of interview (particularly those providing additional context or clarification for narratives) were also separately coded.

While these three layers of analysis were often intricately related, each layer allowed a slightly different understanding of Patti's experiences to emerge. For example, while the first layer of analysis captured the many different ways her sense that she was "bad" was expressed directly and metaphorically in her statements, the second layer clarified the way her "badness" was expressed thematically in her stories, while the final layer suggested the ways the meaning of "badness" could be co-constructed through conversation. Analytical memos (Maxwell, 1996) were written after each layer of analysis was completed to document the emerging categories, as well as the ways these categories seemed connected with each other. Finally, the contents collected into each of the coded categories were analyzed thematically and used to formulate potential understandings of the experience of resilience in general and, more specifically, the ecological nature of trauma and recovery in one woman's life. These analytic methods, including the findings arising from each separate layer of analysis, are discussed in more depth elsewhere (see Sorsoli, in press).

## RESULTS

### Different, Unworthy, and Alone: "Who'd want to hang out with a weirdo like me?"

The main themes across Patti's transcripts indicated the intense degree to which she had internalized feelings of worthlessness and forced isolation. Examining her statements line by line revealed that the three most common kinds of statements in her transcripts involved the sense of being different; bad or inferior in some way; and either hiding or alone. The word "different" was particularly ubiquitous. Patti had a "different definition of home," a "different sense of appropriateness," and a "different" understanding of "happiness." She "looked different," "dressed funny," and had a "gigantic family compared to everybody else." Several times during the interviews she referred to herself as a "freak" or "weirdo." Beyond "different," but often in close proximity in narrative talk, was her perception of herself as bad or inferior. For example, she described herself as "ugly and weird," "skuzzy," "emotionally screwed-up," and a "big fat loser." She often described herself as alone, saying "kids didn't play with me," or "I sat in the corner reading books" and "did not mingle." Her aloneness at home, in spite of her "gigantic family," was disconcerting. "When I'm home," she said, "I just have to sit there and not let anybody know who I am." Although intermingled with other stories and emotions, the sheer preponderance of these kinds of statements across the transcripts was striking.

The separate examination of the stories Patti told about her experiences revealed dramatic swings in mood and deep emotions that she generally kept to herself, including a great deal of anger that tended to erupt suddenly in relationships, exacerbating her ongoing distrust of others. She often narrated fears of being humiliated by her feelings, and suggested that her emotions were "used against [her]," most often by family members. The stories about her family, for example, were frequently about betrayal and/or being "picked at" and "judged" for every "flaw" or "mistake." "If you did not come home with straight A's," she says, "you got told what an idiot you were." Thematically, many of her stories involved struggles within a community, or being singled out or separated from a group, as if a sense of belonging was just beyond her grasp. However, although she told one story about a potentially traumatic childhood experience, the vast majority of her stories seem more emotionally painful than classically "traumatic." Individually, the experiences she described still seemed on the edge of normal everyday experiences of children–she had not been beaten or sexually abused, nor had she been neglected or abandoned–and yet, as a whole her narratives gave the flavor of constant struggles and insecurity.

Examining segments of the interviews in which one narrated experience was contrasted against another clarified that it was not simply what had happened to her, but the way she had made meaning of her experiences, and had transferred these meanings from one situation to another (or not) that had left her psychologically vulnerable. For example, although she felt worthwhile at school, those feelings did little to counter her belief that at home she was just a "big fat loser" and that her sisters had "gotten all the good stuff." In addition, what seemed adaptive in one situation or context, such as hiding every emotion except anger in her family, became maladaptive in other contexts, such as when she tried to talk about her experiences with friends or work out conflicts with room-mates.

Overall, her interviews paint a rather bleak picture of her childhood and later life experiences, even though the words as spoken revealed lit-tle emotion and were surrounded with a great deal of laughter. Never-theless, the relationship between these experiences and racism was not immediately apparent, particularly in her early life, since her academic abilities had a similar tendency to set her apart from her classmates. Ul-timately, however, it was clear that her experiences of discrimination afforded her with many reasons to feel bad or different, and many rea-sons to feel justifiably angry; while her family-life provided few skills that would allow her to cope effectively with the resulting emotional stress. Thus, as illustrated in the following discussion, it was neither her family life nor racism alone but the way societal prejudice intensified the messages she received about herself within her family that was so disruptive. Appreciating both the effect of racism in her life and her re-silience requires integrating the findings arising from the separate, in-tricate layers of this analysis into fuller portrait as follows: first, considering her early relational context and the way those experiences followed her out into the world, and secondly, considering the ways she encountered and understood her experiences of racial prejudice and dis-crimination.

### Resilience and Relational Context: "When I'm at home I'm just a big fat loser"

Patti's earliest memories were of playing with her brothers at home. Describing herself as "the stereotypical nerdy kid," she added, "I do *not* remember anything positive about school. Let's put it that way. It was a miserable experience. I was the kid who sat in the corner reading books. Did not generally mingle. Didn't really fit in with the neighborhood." School was a miserable experience, she explained, not because of the schoolwork, but because she could read long before she went to kinder-garten, which made her feel "weird," as if she did not "fit in." On the other hand, "teachers loved me," she said, "So that part was good. Teachers always loved me, but the kids absolutely hated me." In this example, the way a personal source of resilience like innate intelligence may have both positive and negative relational consequences is very clear.

The contrast between her relationships with adults at school and at home is striking. She mentioned the powerful effect that teachers had on her life, providing her with "continual attention and support," particularly with regard to her artwork. Her parents, however, were described succinctly as "strict" and "old-fashioned." About her relationship with them, she said simply, "There wasn't really a relationship. The relationship was they tell you what to do and you do it." Given the emotional atmosphere, it almost sounded as though she had been raised in factory-like environment. She said,

> We didn't talk about feelings in my family. You weren't entitled to have feelings. You were given all of the appropriate raw materials and guidance to excel. And that's what you were there for. You weren't there to be nurtured and to feel like a normal little kid. You weren't a normal little kid, you were better by God. So it was that sort of attitude, like, we don't have any room for whining around here. We're not raising whiners.

At home, her penchant for the creative arts was met with criticism. She stated clearly that she would never go home and tell her parents that a teacher liked a piece of artwork she made because they would compare it to her sisters' achievements and say, "So what? Your sisters get straight A's." She said, "So fine. It was just mine. Who wanted that to be tainted with that kind of negative, 'so what' kind of thing?" Her creativity in this situation, taking her art underground to protect herself and to preserve its strength, illustrates her resilience as an individual. And yet, it continued to bother her a great deal that her family would judge her art but never "took the trouble to look at it." On the other hand, she mentioned that teachers always "talked" to her and made her feel "interesting and worthwhile." Asking how she felt about her relationships with her teachers in comparison to the way she was treated at home resulted in the following exchange:

> Patti: It was kind of bizarre. It was like, if all of these teachers think that I have something interesting to say and I'm worthwhile, then why is it that nobody in my family does? You know, it was just like, it made no sense.

Lynn: Then how did you make sense of it?

P: I made sense of it by saying that "Well, that's their problem." Like after a while, I really started feeling like I just don't fit in. I'd think, you know, I was born into the wrong family, "oh well." And after a while, it was just something that I accepted. (long pause) There was somebody out there–if nobody out there, if nobody ever thought that I was worth a plug nickel, I think it would be different, but if the only people who constantly criticize you are the people you're related to, you start thinking, well, maybe *they* have a problem, you know?

L: But it seems *more* logical to think that everyone else is wrong.

P: I think in the beginning, when you are really young. But as you get older and there're more people . . . At first it's "Okay, well, maybe in this one school, these teachers are all weird," but then, as you get to another grade, then those teachers think you have some sense too. And then as you eventually move to another school, and you're a little bit older, and those people think you have sense, and you're not even getting A's anymore. Well, there's something going on here, I don't have to get A's for teachers to think that I'm worthwhile. That's another piece of the puzzle. I'm not completely worthless because I don't even have to get A's to try to prove my worthiness.

Patti's realization that because that people beyond her family could see her worth, her family's opinions could be wrong is another testament to her resilience. My skepticism, that from a child's perspective it would be more logical to assume that her family was correct and that everyone else was wrong, is met with acknowledgement, and yet she proceeds to narrate a lengthy experiential process leading to the ultimate understanding of "another piece of the puzzle." The following segment illustrates the way the technique of contrasting her relationships with others with her relationship with her parents continues to illuminate how she makes sense of very different relational experiences, while also highlighting the ways deeper understandings were often co-constructed throughout the course of these interviews:

Lynn: Like you, they (your teachers) saw you as a person.

Patti: Yes.

L: Which would be different than people who couldn't even hear what you said.

P: Right. Right. Definitely.

L: Yeah. So it was as if you and what you did and what you thought was important, not just your grades and your schoolwork.

P: Exactly. It wasn't just how do you fit into this preconceived puzzle, which is pretty much how I always feel in my family, that there was this big jigsaw puzzle with eight little pieces and I was just one of them and I was supposed to fit in that little space. It was like, sorry, I don't know which one it is. And you have some people–the little square puzzle piece that fits exactly where it's supposed to be, all the time. The main thing to me after a while was if you had that many kids and the first one did everything she was supposed to do, exactly when she was supposed to do it and exactly the *way* she was supposed to do it, why can't you just be satisfied with that? Can't you just acknowledge that maybe all the good stuff was used up on her? Why do we all have to do exactly the same thing? She's already done that. That's her gig. Let everybody else have a separate one.

L: It sounds like at least at some point or at some level, there was a sense that she got all the good stuff, or she has the good stuff.

P: Oh yes.

L: So . . . this sense of worthwhile, did that make it all the way into you? How does that fit, how does this sense of being worthwhile that came from the teachers fit with this sense that your sister had all the good stuff and you guys didn't get any?

P: Um . . . well, it fit–it was always, "Gee I wish I'd been born into a different family that thought people like me were okay." *Not* like I felt like wonderful and like I was a great person. I felt wonderful *while* I was talking to teachers or *while* I was at school, and then the rest of the time . . . it's not like you can *live* at school. You'd go home thinking you're somebody and "Oh I forgot, I'm just a big fat loser." So it was like, okay, when I'm home, I'm just a big fat loser, I will sit here and not say anything so then I won't get *any* attention, because it's only going to be negative. After a while, you just sort of go, well, when I'm not home, I can be myself. When I'm home, I just have to sit there and not let anybody know who I am. Because even if I decided to follow in her footsteps and do everything the way she did it, they still found out something wrong with me.

In this interview excerpt, the main themes of "difference" and "badness" are observed, in addition to her desire to be seen and to belong, and her belief that acceptance, even within her family, requires "fit[ting] in that little space," a demand that leaves her with a profound sense of hopelessness because even when she did her best to fit "they still found out something wrong with me." The theme of "aloneness" appears in her decision to just "sit here and not say anything," her way of coping with the negative attention she so often felt she received at home. Her management of the feeling of "badness," a creative splitting of self between a "big fat loser" and this "wonderful . . . great person," can be seen as well, coupled with her sense of being forced into the role of "big fat loser" in her family/community because, unfortunately, "it's not like you can live at school." A similar interaction between themes, having the potential to be seen as good but being forced into a negative role and rejected from a community as a result, occurs later in the interview, when the story is unmistakably tied to race.

One great danger in this context is that the split between home and school, places where she felt bad and good respectively, though a resilient psychological maneuver, is fragile. She feels she must hide how she is treated at home from her teachers because if she told, she would be the "biggest Benedict Arnold ever" or, even worse, her teachers might realize that her family was right "all along." At the same time, she must hide her art successes from her parents because her parents would compare her artwork to her sisters' achievements and still find her lacking. The feeling that she is a fraud and will be "found out" undermines her resilience, and the intervention that her teachers provide is compromised as she retreats from these positive relationships. She also remembered a childhood feeling like she could not be honest with her parents and did not have a relationship with them. When asked if she wanted such a relationship, she said, "I wanted to be left the heck alone. Like just leave me the heck alone. No matter what you did, it was wrong. So you just didn't do anything after a while. It was like, "I'm just sitting here reading a book. Who's going to complain if you're sitting there reading a book? Nobody."

Clearly, Patti's method of coping with her emotions involved with-drawal. She learned to negotiate her early relationships by hiding certain kinds of feelings, such as sadness, and magnifying others, like anger. In fact, feelings were so taboo in her family, she says, that the only emotion you were allowed to express *was* anger. Burdened by a fear that she would be humiliated and deliberately hurt for revealing her feelings, and with no one to model or support emotional modulation, her later relationships were similarly marked by "angry outbursts." She explained that she would let the first "nasty" comment go and then, when "they just push that button at the wrong time, they get blasted for the twelve nasty things they've said in a row." These explosions of anger, accompanied by her firm belief that people should know why she was angry and deal with it accordingly, obviously tended to make her relationships quite difficult.

Listening with an understanding of trauma, certain elements present in Patti's narratives assume a clinical significance. For example, the consistency of her feeling that she is not only "different" but also "bad" and "alone"; her difficulties with affect and impulse control; and her deep distrust of others are striking. And yet, although her narratives allow listeners to glimpse the pervasive stress that must have surrounded her as a child, the experiences she has narrated thus far would not be considered "traumatic" in the classical sense because they do not appear to involve experiences that would necessarily overwhelm psychological coping mechanisms (Herman, 1992b; Terr, 1990) or involve experiences of "actual or threatened death or serious injury" (APA, 1994, p. 463). And yet, what may make these early experiences uniquely threatening is how closely they parallel the many negative cultural assumptions about race, class, and gender that Black and other minority women, as well as others must navigate in America (Jones & Shorter-Gooden, 2003; Sanchez-Hucles, 1999). Listening closely, it becomes clear that even when Patti looks beyond her experiences at home for respite or redemption she encounters a multitude of societal messages, often directed specifically at her race. These messages hold her captive, allowing smaller, everyday, insidious forms of oppression to compound and accumulate.

### Racism and Trauma: "I was transformed into an angry Black woman"

A child during the time when schools were being desegregated, Patti was one of the first Black students to experience "bussing." This was the one experience she narrated that seemed unquestionably traumatic. During the interview, she described the experience in detail. She says,

> I was bussed for a few weeks. And that was just a *horrible* experience. It was an amazing thing to go from school being a safe place in some sense to when you're bussed. We'd have to ride around with a police motorcade guarding us to get to school. And it was bizarre. Sometimes we'd get to school on time and sometimes we wouldn't. Some days they'd send the bus back. It was an amazingly horrendous experience. And we knew that they had tipped over the busses. The high school started first, but they stalled the middle school kids. We were sitting home watching them tip busses over and going, "Okay in a few weeks this'll be us." So it had calmed down a little by the time we started, but if you're 11 years old and you're watching them tip busses over and then you have to go get on one, it's like, "I don't want to go to school." So that was uh . . . not fun.

Of all of her narratives, the experience narrated here comes closest to a "classic" trauma narrative. She describes a "horrible experience" involving a threat to her physical integrity, as well as consciousness of a sudden loss of safety; in this case, both threats are inextricably tied to race. She also describes her feelings of anticipation, helplessness, and dread (although the depth of these feelings, as was typical in these transcripts, is somewhat couched behind unlikely phrases such as "not fun" or "bizarre"). The story itself seems cohesive and complete; if listeners take her final statement in this segment ("so that was uh . . . not fun") as exit speech signaling the end of the story (Reissman, 2002), they may conclude that that story is simply about a traumatic experience associated with desegregation. However, as it was told in the interview, the story had not yet reached its climax–reading forward in the transcript allows us to discover that the story was *also* about the unforeseen gain and loss of a community:

> And *then* when I got there, they put me in an A.P. English class. And there was exactly one Black kid in the class. Oh that was fun! There was just little old me. As if it wasn't bad enough coming here and plus you come on the busses and–it's sort of like a community activity, which is a sad way of having one 'cause at home didn't fit in with my community at all, or my so-called community, the neighborhood, but then when you're on the bus and people are

threatening your lives and suddenly it's like, "Yeah, we're all friends!" So it was weird to go to school and then be separated to go down to A.P. English class.

As the story continues ("and *then* when I got there . . . "), her emphasis indicates that the worst was yet to come. Reading this final segment of the story, listeners come to understand that the climax, the point of her story, is not simply that desegregation was horrible but also about the way the busses created a community where it had never previously existed. As Patti says, "suddenly it's like 'Yeah, we're all friends!'" From the way this story is told, it seems clear that at least part of the tragedy for Patti was that she was once again separated, even from this "sad way of having one" community, because she had been assigned to an A. P. English class. Obviously, the presence and impact of race is still quite evident in the story, unmistakable given the composition of her new English class. At the same time, the phases "exactly one Black kid" and "little old me" signal, yet again, her sense of "aloneness" in the world.

As previously mentioned, although often in the background, the issue of race emerged more clearly from time to time, frequently as a source of disconnections from the people in her life. For example, when she began talking about her experiences in one of her graduate courses, she mentioned that she believed that the instructor was acting inappropriately by bringing race into the class discussions and this was making her extremely angry and uncomfortable. In the following segment, after she describes what happened when she approached the instructor to explain her desire not to be singled out in this manner, I again attempt to make associations between the experience she was describing in that moment and the ways she had described her early experiences in her family earlier in the interview:

> Patti: I told her, I entered this classroom as a graduate student, and an art teacher, and in two weeks, I was transformed into an angry Black woman. That is *not* who I was when I walked into this classroom. Even if that does happen to be a part of who I am, it had nothing to do with this classroom. And I said, what really bothers me the most, is that I am one hell of an art teacher and that's being lost in this 'I'm an angry Black woman.' When I paint I can be an angry Black woman if I want, which I don't, but (laughs) it has nothing to do with my abilities. I got angrier as time went on because I discovered that I was more educated than most of the people in the class. Everybody in that classroom knew more about

modern art than I did, but not a bloody person in that room had a clue about sfumato or chiaroscuro. Not one of them could teach somebody else to understand da Vinci's innovations. And that to me was what I had to contribute that was different from everybody else and instead I was forced to contribute my Blackness. What the hell does Blackness have to do with 15th or 16th century art? Nothing.

Lynn: So, I mean, it kind of is back to . . . you not being seen for who you are.

P: Exactly.

L: Just kind of like how it was in your family.

P: Yes.

L: They didn't see who you were. They forced you to fit as a puzzle piece.

P: Yes. (laughing) Exactly. Right.

L: They were forcing you to be the angry Black woman, that was your little piece and you didn't want to be that.

P: Yes.

L: I can see why that made you very angry.

P: Oh yes! And it's like gee why aren't I a teacher now? Because I wasn't going to be a teacher, I was always going to be "the Black art teacher." You can't just go into a classroom and teach and then run home. You *have* to interact with these people and not anybody had any respect for or wanted to be part of my private life in any way shape or form. I felt I would have no social life. I'm already being set up to not have anything in common personally with my colleagues. For me the only community I ever thought I would be a part of is an academic community and I felt like I was *robbed* of that because people were relating to my race. It was like, people in this room probably like to sit down in the evening and drink a cup of tea. And I like that too. But they don't know that. They think I'm sitting

home, you know, plotting the downfall of the White race or something. And it's not fair. I would have enjoyed having tea with these
people. You know?

In this interview segment, along with the lively sense of humor that
also characterized these interviews, the way her later experiences in the
world mirror her early experiences in her family becomes quite clear.
The sense that nobody "had any respect for or wanted to be part of my
private life in any way shape or form," the feeling of being "set up" to
fail and "robbed" of a community are all familiar elements of her early
life writ large. In this situation, the whole set of elements has also become specifically associated with race and it is clear that, as it can for
many Black women, race has provided both a source and the locus for a
potentially traumatic experience (Daniel, 2000). Moreover, there is the
additional sense that she is trapped in the stories that she learned early in
life, and now, like many trauma survivors, continually relives (Chu,
1991; van der Kolk, 1989).

## *DISCUSSION*

Once we have all of these pieces and a sense for the ways they have
come together in her life, we can see how disruptive they have been. It
becomes clearer that her own personal stories and family environment
colluded with society's stories about race in ways that made her very
vulnerable, and that she has internalized this as being born "wrong,"
creating a situation in which she feels both helpless and hopeless.
Tatum (1997) explains that some experiences having to do with race can
cause important but minor relational disconnections; she deems these
'minor' because typically they are balanced by positive connections at
home and school. However, for Patti, those kinds of disconnections
were not balanced but rather compounded by the ways she felt set apart
from others at home (where she was unlike her sisters) and school
(where she was unlike the other children in her classes). The way her father tried to bolster his children's self-esteem (possibly to combat social
prejudice and/or his own past experiences with racism) (Danieli, 1998;
McAdoo, 1988) was to declare that they were special and to socially
isolate them from others, creating further disconnections. However, because Patti did not feel special and did not feel able to live up to the stan-

dards set by her oldest sister, she was exceedingly vulnerable out in the world, which is where "the whole thing fell apart." She says,

> One of the things we were taught at home was, in a bizarre way, we're special. We're special not in and of ourselves, special because we are a part of this family. In one way that was a good survival strategy, to get us through school and then to college. But we weren't taught that we were special in and of ourselves and that's where the whole thing fell apart once we got out into the world.

Patti was also affected by the ways emotions were taboo in her family. Through the course of our discussions, it was clear that emotions were dangerous and that in her family, showing a range of emotions was not acceptable. As Patti says, "Being mad is acceptable–that's the only thing you ever admit to." Thus, the only time she lets any kind of emotion show is when she is angry. To have feelings, she explains, you need a "reason"; so, for example, "You wouldn't come home and be upset 'cause when you did come home and say you were upset then there was some reason you shouldn't be. There's no point in talking about it so it can be explained to me why it shouldn't be upsetting." There were always good "reasons" to be angry, however, so it was relatively easy to justify, particularly in a society in which racial prejudice can be experienced on a daily basis. Because anger becomes the only emotion she shows, the intellectualization that becomes a family "rule" thus sets her up for being negatively perceived as "the angry black woman," which of course not only leads her to feel increasingly different and isolated but helpless, trapped, and "robbed" of a community.

Patti's experiences in the world, while not the particular brand of "sudden and overwhelming" events that are often associated with trauma, nevertheless seem to have had the cumulative effect of severely disrupting her sense that the world is a safe place and that her self is worthy. The resulting psychological crisis (Janoff-Bulman, 1992) may have fundamentally altered the ways in which she perceives and responds to the world and her relationships, thus leaving her with symptoms similar to survivors of other kinds of complex trauma. The puzzle here is that these symptoms appear to exist in absence of what would traditionally be accepted as a "significant threat" to development. Resilience, meanwhile, is characterized by the existence of a good or positive outcome in spite of a quantifiably serious threat to development (Masten, 2001). As Masten writes, "Individuals are not considered resilient if there has never been a significant threat to their development; there must be current or past hazards judged to have the potential to derail normative development" (p. 228). Without a careful examination of her life history, including ways she has made meaning of her experiences and the ecological system in which she was developing, it would have been fairly easy to conclude that Patti is not a terribly resilient individual.

Taking an ecological perspective of her experiences (Harvey, 1996), however, we can see that her vulnerabilities exist on three interrelated levels: individual, relational, and societal. On the individual level, her emotions, particularly anger and sadness, have occasionally been overwhelming and difficult for her to modulate and as a child her parents' lack of responsiveness almost certainly contributed to her vulnerability in this area. Although her art could have been a personal resource for her, she has in the past tended to hide her passion for it from her family, particularly her parents, who would have "compared" it to her sisters' achievements and in doing so "stolen" its strength.

On a relational level, although she is bright and engaging and obviously has the ability to maintain and develop close relationships, her emotions have occasionally interfered, either because she felt she needed to hide her emotions or because she could not control them. For example, although she felt supported by teachers as a child, this support was limited because she felt she would be betraying her parents if she ever suggested they were anything other than "perfect." At the same time, she lived in fear that her teachers might agree with her family that she had nothing to offer and as a result, felt tremendously at risk of being "found out." As an adult, her family's strict rules about not showing any emotions other than anger also continue to disrupt her interactions in relationships, contributing to her vulnerability on the relational level.

Finally, on the societal level, messages about skin color abound. Patti's skin color, in some cases because she feels she is too light, in others because she feels she is too dark, has made her even more vulnerable to indications that she is less than worthy. Skin color can be a source of significant distress for many Black women, whether or not they fall prey to direct colorism or experience a more generalized negative impact on self-esteem (Jones & Shorter-Gooden, 2000; Keith & Thompson, 2003). Patti attributes being forced out of certain communities to the color of her skin, losses that she feels deeply. However, it is not simply the existence of these distinct vulnerabilities on each level of experience but the ways they reinforce one another that has compromised her sense of worth and well-being, at times leaving her feeling both helpless and "trapped."

Patti's ecological system clearly created a unique set of risks or obstacles to healthy development. If we think about this system itself as a serious hazard for psychological growth, a new understanding of her resilience emerges. For a long while, every available avenue for the development and expression of her resilient capacities was blocked or prevented. It is not that she does not show signs of the impact of her experiences but the fact that she has maintained the ability to *mobilize* her resources and move forward (once certain roadblocks have been removed) that provides the more important confirmation of her resilience. In spite of her challenging youth and subsequent difficulties in relationships, she *has* been able to develop some relationships that sustain and support her emotionally; her resilience thus illustrated by her ability to create for herself a context in which she feels safe and worthwhile, and able to express her emotions. An extremely intelligent, thoughtful, warm, and articulate person, she attributes her success to relationships, saying,

> I think that there are some naturally compassionate people who, maybe instinctively, ferret out those of us who are emotional screw-ups, you know what I mean? It's sort of like if the first time some guy falls madly in love with you, that's a bridge to you eventually falling madly in love with yourself. If you grow up not loving yourself, somebody else has to really love you before it's contagious.

A second important sign of her resilience involves art, a skill and passion that has continued to offer her source of strength across the course of her life, in spite of her family's apparent disdain and disrespect for her accomplishments in this area. Her devotion to art involves a distinct compassion for children who might find themselves feeling as she did as a child. She says that "if one weirdo 11-year-old girl is impressed by [her art] in a way that makes her feel good about herself, I don't care if nobody else ever sees it." Patti has clearly maintained the ability to be touched emotionally in her relationships, as well as the ability to empathize with and reach out to others who might find themselves in similar situations. These are critical resources for future development and their existence illustrates considerable resilience in spite of the presence of certain symptoms of psychological distress.

## CONCLUSION

The complexity of Black women's experiences within the interlocking oppressive systems of gender, race, and class is an issue that many feminists (and feminist therapists) have articulated (e.g., Burstow, 2003; Collins, 1991; Jones & Shorter-Gooden, 2003). As Burstow (2003) writes, "Oppressed people are routinely worn down by the insidious trauma involved living day after day in a sexist, racist, classist, homophobic, and ableist society" (p. 1296). In general, the framework of trauma helps us to understand the potential consequences of this type of psychological "wearing down," even though, like emotional trauma, it does not meet the official psychiatric conceptualizations of trauma as laid out in the diagnostic manual. This case study indicates the additional importance of considering an individual's ecological system as a means of understanding his or her particular psychological risks, resilience, and subsequent development–it is not simply the exposure to multiple stressors that creates vulnerability but also the ways difficult experiences, personal resources, and environmental factors interact.

Although writing about racism is challenging, Patti's story cried out to be told. Taking into account the recurring statements that flavored the interview along with the more lengthy examples and narratives has produced a rich understanding of Patti's life experience that encourages a more generous assessment of the significance of her resilience. This case study involved a rigorous layered approach to analysis that encouraged constant and careful attention to shifts in language and meaning, and a progressive deepening of understanding. The systematic contrast of her words and stories revealed her experiences in a unique context, shedding light on "where it all fell apart" for Patti, and why. It seems clear that in certain systems, race, gender, and/or class may demonstrate serious risks to development; assessing developmental outcomes may thus involve an intricate understanding of the ecological system in which development has occurred. In light of these findings, it also seems clear that accurately assessing resilience may involve more than comparing the seriousness of the experienced risk factors against the quality of developmental outcome but understanding how experiences can affect a person in certain domains or contexts, while leaving other domains relatively unaffected; and, moreover, gauging the kinds of skills still present for adaptation when the right conditions or contexts present themselves.

## NOTE

1. All names, places, dates, and certain other identifying details have been carefully altered throughout this manuscript to protect her confidentiality.

## REFERENCES

Allen, R. L. (2001). *The concept of self: A study of black identity and self-esteem.* Detroit: Wayne State University Press.

American Psychatric Association. (1994). *Diagnostic and statistical manual of mental disorders* (4th ed.). Washington, DC: Author.

Burstow, B. (2003). Toward a radical understanding of trauma and trauma work. *Violence Against Women, 9*(11), 1293-1317.

Chu, J. A. (1991). The repetition compulsion revisited: Reliving dissociated trauma. *Psychotherapy, 28,* 327-332.

Collins, P. H. (1991). *Black feminist thought: Knowledge, consciousness, and the politics of empowerment.* New York: Routledge.

Daniel, J. H. (2000). The courage to hear: African American women's memories of racial trauma. In L. C. Jackson & B. Greene (Eds.), *Psychotherapy with African American women* (pp. 126-144). New York: Guilford Press.

Danieli, Y. (Ed.) (1998). *International handbook of multigenerational legacies of trauma.* New York: Plenum Press.

Edelman, M. W. (1985). The sea is so wide and my boat is so small: Problems facing Black children today. In H. P. McAdoo & J. L. McAdoo (Eds.), *Black children: Social, environmental, and parental environments* (pp. 72-82). Beverly Hills, CA: Sage.

Eyerman, R. (2001). *Cultural trauma: Slavery and the formation of African American identity.* Cambridge, UK: Cambridge University Press.

Garbarino, J., Guttmann, E., & Seely, J. W. (1986). *The psychologically battered child.* San Francisco, CA: Jossey Bass.

Hart, S. N., Binggeli, M. J., & Brassard, M. R. (1998). Evidence for the effects of psychological maltreatment. *Journal of Emotional Abuse, 1,* 27-58.

Harvey, M. R. (1996). An ecological view of psychological trauma and trauma recovery. *Journal of Traumatic Stress, 9*(1), 3-23.

Harvey, M. R., Liang, B., Harney, P. A., Koenan, K., Tumamal-Narra, P., & Lebowitz, L. (2003). A multidimensional approach to the assessment of trauma impact, recovery and resilience: Initial psychometric findings. *Journal of Aggression, Maltreatment & Trauma, 6*(2), 87-109.

Harvey, M. R., Mishler, E. G., Koenen, K. C., & Harney, P. A. (2000). In the aftermath of sexual abuse: Making and remaking meaning in narratives of trauma and recovery. *Narrative Inquiry, 10*(2), 291-311.

Herman, J. L. (1992a). Complex PTSD: A syndrome in survivors of prolonged and repeated trauma. *Journal of Traumatic Stress, 5*(3), 377-391.

Herman, J. L. (1992b). *Trauma and recovery: The aftermath of violence–from domestic abuse to political terror.* New York: Basic Books.

Janoff-Bulman, R. (1992). *Shattered assumptions: Towards a new psychology of trauma*. New York: The Free Press.

Jones, C., & Shorter-Gooden, K. (2003). *Shifting: The double lives of Black women in America*. New York: Harper Collins Publishers, Inc.

Keith, V. M., & Thompson, M. S. (2003). Color matters: The importance of skin tone for African American women's self-concept in Black and White America. In D. R. Brown & V. M. Keith (Eds.), *In and out of our right minds: The mental health of African American women* (pp. 116-135). New York: Columbia University Press.

Masten, A. S. (2001). Ordinary magic: Resilience processes in development. *American Psychologist, 56*(3), 227-238.

Maxwell, J. A. (1996). *Qualitative research design: An interactive approach*. Thousand Oaks, CA: Sage.

McAdoo, J. L. (1988). The roles of Black fathers in the socialization of Black children. In H. P. McAdoo (Ed.), *Black families* (2nd ed., pp. 257-269). Beverly Hills, CA: Sage.

Miles, M. B. & Huberman, A. M. (1994). *Qualitative data analysis: An expanded sourcebook* (2nd ed.). Thousand Oaks, CA: Sage.

Reissman, C. K. (2002). Analysis of personal narratives. In J. F. Gubrium & J. A. (Eds.), *Handbook of interview research: Context and method* (pp. 695-710). Thousand Oaks, CA: Sage.

Rogers, A. G. (1999). Two related layers of psychological trauma in the life-narratives of sexually abused girls. Unpublished manuscript, Harvard University, Graduate School of Education, Cambridge, MA.

Sanchez-Hucles, J. V. (1999). Racism: Emotional abusiveness and psychological trauma for ethnic minorities. *Journal of Emotional Abuse, 1*(2), 69-87.

Shalev, A. Y. (2002). Treating survivors in the immediate aftermath of traumatic events. In R. Yehuda (Ed.), *Treating trauma survivors with PTSD* (pp. 157-188). Washington, DC: American Psychiatric Publishing, Inc.

Sorsoli, L. (2004). Echoes of silence: Remembering and repeating childhood trauma. In A. Lieblich, D. P. McAdams, & R. Josselson (Eds.), *Healing plots: The narrative basis of psychotherapy* (pp.89-109). Washington, DC: American Psychological Association Press.

Sorsoli, L. (in press). Like pieces in a puzzle: Working with layered methods of interpreting personal narratives. In M. Bamberg (Ed.), *Narrative, discourse, interaction: In search of identities*. Amsterdam: John Benjamins.

Sorsoli, C. L. (2003). *Telling: Women's experiences of personal disclosure*. Unpublished doctoral dissertation, Harvard University, Graduate School of Education, Cambridge, MA.

Stake, R. E. (1998). Case studies. In N. K. Denzin & Y. S. Lincoln (Eds.), *Strategies of qualitative inquiry* (pp. 86-109). Thousand Oaks, CA: Sage.

Strauss, A., & Corbin, J. (1998). *Basics of qualitative research: Techniques and procedures for developing grounded theory* (2nd ed.). Thousand Oaks, CA: Sage Publications.

Tatum, B. D. (1997). Racial identity development and relational theory: The case of Black women in White communities. In J. V. Jordan (Ed.), *Women's growth in di-*

*versity: More writings from the Stone Center* (pp. 91-106). New York: The Guilford
    Press.
Terr, L. C. (1990). *Too scared to cry: Psychic trauma in childhood.* New York: Harper &
    Row.
van der Kolk, B. A. (1989). The compulsion to repeat the trauma: Re-enactment,
    revictimization, and masochism. *Psychiatric Clinics of North America, 12*(2),
    389-411.
van der Kolk, B. A. (2002). The assessment and treatment of complex P.T.S.D. In R.
    Yehuda (Ed.), *Treating trauma survivors with PTSD* (pp. 127-156). Washington,
    DC: American Psychiatric Publishing, Inc.
Yin, R. K. (1994). *Case study research: Design and methods* (2nd ed.). Thousand
    Oaks, CA: Sage.

doi:10.1300/J146v14n01_06

# SECTION THREE:
# MULTICULTUAL ASSESSMENT OF TRAUMA, RECOVERY, AND RESILIENCE

# Interpersonal Violence, Recovery, and Resilience in Incarcerated Women

Rebekah Bradley
Katrina Davino

**SUMMARY.** Our first study focuses on interpersonal violence and characteristics of resilience (evaluated by the Multidimensional Trauma Resilience and Recovery [MTRR] interview and rating scales) in a sample of incarcerated women. The second study applies qualitative data analysis to a case study of one participant in group therapy for incarcer-

Address correspondence to: Rebekah Bradley, PhD, Assistant Professor, Department of Psychiatry and Behavioral Sciences, Emory University, Associate Director, Laboratory of Personality and Psychopathology (E-mail: rebekah.bradley@emory.edu, Web: www.psychsystems.net/lab).

[Haworth co-indexing entry note]: "Interpersonal Violence, Recovery, and Resilience in Incarcerated Women." Bradley, Rebekah, and Katrina Davino. Co-published simultaneously in *Journal of Aggression, Maltreatment & Trauma* (The Haworth Maltreatment & Trauma Press, an imprint of The Haworth Press, Inc.) Vol. 14, No. 1/2, 2007, pp. 123-146; and: *Sources and Expressions of Resiliency in Trauma Survivors: Ecological Theory, Multicultural Practice* (ed: Mary R. Harvey, and Pratyusha Tummala-Narra) The Haworth Maltreatment & Trauma Press, an imprint of The Haworth Press, Inc., 2007, pp. 123-146. Single or multiple copies of this article are available for a fee from The Haworth Document Delivery Service [1-800-HAWORTH. 9:00 a.m. - 5:00 p.m. (EST). E-mail address: docdelivery@haworthpress.com].

Available online at http://jamt.haworthpress.com
doi:10.1300/J146v14n01_07

ated women with a history of childhood sexual abuse. Despite extensive history of both frequent and severe abuse, the women displayed a high degree of resilience across multiple domains, including, in particular, the ability to derive meaning from traumatic events and to place the memories into context, ability to form meaningful relationships with others, and ability to regulate affect. These findings were replicated in study two, which illustrates the process of recovery from a poly-traumatic history. doi:10.1300/J146v14n01_07 *[Article copies available for a fee from The Haworth Document Delivery Service: 1-800-HAWORTH. E-mail address: <docdelivery@haworthpress.com> Website: <http://www.HaworthPress.com> © 2007 by The Haworth Press, Inc. All rights reserved.]*

**KEYWORDS.** Trauma, abuse, incarcerated women, recovery, resilience, MTRR

In the last fifteen years, the number of incarcerated women in the United States has increased dramatically. According to the U.S. Department of Justice (1999), 950,000 women (i.e., approximately 1% of the U.S. female population) are currently in custody, care or control of corrections at the federal, state or local levels. Moreover, women are the fastest growing group of people involved in the criminal justice system (Powell, 1999). Incarcerated women, as compared to the general population of women, are disproportionately likely to have experienced interpersonal victimization prior to incarceration (Chesney-Lind, 1997), although similar rates of abuse are reported by homeless and housed poor women (Browne & Bassuk, 1997). Browne, Miller, and Maguin (1999) conducted one of the most comprehensive studies to date examining the prevalence of pre-prison interpersonal violence (IPV) among incarcerated women. Their sample included 150 women incarcerated in a New York state prison. They reported a 59% rate of childhood sexual abuse (CSA), a 70% rate of child physical abuse by a caretaker, a 49% rate of rape as an adult, and a 75% rate of "severe" physical abuse by an intimate partner as an adult. Further, they found that the IPV reported by these women was more severe, frequent, ongoing, and, for childhood abuse, began at relatively young ages, as compared to rates reported in other populations. The relationship between interpersonal victimization and later incarceration is part of a larger social structure of gender, race, and class inequities. Poverty is associated with an increased risk for interpersonal victimization (e.g., Browne & Bassuk, 1997; Goodman, 1991) as well as for incarceration (Chesney-Lind, 1996). African American women are over-represented among both poor women (Amott & Matthaei, 1996) and incarcerated women (Greenfeld & Snell, 1999).

These high rates of trauma are also linked to higher rates of trauma related symptomatology. In assessing incarcerated women, Teplin, Abram, and McClelland (1996) reported a 33.3% lifetime prevalence of Posttraumatic Stress Disorder (PTSD). Jordan, Schlenger, Fairbank, and Caddell (1996) found that 30% of their sample reported both a history of a traumatic event and experiencing six or more PTSD symptoms in the past six months. Powell (1999) found that mentally ill female inmates were more likely to report a history of abuse (60%) as compared to non-mentally ill female inmates (33%).

Given the wide array of adversities (gender and race discrimination, poverty, IPV) incarcerated women are likely to face, it is important to understand both the types and degree of symptoms they experience and the ways in which they may be resilient in the face of these obstacles. Over the last twenty years, researchers have called for a focus on resilience or hardiness concomitantly with the study of negative outcomes (see, e.g., Seligman & Csikszentmihalyi, 2000; Tsuang, 2000). As compared to other aspects of trauma (e.g., prevalence, impact, and treatment effectiveness), relatively less attention has been directed toward the definition of resilience in the wake of traumatic events, including both hardiness in the face of traumatic events and the ability to improve with assistance.

A number of assessment instruments have been developed to assess the impact of traumatic events. Although PTSD is the framework most commonly utilized for understanding the impact of traumatic events including IPV (see, e.g., Widom, 1999), assessment instruments have also been developed to assess a broader range of sequelae often associated with IPV (e.g., difficulties in regulation of affect and impulses, regulation of attention and consciousness, self-perception, and relationships with others; Briere, 1995, 1996; Pelcovitz et al., 1997). In addition, some research has been directed at assessment of resilience in women with a history of IPV (see, e.g., Grossman, Cook, Kepkep, & Koenen, 1999; Lam & Grossman, 1997; Liem, James, O'Toole, & Boudewyn, 1997). Of particular relevance to this paper, Harvey (1996) proposes an ecological perspective on trauma recovery and resilience. This framework, which includes both theoretical background and the development of several assessment instruments, proposes that individual differences in trauma impact, recovery, and resiliency are variably expressed across eight interrelated domains of psychological experience (i.e., authority over the remembering process, integration of memory and affect, affect tolerance and regulation, symptom mastery and positive coping, self-esteem, self-cohesion, safe attachment, and meaning) and describes criteria definitive of resilience and recovery in each of these domains.

The studies presented here aim to evaluate resilience to IPV in a group of incarcerated women. First, we use Harvey's multi-dimensional framework to assess the level and characteristics of resilience in a group of 164 incarcerated women. Second, we apply qualitative data analysis to a life narrative written by a woman who participated in a group therapy program for incarcerated women with a history of sexual abuse. In both cases, the goal is to provide a more rich description of resilience as it manifests in incarcerated women with a history of IPV.

## STUDY ONE:
## IPV AMONG INCARCERATED WOMEN:
## IMPACT AND RESILIENCE AS MEASURED
## BY THE MULTIDIMENSIONAL TRAUMA RESILIENCE
## AND RECOVERY INTERVIEW

### Method

#### Procedure

One hundred and sixty-four women incarcerated in a medium security women's prison in South Carolina were interviewed as part of a study of "women's life experiences." The prison facility served as the "special needs" prison for women in the state, meaning that all female prisoners in need of chronic medical or psychological care were housed there. Participants were recruited in three ways: (a) individuals referred by prison mental health staff; (b) individuals selected at random from a list of inmates and asked to participate in an interview; and (c) individuals who had heard of the study from other participants and requested participation. The interviews normally lasted 2-3 hours and involved administration of: (a) the Multidimensional Trauma Resilience and Recovery Interview (MTRR-I), (b) interviews regarding history of physical and sexual assault in childhood and adulthood, and (c) a set of self-report measures. Only the data from the MTRR-I and the history of physical and sexual trauma are presented in this paper. The data in this study were confidential and coded anonymously. The study was approved by prison and university human participants review committees.

## Participants

Of the approximately 200 women recruited for the study, 175 agreed to participate in an interview. Of the 175 interviews, 164 yielded complete, valid protocols. The sample included 61% African American, 38% Caucasian, and 1% Latina women, most of whom had a high school education or less (72%). They reported relatively low household incomes (35% less than $12,000/year; 74% less than $36,000/year). Most had children (86%) and were currently not married (81%). Sixteen percent of the participants reported that they were HIV positive, which was the most prevalent medical condition in the sample.

## Measures

*MTRR-I and MTRR-99.* The MTRR-I is a semi-structured clinical research interview assessing impairment, recovery, and resiliency in trauma survivors. Designed to gather a life-history narrative that is guided by questions specific to the assessment of resilience to and recovery from traumatic experience(s), it addresses trauma history, family background, current relationships, work functioning, specific posttraumatic symptoms as well as affect regulation capacities, beliefs about self and others, coping abilities, change over time, sense of purpose/meaning, and beliefs about the future. The MTRR-99 is used in conjunction with the MTRR-I to generate quantitative data. Essentially, the MTRR-99 is a clinician-rating measure designed for use by experienced and trained clinical observers to rate recovery from trauma across the eight "domains" of functioning highlighted in Harvey's (1996) ecological framework. Ratings are made on a five-point Likert-type scale ranging from *not at all descriptive* to *highly descriptive*. Data supports both the reliability and validity of the MTRR (see Harvey et al., 2003; Liang, Tummala-Narra, Bradley, & Harvey, this volume; see Appendix B at the end of this volume).

In this study, interviewers included a doctoral candidate in clinical psychology, six other graduate students in clinical psychology, and one advanced undergraduate student. The primary interviewer (Davino) completed 87 of the interviews. All of the interviewers received training in the impact of trauma on mental health, and in the administration of the interview protocols. Four taped MTRR interviews were conducted by the primary interviewer at a battered women's shelter, then listened to and scored by each interviewer. Scoring of these training tapes was reviewed and discussed until consistency of scoring between interviewers was achieved. These four interviews were not included in the data set for this study. In addition, in twenty cases we conducted interviews with two raters present (in each case, the primary interviewer either conducted or observed each interview). It was not possible to tape the interviews because of restrictions in the prison environment; however, immediately following each observed interview the interviewers separately rated the MTRR-99 items. Based on these 20 pairs of interviews, inter-rater reliabilities for each subscale were adequate ($M =$ .67, $SD = .08$.)

*History of sexual trauma.* History of sexual assault was assessed using a series of questions developed based on the work of Russell (Russell, 1983; Russell, Schurman, & Trocki, 1988) and Resnick, Kilpatrick, Dansky, Saunders, and Best (1993). Women were asked about three types of non-consensual contact sexual experiences over their lifespan (i.e., intercourse; oral sex; touching) and one additional question about consensual sexual contact prior to age 13. A woman was considered to have had an experience of CSA if she reported any unwanted contact sexual experiences before age 18 or if she reported "consensual" contact sexual experiences before age 13 when the other person was five or more years older than she. This is consistent with Wyatt's (1985) definition except that non-contact sexual abuses were excluded and only unwanted experiences were included after the participant reached age 13. A woman was considered to have experienced sexual assault in adulthood if she reported any nonconsensual contact sexual experiences when she was age 18 or older.

Women who reported any experiences of child or adult sexual assault were asked about their age at the time of the assault, how often they had experienced each type of sexual assault, and their relationship to the person who perpetrated each child sexual assault or adult sexual assault. Duration was defined as the time period during which a specific type of contact occurred repeatedly with the same perpetrator.

*History of physical trauma.* Histories of physical assault in child and adult relationships were assessed using the Conflict Tactics Scale (Straus, 1979, 1990). Women were asked about experiences ranging from threat of physical assault and being spanked to being beat up or threatened with a knife or gun. They were asked to report how often they had experienced each type of violence before age 18 by "an adult who raised you" or at 18 or older by a "spouse or partner" on a 5-point scale (ranging from *never* to *over 50 times*). They were also asked about the severity of injury resulting from the most "typical" assault and the "worst" assault. This was rated on a 4-point scale including: (a) no injury; (b) mild (bruise, minor cuts, abrasions); (c) moderate (black eyes, broken bones, swelling in bruised areas, serious cuts, losing hair, sprains, lost teeth); and (d) severe (knocked unconscious, required hospitalization, stab or bullet wound, burn, concussion, internal injury). A woman was considered to have had an experience of childhood physical abuse if she reported having been hit with an open hand harder than a slap or spanked at least three times, hit with a fist at least three times, kicked, hit with an object, beaten up, choked, smothered, burned or scalded, or threatened or assaulted with a gun or knife by the adults who raised her. This definition is consistent with that used in the Second National Family Violence Survey (Wolfner & Gelles, 1993) except that frequency criteria were included for being hit with an open hand or hit with a fist in this study, and a more restricted criterion was used for being hit with an object. Being hit with some objects (e.g., a belt or a switch), especially on the buttocks or legs, was extremely common in this sample. These experiences were not considered childhood physical abuse unless the woman felt that they were abusive or in excess of behavior she considered normative.

The Conflict Tactics Scale was administered in interview form. Participants were asked to specifically consider all of the adults who were in a parental/caregiver role, with an acknowledgment that more than one or two adults might have had this role in their lives at any point in time and that multiple adults might have had this role over the course of their childhood. In order to be considered childhood physical abuse, an adult who was in a significant care giving role must have perpetrated the violence. Participants were considered to have had an incident of adult physical abuse if they reported having been hit with an open hand harder than a slap at least three times, with a fist at least three times, hit with an object, choked, smothered, burned/scalded, or threatened or assaulted with a gun or knife by an intimate romantic partner.

## Results

### History of IPV

*CSA.* Sexual abuse was highly prevalent, with 79% of the sample reporting at least one incident of CSA. The majority of the women who reported an experience of CSA reported being abused by more than one perpetrator (69%). Most of the women who reported CSA reported that the onset of sexual abuse was at an early age, with 55% reporting abuse beginning prior to the age of nine. Sixty-nine percent of the women who reported CSA reported experiencing unwanted sexual intercourse. The distribution of CSA frequency was bimodal, with 28% of participants reporting one-time CSA and 26% of the participants reporting more than 100 incidents of sexual abuse perpetrated by one person.

*Child Physical Abuse (CPA).* Sixty-two percent of the women reported at least one incident of CPA. Most of the women who reported CPA reported being abused beginning at an early age, with 72% being abused beginning prior to the age of nine. The CPA reported by participants was severe, with 23% of the abused women reporting being threatened with a knife or gun by a parental figure prior to the age of 18. The CPA behaviors that participants reported experiencing most frequently were "hit harder than a slap or a spank," and "hit with an object." The CPA reported by the participants was also relatively long in duration: 65% of the participants reported at least one CPA relationship that lasted more than 5 years.

*Adult Sexual Assault (ASA).* Sixty-eight percent of the women reported that they had experienced ASA. The most common ASA perpetrator was an intimate romantic partner (56%).

*Adult Physical Abuse (APA).* Eighty-four percent of the women reported APA, with 62% reporting more than one perpetrator. The women reported severe APA, with 64% of the women reporting APA experiences reporting being threatened with a knife or gun by an intimate/romantic partner. APA relationships were also long in duration, with 70% of the women reporting that their longest APA relationship lasted between 1 and 10 years. The APA behaviors that participants reported experiencing most frequently were "hit harder than a slap" and "hit with a fist or kicked."

*Overlap of Abuse Types.* The four categories of abuse experience are highly interrelated in this sample, suggesting that one experience of abuse may increase the risk for continuing to experience abuse. Forty-two percent of the women in this study reported that they had experienced all four types of abuse (i.e., CSA, CPA, ASA, APA). Conversely, only 5% of the participants had experienced no abuse of any of the four types.

## MTRR Scores

First, we looked at the average scores of the entire sample on each of the eight domains of the MTRR, which were as follows: (a) Authority over the remembering process ($M = 3.60$, $SD = .87$), (b) Integration of memory and affect ($M = 3.57$, $SD = .96$), (c) Affect tolerance/regulation of trauma affect ($M$ = 3.18, $SD$ = .93), (d) Symptom mastery and positive coping ($M$ = 3.44, $SD$ = .74), (e) Self-esteem/self-care and self-regard ($M$ = 3.78, $SD$ = .83), (f) Self-cohesion ($M$ = 4.13, $SD$ = .87), (g) Safe attachment ($M$ = 3.28, $SD$ = .80), and (h) Meaning ($M$ = 2.90, $SD$ = .83). In order to better understand these scores, we looked at them in the context of norms established by Harvey and colleagues (Harvey et al., 2003) based on a sample of patients seeking treatment in a trauma treatment program at a large, public urban hospital. The comparison suggests a high level of resiliency despite the extent and severity of trauma reported in this sample. Mean domain cores for this sample were either above those of the largely recovered groups (authority over memory, symptom mastery and positive coping, self-esteem, self cohesion, and safe attachment) or between the means for the partially recovered and the largely to fully recovered groups (integration of memory and affect, affect regulation, and meaning).

*Profiles of Resilience*

To provide a more descriptive portrait of resilience among the women in this sample, we created a composite description of the women in the sample using the MTRR-99. Specifically we averaged the MTRR-99 items across all of the women and then arrayed the items in descending order of magnitude. The items with scores of 3.5 and higher are presented in Table 1. These results confirm that, despite histories of multiple traumatic experiences, the women in this sample displayed many resilient characteristics. In fact, of the 25 highest ranked items, only three items (inability to trust others, difficulty sleeping, and tendency to become involved in repeated abusive relationships) reflect problems in adaptive functioning. The other items describe adaptive responses to trauma including ability to remember past experiences clearly, ability to recall positive and negative past events, a capacity to experience broad range of emotions, altruistic feelings towards others and positive spirituality.

As a second step in the analysis, we wanted to look at how the profiles of most resilient women (defined at the top quartile of women in overall MTRR-99 score, which is obtained by averaging across the scores on the eight domains). To do this, we first standardized the MTRR-99 across all participants ($M$ = 0, $SD$ = 1). Next, we selected the women ($N$ = 41) whose overall MTRR-99 score (the average across all 99 items) fell into the top quartile and averaged the MTRR-99 item scores of these women. Third, we arrayed the MTRR-99 items of the women in the top quartile in descending order of magnitude, thus producing a composite portrait of the

## TABLE 1. Composite MTRR-99 Description (*N* = 164)

| MTRR-99 ITEMS | M | SD |
|---|---|---|
| Is comfortable with her sexual orientation | 4.41 | 1.13 |
| Has relatively continuous memory for adulthood | 4.31 | 1.07 |
| When recalling painful or traumatic events, she is able to remember feelings experienced at the time | 4.22 | 1.11 |
| Experiences altruistic inclinations towards others | 4.16 | 1.03 |
| Has an occupation appropriate to her abilities and talents | 4.03 | 4.22 |
| Responds empathically to other people's needs | 4.01 | 4.16 |
| Recognizes and avoids anxiety provoking situations | 3.94 | 4.03 |
| Has assumed control over dissociative capacities that once compromised psychological status and daily functioning | 3.88 | 4.01 |
| Is able to experience a wide range of emotions, specifically: anger, fear/anxiety, sadness, pleasure, anticipation, joy and hope | 3.85 | 3.94 |
| Is distrustful even when trust is warranted | 3.82 | 1.31 |
| Enjoys work and is able to be task-involved despite outside stressors | 3.78 | 4.41 |
| Has relatively continuous memory for events in childhood and adolescence | 3.73 | 4.31 |
| Is able to feel a realistic sense of hope and optimism about the future | 3.72 | 4.22 |
| Acts on altruistic inclinations towards others | 3.69 | 4.16 |
| Functions adaptively after retrieving painful memories, including memories of traumatic events | 3.68 | 4.03 |
| Recognizes and avoids situations that are demeaning, humiliating or unnecessarily painful | 3.65 | 4.01 |
| Is troubled by disturbed sleep | 3.62 | 3.94 |
| Is able to draw comfort and meaning from a coherent set of religious, spiritual or moral values | 3.62 | 3.88 |
| Can recall painful events, including traumatic events, with detail and clarity | 3.62 | 3.85 |
| Find meaning in life (and in past suffering or trauma) | 3.58 | 1.43 |
| Can remember and can relate to others a relatively complete story of his or her life, from childhood to present | 3.58 | 1.36 |
| Seldom re-experiences extreme trauma-related affects such as terror, rage, overwhelming arousal, or utter helplessness | 3.56 | 1.45 |
| Memories of painful or traumatic events integrate feelings from the past with new (and possibly different) feelings about the past | 3.52 | 1.33 |
| Can recall both positive and negative experiences from childhood and adolescence | 3.51 | 1.35 |
| Gets involved in emotionally, physically or sexually abusive relationships in the role of victim | 3.50 | 1.14 |

most resilient women by examining the items with the highest mean rankings. The reason to standardize the MTRR-99 items prior to averaging the profiles of the resilient women is that doing so tends to amplify values for positive scores on low base rate phenomena. Using this method, items that may be highly descriptive of resilient women but that are also highly prevalent among all of the women in the sample and hence not specific to resilient women will tend to be eclipsed by items that are more specific to resilience. For example, the use of spirituality as a coping mechanism is common among all of the women in the sample and when using scores that are non-standardized it ranks highly in a composite description of both women in the top and bottom quartiles in terms of MTRR total scores. However, when we use the standardized scores, this item no longer ranks highly among the resilient women. Neither manner of aggregating the data is more "correct"; rather, we chose to use standardized scores because our question was which items separate more resilient women from less resilient women.

The items most descriptive of the more resilient women are presented in Table 2. The profile of resilient women is marked by high functioning in three areas: integration of traumatic memories into a coherent part of one's life story and sense of self (rather than experiencing them as fragmented and intrusive memories), ability to form intimate and healthy relationships with others, and capacity to regulate affect and actively engage in self-care activities. These items appear qualitatively more adaptive than those in the whole sample. First, even through women in the sample as a whole appeared to have continuous memories of their lives, including both traumatic and non-traumatic events, the women in the most resilient group appeared to have more actively processed the trauma (e.g., "memories of painful or traumatic events integrate feelings from the past with new [and possibly different] feelings about the past"). Second, although the women in whole sample have altruistic reactions to others and are able to respond to others with empathy, they also have difficulty trusting others. The more resilient women seemed to be able to engage actively in intimate relationships. Similarly, while the women in the whole sample were able to experience a full range of emotions, the more resilient women had developed strategies and self care routines for managing painful affect.

One question raised with respect to resilience is to what extent the resilience is likely to be related to less severe history of interpersonal violence. We looked at the prevalence of each type of abuse in women we identified as most resilient. Among these women, the frequencies of CSA (54%), CPA (37%), ASA (37%), and APA (64%) is lower than

TABLE 2. Composite MTRR-99 Description of Women in the Top Quartile on MTRR Total Score (*N* = 41)

| MTRR-99 ITEMS | $M^a$ | SD |
|---|---|---|
| Appears to have come to terms with painful or traumatic events of the past | 1.10 | 0.70 |
| Has generally positive experiences with members of the opposite sex | 1.02 | 0.78 |
| View of self incorporates but is not dominated by painful or traumatic experiences | 1.00 | 0.60 |
| Seldom re-experiences extreme trauma-related affects such as terror, rage, overwhelming arousal, or utter helplessness | 0.98 | 0.11 |
| Maintains a realistic view of situations even when emotions are strong | 0.93 | 0.63 |
| Has generally positive experiences with members of own sex | 0.93 | 0.73 |
| Functions adaptively after retrieving painful memories, including memories of traumatic events | 0.92 | 0.25 |
| Engages in safe, pleasurable and consensual sex | 0.92 | 0.47 |
| Find meaning in life (and in past suffering or trauma) | 0.89 | 0.25 |
| Is able to enter into and maintain safe and mutually satisfying relationships with intimate partners | 0.88 | 0.92 |
| Is able to experience each of these emotions in a range of intensities | 0.84 | 0.60 |
| Can reflect upon painful events, including traumatic events, with varied and appropriate feeling | 0.82 | 0.68 |
| Forms and maintains safe and mutually satisfying friendships | 0.81 | 0.80 |
| Uses humor appropriately and effectively to manage stress | 0.80 | 0.66 |
| Recognizes and avoids situations that are demeaning, humiliating or unnecessarily painful | 0.78 | 0.53 |
| Is able to regulate unpleasant affects without resorting to self-harming, self-destructive behaviors (e.g., substance abuse, cutting, etc.) | 0.77 | 0.74 |
| Is able to feel a realistic sense of hope and optimism about the future | 0.77 | 0.35 |
| Can choose to recall or to put aside memories of painful events, including traumatic events | 0.76 | 0.68 |
| Exhibits self-care by maintaining healthy sleeping and eating routines | 0.75 | 0.77 |
| Exhibits self-care by engaging in a well-balanced variety of personally meaningful activities | 0.75 | 0.84 |
| Feels like an integrated person whose actions and emotions fit together coherently | 0.75 | 0.63 |
| Memories of painful or traumatic events integrate feelings from the past with new (and possibly different) feelings about the past | 0.75 | 0.66 |

[a]obtained by first standardizing the MTRR times on the full sample and then averaging the value of the item across women in the top quartile on MTRR total scores.

those in the overall group of women (although still high). Additionally, in this group fewer women (14.6%) reported that they had experienced all four types of abuse, and more of the resilient women (17%), compared to the sample as a whole, had experienced no abuse of any of the four types.

## STUDY TWO

In this study, we applied qualitative data analysis to a "life story" narrative created by a woman who identifies as a "survivor" of both child abuse and abuse as an adult (and who also qualifies as mostly recovered based on her MTRR scores). We used the results of this analysis to place this story of recovery the context of the MTRR domains.

### Method

Some of the women completing the first study were referred to a group psychotherapy program for women with a history of CSA (see Bradley & Follingstad, 2003 for more details of this study). As part of the therapy process, women wrote a "life story" by completing a series of writing assignments (see Table 3). For this study, we examined the writing completed as part of the group by one participant. This woman completed two cycles of the group therapy; thus, she completed each of the writing assignments twice over the course of a six month time period. We chose this woman because her MTRR data (rated following the completion of the second group, by a rater blind to the group therapy process) placed her in the largely to fully recovered range based on Harvey's (Harvey et al., 2003) norms.

### Background Information

Here we present a brief case summary based on both the woman's MTRR data and group participation. We obtained her permission to use this case study (details of the case have been changed to protect her identity). The woman is a 29-year-old HIV+ African American woman. She is separated with one daughter and has a high school education. Prior to her incarceration, she held a variety of jobs ranging from store clerk to administrative assistant. She states that she does not remember much about her childhood, which she describes as "lonely." She reports that she felt as though she never had a childhood and that she ran away often. She de-

### TABLE 3. Summary of Group Writing Assignments

| Number | Description |
|---|---|
| 1 | Write about who you were when you were young |
| 2 | Write about the community you grew up in |
| 3 | Write about your adult life. As you write imagine you are traveling back in time to describe your adult self to your child self |
| 4 | Write about how you think that your younger self came to be your adult self |
| 5 | Write a letter to the group about your feelings of anger and how you deal with them |
| 6 | "Write a letter to God/Higher power about your life and your relationship with God/Higher power" and "Write a letter from God/Higher Power to yourself about who you are and your relationship with God/Higher Power" |
| 7 | Write a letter to the group about the lessons you have learned in your life |
| 8 | Looking at last week's assignment, pick a particular person and write a letter sharing your wisdom with them (you don't have to send this letter) |
| 9 | Write notes to each of the other group members |

scribes the early part of her life as marked by poverty and remembers leaving school to work in agricultural fields. She reports she still blames herself for the things that happened to her as a child, but she does not think it fully controls her life anymore. She has a history of drug use and of prostitution. She reports repeated physical and sexual assault as both a child and as an adult. Some excerpts from the writing assignments she completed as part of the therapy group are presented in Figure 1.

## Results

Following the recommendations of Miles and Huberman (1994), we conducted data analysis in two consecutive phases: data reduction and data display. They also identify a third stage of conclusion-drawing/verification, but given that this was an evaluation of a single case study that constituted an initial analysis of a larger set of data we did not complete this stage of data analysis.

### Data Reduction

Codes are labels for retrieval and storage of data based on units of meaning (Miles & Huberman, 1994). Our first goal was to arrive at a set of categories that could be used to apply to the text. Following the procedures set out by Strauss and Corbin (1990), we used open-ended coding in which we reduced the full data set to subsections of labeled text. The data were reviewed line-by-line with initial codes noted in the mar-

FIGURE 1. Examples of Writings Created as Part of Life Narrative

*Write about the traumatic experiences of your younger self:*
1) Growing up I was lonely-isolated
2) Dark closets-locked inside
3) Raped
4) Hiding places
5) Can't breath
7) The dark-scary, a long time
8) Scalding hot water

Heavenly father . . . I pray for peace, no matter what situation I find myself in, Because I know that you will make a way out of no way.

I realize today I must be truthful in order to find healing and I thank you for revealing this.

When I was young I was a very lonely child, and I longed to have friends. In reality I was desperate to be accepted and I allowed many individuals to have their way to be a part of the click.

I had been in a deep state of mourning my life though I was still physically alive, spiritually and emotionally I was dead, I had given up on hope, faith and life in many areas. . . .

But I have finally surrendered to a lot though I still have a lot to face, accept and deal with I know that there must be a God, that you are real. . . .

I have high hopes of getting my life together. I want to live again; I'm tired of existing. I have goals, hopes, and dreams I want to become reality. . . . . . .My life is already gaining meaning, and I'm finding happiness and peace.
. . .There was a time I didn't care, today I do. . . . I think about ordering my days. . . .

gins. The goal at this stage was to arrive at potential coding categories rather than agreement about the specific code of a given line of text. In order to arrive at a comprehensive list of codes with the aim of achieving saturation of the data before beginning reduction of codes, each of the four coders first evaluated the writing assignments independently and generated a list of codes. The four coders met in pairs to compare coding categories. Specifically, the coders began with the first codes on their list. If the content and meaning of the codes were similar, they were reduced to one code; if not, then each constituted a separate category. This process was repeated for each of the categories generated between the two coders. Once each pair agreed upon a set of common codes, this procedure was repeated with the two pairs of coders meeting together (see Table 4). Once the initial set of codes was established, each of the coders again evaluated the text independently and labeled each line with appropriate code(s). We used the following formula: total number of agreements/total number agreements + disagreements. The reliabilities ranged from .81-.92.

The second stage of data reduction involved a procedure Miles and Huberman (1994) refer to as "pattern coding," by which initial codes are distilled into higher order units of meaning, referred to here as themes (this procedure is theoretically analogous to factor analytic techniques for reducing quantitative data). We used the same procedure for

## TABLE 4. Codes by Themes

| Codes | Codes included |
|---|---|
| Alone | Lack of trust, Isolation, Alone, Abandonment, Rejection |
| Anger | Rebellion, Pride, Anger, Hypocrisy |
| Need for Social Acceptance | Need for Social Acceptance, Do anything to fit in |
| Harmed by others | Power of others over her, Others took advantage, Used, Harm by others, Harm by others as a child, Harm by others as an adult |
| Vulnerable | Weakness, No sense of self, Vulnerable to being hurt, Uncertainty |
| Dominance/Control of Others | Harm to others, Her power over others |
| No Self Respect | Stealing, Prostitution, No self respect |
| Sadness | Hopeless, Grief, Sad, Loss |
| Self Harm/Death | Self Harm, Suicide, Death, HIV+ |
| Self Admonition | Remorse, Guilt, Shame |
| Spiritual Death/Need to fill a void | Drugs, Numb, Self medication, Spiritual death, Existing |
| Connection | Want to talk/confide/communicate, Love for others, Try to find love |
| Process of Self Acceptance | Thankful, Struggles, Forgiveness of Others, Learning From Mistakes, Acceptance, Recognition of own part in problems, Peace with Self, Forgiveness of Self |
| God/Quest | Truth, God, Search for Meaning, Life |
| Survivor | Optimism, Strength, Hopes, Victory/Triumph |

identifying themes as we used for identifying initial codes. In this case, the definition of a theme was that it subsumed two or more codes. Again, after the initial set of codes had been agreed upon the text was recoded line by line with themes. In this case, the inter-rater reliability ranged from .84-.91.

### Data Display

The goal of data display (which may include a variety of methods including matrices, charts, and vignettes) is to further organize and reduce data in a way that allows for further data analysis and for drawing and evaluating conclusions (similar to the use of histograms or stem and leaf displays in quantitative data analysis). We summarized our data at two levels. First, we identified a causal pattern among the themes. Working again from the individual level to the group level, each pair of themes was evaluated to determine if there was a causal or reciprocal relationship between the two themes. As before, the coders worked first individually and then each pair worked together until consensus was gained regarding the relationship between each pair of themes. This procedure was then repeated with the two pairs. Figure 2 represents a causal network display (Miles & Huberman, 1994). The arrows represent casual relationships among themes that emerged during the data coding process. The double-headed arrows represent reciprocal relationships among themes (i.e., relationships in which the coders identified bi-directional causality between the two themes). In order to evaluate the reliability of the coding at these two steps, an outside coder who was blind to the initial coding process was provided with a list of the themes and the codes comprising them. This rater then read the life narrative and identified themes with causal connections. Agreement between this so-

FIGURE 2. Casual Connection Among Themes

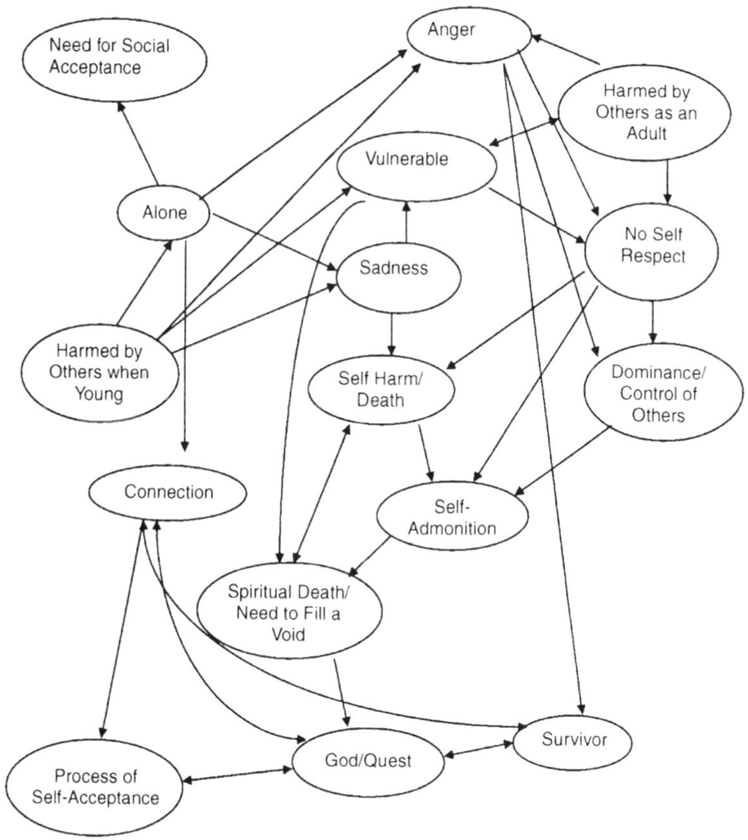

lution and the solution arrived at by the larger group was evaluated with
the total number of agreements/total number agreements + disagreements. The resulting coefficient was .78, indicating relatively robust
inter-rater reliability.

In a final analytic step, we again coded the narrative, taking into account both time and increased parsimony. Specifically, because the data
being coded was a life narrative of recovery, we wanted to identify the
ways in which the most central themes appeared in the story over time.
As above, we worked individually to place themes into an order based
on both time and causality. In this case, we were guided by the decision
to look at themes that seemed the most directly related casually and with
respect to time frame over the development of the life narrative. In this
case, rather than in the hierarchical coding process from individual to
group, we worked as group using discussion, comparison, and returning
to the original data repeatedly to arrive at a consensus. In this process,
we excluded a few themes and collapsed other themes into single categories (e.g., two initial codes, "numb" and "existing," were grouped
into the larger spiritual death theme). The results of this analysis (see
Figure 3) present a process of moving from victimization and related
negative emotions to avoidance of emotions, emotional/spiritual empti-
ness, and numbness, to an ability to connect to others and to achieve
self-awareness and a sense of meaning.

Clearly, many of the themes identified through the coding process
were consistent with the framework of the MTRR. In order to more
clearly specify these relationships, the first author organized the identified themes using the framework of the MTRR domains. The goal was
to understand the changes in life story as viewed by the MTRR narratives. The results presented in Table 5 reflect increased capacity to experience and manage emotions, increased sense of meaning, improved
self-esteem, and a marked increased in coherence of the life narrative.
As an example, the initial description of the participant's childhood was
a bulleted list of traumatic events, and in a later group writing assign-
ment in which she wrote letter to her daughter, she is able to make
causal connections and place her experiences of violence in context.

## DISCUSSION

The data presented in this study have two primary implications for
understanding risk and resilience in incarcerated women. First the results of this study are consistent with the finding that incarcerated

FIGURE 3. Themes Across Time

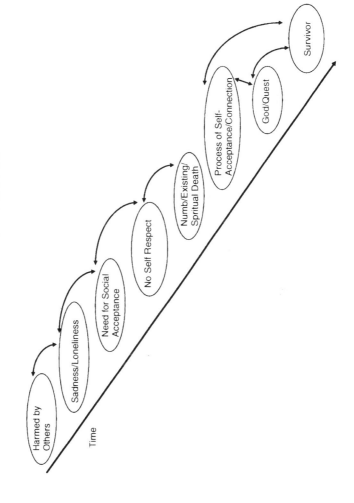

TABLE 5. Changes in Life Story as Viewed by MTRR Themes

| MTRR Domain | Initial | Current |
|---|---|---|
| **I and II:** Authority over the remembering process. Integration of Memories and Affect | Fragmented memories of the past. Avoidance of negative affect preferring to remain "numb" | More coherent understanding of past events. Increase tolerance for affect related to memories of past events |
| **III and IV:** Affect Tolerance and Symptom Mastery | Unable to tolerate negative emotions particularly feelings of loneliness and anger without engaging in self harmful behaviors (e.g., drugs) | More able to tolerate negative emotions without resorting to self-harm |
| **V and VI:** Self Esteem and Self-Cohesion | Image of self as vulnerable and weak. Thinks of self as "bad" and feels high level of shame | Increase in tolerance for own flaws; increased ability to identify positive aspects of self. Identification of self as "survivor" |
| **VII:** Safe Attachment | Alone, Desperate for attention from others | Desire for connection for others at times (though still has part of her that wants to avoid all connections) |
| **VIII:** Meaning | Little sense of meaning and belonging | Sense of life as having a higher meaning, able to identify ways in which would like to help others, strong relationship with God |

women have experienced IPV, often occurring throughout the lifespan and often severe and frequent. And although research suggests that these experiences are related to many negative outcomes (e.g., PTSD and substance abuse), less research has focused on sources and manifestations of resilience in this population. The data we collected using the MTRR clearly shows that the women demonstrate a high level of resilience despite their experiences of abuse that is usually compounded by poverty and the "double jeopardy" of being a woman in a racial/ethnic minority group. The composite description of the resilient women in which adaptive function items greatly outnumbered non-adaptive items confirmed this finding.

The profile of resilience drawn from the most resilient women (using total MTRR score) includes several notable aspects. First, while still reporting strikingly high levels of prior abuse (83% reported at least one type), these women had relatively lower rates and they were less likely to report experiencing all four types of abuse. Thus, this data suggests that extent of abuse contributes to resilience. This may be reflected in one of the characteristics marking the more resilient women: the capacity to establish close and healthy relationships with both men and women. Having experienced less abuse, these women presumably have increased ability to trust and relate well to others. A second notable characteristic of the more resilient women is the ability to place their traumatic experiences in the context of their full life narrative (the trauma is part of the story rather than trauma defining the narrative). Lastly, this group of women showed an ability to actively and effectively manage negative affect.

The case study presented similar themes. Increased capacity for relatedness was one of the elements of recovery in this case. Because this data was presented as part of a life story, we were able to draw preliminary hypotheses about connections between elements of the recovery process as they emerged over time. In this case, damaged relationships with others (often marked by violence) were both the source of many of the problems and ultimately a touchstone in recovery. The recovery process in this case also reflected increased ability to manage strong emotions and the ability to integrate traumatic material into a meaningful narrative. This case also highlights the centrality of improvement of a damaged conception of self in the recovery process.

Clearly these three areas (relationships, affect regulation, integration of traumatic experiences and self-esteem) should be included when developing interventions to increase resiliency and promote recovery among incarcerated women. In fact, several extant studies focus on these areas (see, e.g., Bradley & Follingstad, 2003; Zlotnick, Najavits, Rohsenow, & Johnson, 2003). Also, the ecological model posited by Harvey (1996) underscores the importance of taking social context into account when understanding the impact of traumatic experiences. In the case of incarcerated women, it is clear that gender, race, and SES are macro-social variables that, although not the focus of this study, are central to understanding the experiences of incarcerated women (see, e.g., Bradley & Davino, 2002; Richie, 1996).

There are a number of limitations to this study. First, the location of this study in a prison environment specifically for women with physical and mental health problems limits the generalizability of the findings to other samples of incarcerated women. For example, it is likely that the rates of IPV would be lower in a broader sample of incarcerated women (although based on other research, still higher than those of a general population of women). In addition, given the high rates of multiple experiences of physical and sexual abuse that began at a young age and with a high level of severity, it was not possible to conduct meaningful analyses with respect to magnitude of abuse (e.g., it would not necessarily make theoretical sense to place the impact of rape at a young age and ongoing physical abuse by a caretaker on the same continuum). The profile of resilience presented here reflects the women who are most re-silent when averaged across all eight domains of the MTRR. It is likely that with a larger number of participants we would be able to identify patterns of resilience that are obscured by the use of an average score. Third, the data were based on clinician rating measures of resilience. While having only one method of assessment in research on the impact of IPV (usually self report) is modal in the literature, it would be ideal to triangulate data from multiple sources. Also, there are distinct benefits to using clinician ratings for assessment of women with a history of trauma that are discussed more thoroughly in other articles (Harvey et al., 2003; Liang et al., this volume). Fourth, the qualitative data analyses presented in this study are preliminary analyses. A project that will examine a series of case studies, thus allowing for validation of the data, is planned. Finally, future studies need to more explicitly analyze race, SES, and gender (as well as other macro level variables). Clearly, this study represents initial research in an under-researched area (resilience to trauma) with an under-researched group of women.

## REFERENCES

Amott, T., & Matthaei, J. (1996). *Race, gender and work: Multi-cultural economic history of women in the United States.* Boston: South End Press.

Bradley, R. G., & Davino, K. M. (2002). Women's perceptions of the prison environment: When prison is "the safest place I've ever been." *Psychology of Women Quarterly,* 26(4), 351-359.

Bradley, R. G., & Follingstad, D. R. (2003). Group therapy for incarcerated women who experienced interpersonal violence: A pilot study. *Journal of Traumatic Stress,* 16(4), 337-340.

Briere, J. (1995). *Trauma Symptom Inventory (TSI) professional manual.* Odessa, FL: PAR.

Briere, J. (1996). *Therapy for adults molested as children: Beyond survival.* New York: Springer.

Browne, A., & Bassuk, S. (1997). Intimate violence in the lives of homeless and poor housed women: Prevalence and patterns in an ethnically diverse sample. *American Journal of Orthopsychiatry,* 67(2), 261-278.

Browne, A., Miller, B., & Maguin, E. (1999). Prevalence and severity of lifetime physical and sexual victimization among incarcerated women. *International Journal of Law and Psychiatry,* 22, 301-322.

Chesney-Lind, M. (1996). Sentencing women to prison: Equality without justice. In M. D. Schwartz & D. Milovanovic (Eds.), *Race, gender, and class in criminology: The intersection* (pp. 127-140). New York: Garland Publishing, Inc.

Chesney-Lind, M. (1997). *The female offender: Girls, women, and crime.* Thousand Oaks, CA: Sage Publications.

Goodman, L. A. (1991). The prevalence of abuse among homeless and housed poor mothers: A comparison study. *American Journal of Orthopsychiatry*, 6(4), 489-500.

Greenfeld, L. A., & Snell, T. (1999). *Women offenders* (NCJ 175688). Washington, DC: U.S. Department of Justice.

Grossman, F. K., Cook, A. B., Kepkep, S. S., & Koenen, K. C. (1999). *With the phoenix rising: Lessons from ten resilient women who overcame the trauma of childhood sexual abuse.* San Francisco: Jossey-Bass.

Harvey, M. R. (1996). An ecological view of psychological trauma and trauma recovery. *Journal of Traumatic Stress*, 9(1), 3-23.

Harvey, M. R., Liang, B., Harney, P., Koenen, K., Tummala-Narra, P., & Lebowitz, L. (2003). A multidimensional approach to the assessment of trauma impact, recovery and resiliency: Five psychometric studies. *Journal of Aggression, Maltreatment & Trauma*, 6(2), 87-109.

Jordan, B., Schlenger, W. E., Fairbank, J. A., & Caddell, J. M. (1996). Prevalence of psychiatric disorders among incarcerated women: Convicted felons entering prison. *Archives of General Psychiatry*, 53(6), 513-519.

Lam, J. K., & Grossman, F. K. (1997). Resiliency and adult adaptation in women with and without self-reported histories of childhood sexual abuse. *Journal of Traumatic Stress*, 10, 175-196.

Liang, B., Tummala-Narra, P., Bradley, R., & Harvey, M. R. (2007). The Multidimensional Trauma Recovery and Resiliency instrument: Preliminary examination of an abridged version. *Journal of Aggression, Maltreatment & Trauma*, 14(1/2), 55-74.

Liem, J. H., James, J. B., O'Toole, B. A., & Boudewyn, A. C. (1997). Assessing resilience in adults with histories of childhood sexual abuse. *American Journal of Orthopsychiatry*, 67, 594-606.

Miles, M., & Huberman A. (1994). *Qualitative data analysis* (2nd ed.). London: Sage Publications.

Pelcovitz, D., van der Kolk, B., Roth, S., Mandel, F., Kaplan, S., & Resick, P. (1997). Development of a criteria set and a structured interview for disorders of extreme stress. *Journal of Traumatic Stress*, 10, 3-16.

Powell, T. A. (1999, August). *Women inmates in Vermont.* Paper presented at the annual meeting of the American Psychological Association, Boston, MA.

Resnick, H. S., Kilpatrick, D. G., Dansky, B. S., Saunders, B. E., & Best, C. L. (1993). Prevalence of civilian trauma and posttraumatic stress disorder in a representative national sample of women. *Journal of Consulting and Clinical Psychology*, 6, 984-991.

Richie, B. E. (1996). *Compelled to crime: The gender entrapment of battered Black women.* New York: Routledge.

Russell, D. E. H. (1983). The incidence and prevalence of intrafamilial and extrafamilial sexual abuse of female children. *Child Abuse and Neglect*, 7, 133-146.

Russell, D. E. H., Schurman, R. A., & Trocki, K. (1988). The long-term effects of incestuous abuse: A comparison of Afro-American and White American victims. In G. E. Wyatt & G. J. Powell (Eds.), *Lasting effects of child sexual abuse* (pp. 119-134). Newbury Park: Sage Publications.

Seligman, M. E. P., & Csikszentmihalyi, M. (2000). Positive psychology. *American Psychologist,* 55, 5-14.

Straus, M. A. (1979). Measuring intrafamily conflict and violence: The conflict tactics scales. *Journal of Marriage and the Family,* 41, 75-88.

Straus, M. A. (1990). The Conflicts Tactics Scale and its critics: An evaluation of new data on validity and reliability. In M. A. Straus & R. J. Gelles (Eds.), *Physical violence in the American family* (pp. 49-73). New Brunswick, NJ: Transaction Books.

Strauss, A., & Corbin, J. (1990). *Basics of qualitative research.* Newbury Park: Sage.

Teplin, L. A., Abram, K. M., & McClelland, G. M. (1996). Prevalence of psychiatric disorders among incarcerated women: I. Pretrial jail detainees. *Archives of General Psychiatry,* 53(6), 505-512.

Tsuang, M. T. (2000). Genes, environment and mental health wellness. *American Journal of Psychiatry,* 157, 489-491.

United States Department of Justice. (1999). *Correctional populations in the United States.* Report available from, http://www.ojp.usdoj.gov/bjs/pubalp2.htm#cpus

Widom, C. S. (1999). Posttraumatic stress disorder in abused and neglected children grown up. *American Journal of Psychiatry,* 156(8), 1223-1229.

Wolfner, G. D., & Gelles, R. J. (1993). A profile of violence toward children: A national study. *Child Abuse and Neglect,* 17, 197-212.

Wyatt, G. E. (1985). The sexual abuse of Afro-American and White-American women in childhood. *Child Abuse and Neglect,* 10, 241-251.

Zlotnick, C., Najavits, L. M., Rohsenow, D. J., & Johnson, D. M. (2003). A cognitive-behavioral treatment for incarcerated women with substance abuse disorder and posttraumatic stress disorder: Findings from a pilot study. *Journal of Substance Abuse Treatment,* 25(2), 99-105.

doi:10.1300/J146v14n01_07

# Exposure to Violence
# and Expressions of Resilience
# in Central American Women Survivors
# of War

Angela Radan

**SUMMARY.** This article focuses on expressions of resilience in a sample of 30 women from El Salvador and Guatemala who survived multiple types of violence, including war trauma, before taking refuge in the US. Traumatic impact, recovery, and resilience were assessed using the Multidimensional Trauma Recovery and Resilience Interview (MTRR-I) and rating scale, MTRR-99. Exposure to violence was assessed by the Harvard Trauma Questionnaire and the MTRR-I. The study established that the women had suffered multiple and extreme forms of violence prior to and en route to the United States and yet were highly resilient on multiple MTRR domains when compared with a US sample. Implications for future research for assessment of trauma exposure and resilience among war-afflicted populations are discussed. doi:10.1300/J146v14n01_08 *[Article copies available for a fee from The Haworth Document Delivery Service: 1-800-HAWORTH. E-mail address: <docdelivery@haworthpress.com> Website: <http://www.HaworthPress.com> © 2007 by The Haworth Press, Inc. All rights reserved.]*

---

Address correspondence to: Angela Radan, PhD, Latino Mental Health Program, 119 Windsor Street, Cambridge, MA 02139.

[Haworth co-indexing entry note]: "Exposure to Violence and Expressions of Resilience in Central American Women Survivors of War." Radan, Angela. Co-published simultaneously in *Journal of Aggression, Maltreatment & Trauma* (The Haworth Maltreatment & Trauma Press, an imprint of The Haworth Press, Inc.) Vol. 14, No. 1/2, 2007, pp. 147-164; and: *Sources and Expressions of Resiliency in Trauma Survivors: Ecological Theory, Multicultural Practice* (ed: Mary R. Harvey, and Pratyusha Tummala-Narra) The Haworth Maltreatment & Trauma Press, an imprint of The Haworth Press, Inc., 2007, pp. 147-164. Single or multiple copies of this article are available for a fee from The Haworth Document Delivery Service [1-800-HAWORTH, 9:00 a.m. - 5:00 p.m. (EST). E-mail address: docdelivery@haworthpress.com].

**KEYWORDS.** Central America, trauma, resilience, recovery, MTRR

War and violence have drawn the attention and outrage of social scientists and the general public because of the devastation and pain they inflict on victims. Trauma researchers have made an enormous contribution to our understanding of war trauma by documenting the multiple negative effects of victimization. These efforts have informed our understanding of trauma and guided the design of interventions to alleviate victim distress. A "medical model" approach emphasizing individual psychopathology, diagnosis, and treatment has played a prominent role in this area of study. Too often this approach has failed to take into account the context in which both violence and recovery from violence take place and/or the resilience exhibited by some survivors. Awareness of environmental influences and attention to social, cultural, and political context, however, are crucial to understanding the experience of war-afflicted populations.

## THE CONTEXT OF WAR:
## THE CONTRIBUTIONS OF LATIN AMERICAN
## PSYCHOLOGISTS

Latin America has survived decades of repressive regimes, and many Latin American social scientists have incorporated these violent realities into their work. Chilean psychologists, for example, emphasize that a full understanding of trauma requires an integration of the subjective experience of the survivor and the sociopolitical dimensions of the violence to which survivors have been exposed (Becker, Lira, Castillo, Govez, & Kovalsky, 1990). The writings of Ignacio Martín-Baró, a Jesuit priest and psychologist assassinated in El Salvador in November 1989, are particularly relevant to understanding war trauma. Defining war as a psychosocial trauma, affecting "a whole population, and not only as individuals but precisely in their social character, that is, as a totality, as a system," Martín-Baró (1990, p. 3) suggests that people's reactions to trauma must be viewed in the context of social relationships.

Martín-Baró (1994a, 1994b) is critical of prevailing theories of psychological trauma, suggesting that they rely on assumptions that do not hold for the reality of Central America. One such assumption is that war affects everybody in the same way, while in reality war impacts different sectors of the population differently. One sector, comprised of an elite and privileged minority, may actually benefit from wars that preserve the status quo. Another, which in Central America includes the popular majority, has much less access to power and resources, is severely and negatively impacted by war, and suffers its consequences in a more direct and generalized way. A second assumption questioned by Martín-Baró (1994b) is the unexpectedness of traumatic experiences. In Guatemala and El Salvador, the violence of war was a daily occurrence. Even after peace accords were signed in both countries, violence continued to be a part of people's everyday experience. Finally, Martín-Baró (1990) questions the conceptualization of trauma as an individual experience. In fact, war is a form of violence that is produced socially and affects all social relations. Besides its direct impact, war has consequences at multiple ecological levels, causing, for example, the corruption of institutions, the destruction of a country's natural resources, and helping to bring about the loss of national sovereignty, growing militarization, and the acceptance of violence as part of daily life.

## AN ECOLOGICAL PERSPECTIVE

An ecological view of psychological trauma (Harvey, 1996) offers a useful framework for examining the impact of war on its victims and the role of social context in mediating that impact. Based on the assumptions that psychological attributes of human beings are best understood in the ecological context of human community, this framework acknowledges that individuals react differently to similar events as a result of complex interactions among person, event, and environmental factors (Harvey, 1996). Within this framework, resilience is viewed as a multidimensional phenomenon. Individuals may exhibit considerable strengths in some areas of functioning even while exhibiting considerable impairment in others.

The multidimensional definition of resilience articulated in Harvey's (1996) ecological model has been operationalized in the form of two assessment tools, the Multidimensional Trauma Recovery and Resiliency Scale (MTRR) and companion interview (MTRR-I), which have been used in both quantitative and qualitative studies of trauma impact, recovery, and resilience (Harvey, Mishler, Koenen, & Harney, 2000; Liang, Tummala-Narra, Bradley, & Harvey, this volume). In an initial series of psychometric studies with traumatized patients, these measures demonstrated promising psychometric strengths (Harvey et al.,

2003). In reporting these data, the investigators articulated the need for studies examining the utility of the measures with untreated survivors and with survivors from other than mainstream segments of the culture. The current study was undertaken with these issues in mind. Specifically, it applied the ecological framework to the experience of Central American women refugees of war and utilized a Spanish-language version of the MTRR-I and MTRR-99 (Liang et al., this volume) to assess trauma impact, recovery, and resilience in a group of participants drawn from this largely untreated, multiply violated population.

## WAR AND POST-WAR EXPERIENCES OF THE GUATEMALAN AND SALVADORAN WOMEN

Central American women have suffered enormous exposure to violence in the context of war. Many have had to endure the knowledge or experience of their loved ones being tortured and victimized. Many have been attacked and violated, becoming victims of rape and sexual assault in uncounted numbers (Allodi & Stiasny, 1990; Aron, Corne, Fursland, & Zelwer, 1991; Fornazzari & Freire, 1990). In the context of war, rape is used not only to harm and humiliate the victim, but also to torture family members and friends (Friedman, 1992). Aron et al. (1991) differentiate between rape as a crime and government-sanctioned rape as a weapon of torture. In the latter case, the political sanctioning of rape normalizes the crime and converts it into a form of political control, effectively granting war combatants permission to violate women. Thus, the "sexist structures and policies that render women and their special needs invisible are reinforced rather than diminished under conditions of state-sponsored violence" (Lykes, Brabeck, Ferns, & Radan, 1993, p. 527).

The fact that these acts are sanctioned by the government has profound impact on the psyche of the population. The women of Guatemala and El Salvador have faced enormous fear and terror due not only to the violence directed at them, but also to the impunity of perpetrators. That women are abused by the military has equally serious implications. They are unable to call for help, press charges, or seek justice. Indeed, victims can actually get killed if they try to resist or look to others for support. Thus, during war women face an ongoing catastrophe (Aron et al., 1991). State sponsored violence and terror is accompanied by silencing, not only of individuals but of the community as well (Lykes et al., 1993).

Domestic violence is another form of violence experienced by women survivors of war. As in other parts of the world, battering and violence against women is a common occurrence in Central America, and it does not abate when women flee with their families in search of refuge. Indeed, work with refugee women suggests that refugee men who have suffered their own experience of war and who believe they have failed to protect themselves and their families may become perpetrators. Wife abuse becomes a way of recovering control and power (Friedman, 1992), adding another layer of victimization to the experiences of refugee women.

In addition, Central American women and girls who are forced to leave their countries due to war are vulnerable to violence during their flight. Many Central American women refugees report having been raped by "coyotes," men paid money in exchange for a safe escort to another country (Friedman, 1992). Those who make it to refugee camps run the risk of being subjected to violence by camp authorities and military guards who are supposed to provide safe haven (Friedman, 1992).

The migration of Central Americans to the United States represents not only a flight for safety but also "involves breaking life-long ties with family members, friends, community and cultural patterns" (Salgado de Snyder, Cervantes, & Padilla, 1990, p. 442). Thus, family disintegration is another hardship experienced by women refugees (Roe, 1986). Having lost family members to war, they also face the agony of having to leave behind family, children, homes, and belongings. Like other war refugees, Central American women suffer psychosocial adjustment difficulties when they migrate to the United States. Some become skeptical and hesitate to invest in the future, while others focus on the past, long for the future, and cannot rely on the present (Roe, 1986).

When considering the post-war status of Central American women in the United States, a number of factors require attention, including time in the U.S., age, occupational skills and education, exposure to traumatic events (before, during, or following migration), knowledge of English, access to family supports, social contacts, and level of maintenance of ethnic identity in the United States (Roe, 1986), as well as adjustment to the new culture and, of course, gender. Women refugees are vulnerable to gender-based discrimination, exploitation, and violence, and are at risk not only in the communities from which they are fleeing, but also in their adopted homelands and while en route from one to the other. At all times, women "continue to remain responsible for the survival of their children and other members of their families, and for the preservation of their cultural heritage" (Brautigan, 1996, p. 361).

Despite the obstacles and traumatic experiences they have encountered, many Central American refugee women say that their new life has also meant new opportunities and the equally new experience of personal safety. The stories shared by Central American women in clinical settings reveal not only the horrors to which they have been exposed but also how exile may provide opportunity to get away from both abusive partners and oppressive environments. For example, some women report having greater control over their lives and more independence and decision-making power in matters relevant to their lives. Others have benefited from new opportunities to pursue their education and a new sense of security. An environment that fosters safety offers a first step toward recovery from experiences of violence. One of the participants in the study reported here expressed the following: "Had I stayed in my country I would have led a life of misery and poverty. I would not be able to be independent and provide a safe place for my children. Here I was even able to get a degree."

## THE STUDY:
## EXPOSURE TO VIOLENCE AND EXPRESSIONS OF RESILIENCE AMONG CENTRAL AMERICAN WOMEN REFUGEES OF WAR

The current study applies an ecological perspective and an ecologically-informed assessment approach to the study of resilience in Central American women with histories of exposure to war trauma and other forms of violence. Guatemalan and Salvadoran women who had left their homelands as a result of and in the wake of the wars in their home countries were interviewed extensively using a Spanish-language translation of the MTRR-I developed by Harvey et al. (1994). The study assessed these women's lifetime exposure to interpersonal and political violence and sought to document their resilience (individually and as a group) in multiple areas of functioning. In addition, the study examined the cross-cultural applicability of the ecological framework and the cross-cultural utility and inter-rater reliability of the MTTR measures used in the study.

### Methods

#### Participants

Thirty women from El Salvador and Guatemala (15 from each country) who had migrated to the United States to flee war or to escape the precarious economies that their countries of origin were experiencing as a result of war participated in the study. The women were chosen to participate regardless of their immigration status in the United States.

The sample interviewed was comprised of mostly low-income women. Nineteen of the women had never been in therapy; six had sought psychological care in the past, and five were in treatment at the time of the interview. The women ranged in age from 21 to 58 ($M = 37, SD = 10.5$). Half were married, seven lived in common law relationships, four were divorced, and four were single at the time of their interviews.

Most of the women had had some schooling. Two had never been to school and were illiterate, seven had had some level of primary education, seven had had several years' secondary education, one had had vocational training, and seven had had some university education, either in their home countries or in the U.S. One participant had completed two graduate degrees. All of the participants had obtained some kind of employment. Regardless of their educations, the most common forms of employment for these women were: cleaning (either private homes or businesses), childcare, cosmetology, and factory work.

## Measures

The instruments used in this study were the Spanish language MTRR-I, the MTRR-99 rating scale, and the Harvard Trauma Questionnaire (HTQ; Mollica et al., 1991). All instruments with the exception of the MTRR-99 were translated into Spanish and back-translated into English by a second bilingual and bicultural translator with clinical training and experience working with Central American trauma survivors. English language versions of both MTRR measures are included in this volume (see Appendices A and B).

*The MTRR measures.* The MTRR-I was developed to assess trauma impact, resilience, and recovery through open-ended questions regarding an individual's life history, including his or her trauma history (Harvey et al., 1994). Information gathered from the interview is rated by the MTRR-99 scale (see Appendix A at the end of this volume), which yields an overall composite score as well as individual scores on each of eight recovery domains: authority over the remembering process, integration of memory and affect, affect tolerance, symptom mastery, self esteem, self cohesion, safe attachment, and meaning-making. Possible mean scores range from 1.00 to 5.00 for each of the dimensions. Preliminary psychometric data indicate that this instrument is able to draw statistically significant distinctions between individuals at different stages of recovery from traumatic events (Liang et al., this volume).

*The Harvard Trauma Questionnaire* (Mollica et al., 1991). The HTQ measures type and severity of traumatic experiences. It consists of four parts. Part I describes a range of traumatic events that respondents may have experienced. Part II asks respondents to describe the most traumatic events experienced in country of origin and in a host country. Part III explores the possibility of head injury and Part IV focuses on symptoms of Post Traumatic Stress Disorder or symptoms associated with exposure to overwhelming stress. For the purposes of this study, only Part I was used to measure exposure to trauma. It is comprised of 17 items describing possible traumatic experiences. Respondents are asked to indicate if they have: "experienced" (3), "witnessed" (2), "heard about" (1), or "not experienced" (0) indexed events. A total score, ranging from 0 to 51 is calculated by summing 17 item scores, with a score of 51 representing the most severe exposure.

## Procedures

*Recruiting participants.* Participants were recruited from both formally established and loosely structured and informal groups for Central Americans in the Boston area. Whenever possible, the investigator visited the groups and made a personal appeal inviting women to participate. A description of the research project was provided in Spanish. As the study progressed, participants themselves were asked to refer others who might be interested in participating,

*Interviewing participants and administering the measures.* Once a person agreed to participate, she was given the consent form and an appointment was arranged at a time and place convenient to the participant. The interview was expected to take between two to three hours, but some lasted up to four and a half hours. All interviews were conducted by the author in Spanish and were audiotaped and later transcribed. The HTQ was administered orally (in Spanish) because a given participants' level of literacy was unknown prior to HTQ administration and to ensure consistency in data gathering

During the course of each interview, the author was careful to assess the emotional impact of the interview on the participant and was prepared to provide clinical assistance and make appropriate referral to clinical care. In fact, only one participant required such assistance. In addition, a list of local Spanish language mental health services was provided.

Participants were offered $10 in appreciation for their participation. Eleven rejected payment. In these cases, the interviewer brought baked goods, a small plant, or a toy for a child as a token of appreciation. In general, the participants described their participation in the study in positive terms, felt it was important to speak their truth, and were very enthusiastic in finding new people for the study.

*Data analysis.* All interviews were rated by the principal investigator and 20% of them were rated by a second bilingual and bicultural rater in order to assess inter-rater reliability. Both researcher and second rater received training on the use of the MTRR measures. The intraclass correlation coefficient (ICC) was used to measure the reliability. Results indicated generally high interrater reliability and consistency between raters in how the measures were scored.

Following data collection, an initial analysis was conducted to determine if differences existed between the Guatemalan and El Salvadoran women on any of the measures. Following a determination that both the HTQ and MTRR data for the two groups could be combined, analysis focused on: (a) the nature of traumatic experiences reported by the women in response to questions from both the HTQ and the MTRR-I, and (b) an examination of the MTRR overall and domain scores.

## Results

### Comparisons of Guatemalan and El Salvadoran Women

No significant differences were found between the Guatemalan and El Salvadoran women in terms of age, age of arrival and length of stay in the United States, education, and/or MTRR-99 scores. T-tests for independent samples did indicate, however, that the Guatemalan women had been in the U.S. for a significantly longer period of time, possibly reflecting the earlier beginning of armed conflict in Guatemala and correspondingly earlier migration dates for the Guatemalan women. The Guatemalan women were also older, but these results were marginally significant.

In terms of their MTRR scores, no major differences were found between the two groups, with the exception of significantly higher scores obtained by the Guatemalan women on authority over memory domain. It is very likely that this finding has to do with the fact that the Guatemalan women had been in the U.S. longer and were more removed from the traumatic events experienced in their country. No other significant differences were found between the group of women from Guatemala and El Salvador. The two groups of women were considered comparable and were merged for analysis.

## Exposure to Traumatic Events

Table 1 presents data gathered using the HTQ concerning the range and extremity of exposure to violence among this group of Central American women. As indicated, the women as a group endorsed having experienced, witnessed, or heard about every experience indexed by the HTQ, including lack of food or water, ill health without access to medical care, lack of shelter, imprisonment, serious injury, combat situation, brainwashing, rape/sexual assault, enforced isolation from others, being close to death, forced separation from family members, murder of family or friend, unnatural death of family or friend, murder of stranger or strangers, being lost or kidnapped, torture, and any other situation that was frightening or where the person felt their life was in danger.

An unanticipated finding of this investigation was the extent to which women in the study revealed much more about the nature and extremity of their trauma histories during the interview than when responding to the HTQ. For example, when asked about particular types of traumatic experiences using the HTQ, many participants would acknowledge that they had "witnessed" or "heard about it" the designated event, but in the interview would describe a situation in which they clearly identified themselves as direct victims. This finding is discussed in greater detail in the discussion.

## Multidimensional Profiles of Resilience

Mean scores for the Guatemalan and Salvadoran women on each of the eight MTRR domains are depicted in Table 2. As indicated, these mean scores ranged from 3.38 to 4.11, suggesting a relatively high level of overall recovery or resilience when compared to the mean scores reported by on a North American clinical sample (Harvey et al., 2003; Liang et al., this volume). These results reflect the resilience of this group of women as a whole and their ability to recover without aid of clinical care. For the majority of these women, psychotherapeutic care was never an option.

When working with group means, there is a danger of masking the pathology of individual participants with the lowest scores. Therefore, participants with a composite score of 3.00 or less (out of 5.00) were identified as largely unrecovered and those with overall mean scores above 3.00 as

## TABLE 1. Responses to Items of the Harvard Trauma Questionnaire

| Item | Experienced | Witnessed | Heard | No |
|---|---|---|---|---|
| Lack of food or water | 2 | 5 | 23 | 0 |
| Ill health without medical care | 4 | 7 | 16 | 3 |
| Lack of shelter | 5 | 11 | 11 | 3 |
| Imprisonment | 6 | 17 | 3 | 4 |
| Serious injury | 6 | 10 | 10 | 4 |
| Combat situation | 9 | 12 | 9 | 0 |
| Brainwashing | 6 | 5 | 5 | 14 |
| Rape | 10 | 8 | 12 | 0 |
| Forced isolation from others | 3 | 6 | 8 | 13 |
| Being close to death | 3 | 6 | 18 | 3 |
| Separation from family members | 2 | 7 | 15 | 6 |
| Murder of family or friend | 6 | 0 | 22 | 2 |
| Unnatural death of family | 0 | 4 | 14 | 12 |
| Murder of stranger | 6 | 5 | 17 | 2 |
| Lost or kidnapped | 6 | 18 | 4 | 2 |
| Torture | 11 | 10 | 5 | 4 |
| Frightening situation | 3 | 2 | 21 | 4 |

## TABLE 2. Group Mean Scores on the Domains of the MTRR

| | M | SD | Min | Max |
|---|---|---|---|---|
| Authority over Memory | 3.54 | .64 | 2.36 | 4.86 |
| Integration Memory and Affect | 3.90 | .76 | 1.90 | 5.00 |
| Affect Tolerance | 3.54 | .65 | 2.18 | 4.72 |
| Symptom Mastery | 3.58 | .68 | 2.35 | 4.65 |
| Self Esteem | 3.88 | .77 | 2.03 | 4.80 |
| Self Cohesion | 4.11 | .78 | 2.33 | 5.00 |
| Safe Attachments | 3.52 | .70 | 2.23 | 4.73 |
| Meaning Making | 3.38 | .90 | 1.66 | 4.87 |

largely to fully recovered. As indicated in Table 3, only six participants had a composite score of 3 or less. In addition, although individual participants might have had overall MTRR scores above 3.00, they could also have received lower scores on particular domains (see Table 3). As indicated, the domains of symptom mastery, safe attachment, meaning, and affect tolerance were the domains on which a third or nearly a third of these participants had scores below the 3.0 level. It is important to emphasize, however, that the majority of the women in this study fell in the category of "almost fully recovered" in and across all domains.

## DISCUSSION

This study focused on histories of violence and expressions of resilience in 30 Central American women refugees of war trauma and on the relationship between social support and expressions of resilience in this population. A major finding of the investigation is the degree of resilience attained by the women who participated in this research. In general, results indicate that despite the risks of extreme poverty, lack of opportunities for education, prior experiences of physical and/or sexual abuse, and the trauma of being a witness to and, in some cases, a direct victim of war-related violence, the majority of the women interviewed have been able to overcome adversity, survive both the horrors of war and the dangers of flight, and build satisfying lives in their new homelands.

TABLE 3. Scores of Unrecovered Participants on the MTRR and its Domain

|  | Frequency | *M* | *SD* | Min | Max |
|---|---|---|---|---|---|
| MTRR | 6 | 2.82 | 0.14 | 2.65 | 2.97 |
| Authority over memory | 5 | 2.73 | 0.28 | 2.36 | 3.00 |
| Integration memory and affect | 4 | 2.65 | 0.52 | 1.90 | 3.00 |
| Affect tolerance | 7 | 2.64 | 0.28 | 2.18 | 2.91 |
| Symptom mastery | 9 | 2.73 | 0.25 | 2.35 | 3.00 |
| Self esteem | 4 | 2.47 | 0.32 | 2.03 | 2.80 |
| Self cohesion | 4 | 2.69 | 0.28 | 2.33 | 2.92 |
| Safe attachments | 9 | 2.71 | 0.27 | 2.23 | 3.00 |
| Meaning making | 10 | 2.33 | 0.44 | 1.67 | 3.00 |

Of the 30 women interviewed, only six had overall MTRR mean scores of 3.0 or less, while 24 had overall scores greater than 3. The highest mean scores for the Central American women refugees in this study were in the domains of self cohesion, integration memory and affect, and self esteem, indicating that they possessed a sound level of psychological integration, the ability to recall the past with varied and appropriate feelings, and a fundamental sense of positive self worth.

Despite their generally high scores, a third of the women in the sample were still struggling to make meaning of their experiences and nearly a third had scores below 3.0 in the symptom mastery and safe attachment domains. Nine of the women were still struggling with symptoms related to their traumatic pasts, which might be related to the fact that most of the participants had never received psychotherapeutic care as a result of their experience. In addition, their ability to build safe attachments may well reflect the experience of forced migration and a sense of alienation in the new home country.

An important and unexpected finding of this investigation was that of the MTRR-I's sensitivity to and ability to assess the nature and degree of traumatic exposure suffered by research participants. Comprised of open-ended questions that invite the respondent to provide a detailed, free-flowing narrative of personal history and experience, the MTRR-I may provide a means of more accurately assessing traumatic exposure. Certainly in this investigation, the responses women gave to questions posed by the MTRR-I gave a more complete and complex understanding of what the women had survived and overcome than did other measures. Thus, when their responses to a quantitative measure of traumatic experience (HTQ) are compared with their responses to the MTRR-I questions, it is clear that a majority of women under-reported their experiences of direct victimization on the HTQ.

For example, some of the women who denied experiencing lack of food or water when responding to the HTQ later shared the following:

Participant #11: On our way to this country, we were eating only every three days.

Participant #13: At night the shootings would start and we had to get under the houses, without water without electricity. We would come out the next day and we would find rows of dead people in the trenches. The military would force us to dig trenches around the houses and if we refused, we would get killed. We experienced hunger and thirst.

A similar discrepancy was found when responses to the HTQ item "Being close to death." Women who reported only hearing about such experiences on the HTQ later described the following:

> Participant #10: We were fleeing and the children were coughing. We had to cover their mouths so that the soldiers would not hear us.

> Participant # 16: The guerrilla was using me as a human shield.

The findings were similar when the indexed event was exposure to the murder of a family member or friend. Although only 6 women reported having had this experience when responding to the HTQ, 16 women discussed such experiences in the context of the interview. Following are descriptions of what some of them experienced:

> Participant #15: I found my uncle, he was dead, he was being eaten by animals.

> Participant #24: A female friend of mine was burned. Two male friends were found dead, it was the police.

In viewing these findings it is important to remember that violence and trauma were part of the daily life experiences of Guatemalan and Salvadoran women who, like the women in this investigation, suffered horrific exposure before fleeing their homelands. For these women, the violence was not experienced as an isolated event, and was not reported as such.

This finding suggests that the nature and severity of complex and sustained traumatic experiences may defy accurate assessment by multiple-choice, quantitative measures. Indeed, they illustrate Martin-Baró's (1994c) concept of "normal abnormality." Central Americans have suffered decades of war and countless episodes of violence, episodes that become part of the everyday life of an entire population and are not registered as isolated events with distinct effects. It is only in testimonies and extended narratives of lives lived that we begin to accurately glimpse the full range of horrors that survivors have experienced.

It may be, too, that not identifying a given experience as traumatic but instead blending it into a larger narrative of everyday life is a form of coping that enabled these women to continue with their lives in an environment of repetitive and unpredictable violence. However, it is also likely that the structure of the MTRR-I, with its open-ended questions that together provide multiple opportunities for personal disclosure and reflection, helped the women interviewed in this investigation feel more comfortable with the disclosure and more in control of what and how they were sharing. As a group, the women indeed seemed less guarded in the interview than when they were asked about trauma in their lives using the items of the HTQ.

An important aspect of the MTRR-I is that it invites the respondent to provide both a complete history of personal experience and a personal assessment of how she understands and is now coping with her experience. What is considered a "traumatic" experience varies widely both individually and cross-culturally. Instead of asking about particular events that are believed to be traumatic, the MTRR-I invites interviewees to identify and describe what they themselves perceive to be "painful or traumatic" experiences. It offers a respectful means of eliciting not only the nature of their experiences but also how they have coped with and made meaning of these experiences.

As is true of any other instrument that is used cross-culturally, difficulties were also encountered in using the MTRR-I with this population. For instance, the MTRR-I questions regarding sexual activity appeared to have made women in this study quite uncomfortable. Some declined to answer these questions. Because sexuality is a topic that is not openly discussed in Central American culture, it may be that researchers will need to modify either the MTRR-I questions about women's sexual experiences or the ways in which questions concerning this topic are posed.

Of the eight domains of psychological functioning assessed by the MTRR measures, only self-cohesion proved to be cross-culturally problematic. The translation of items related to self-cohesion was particularly difficult. Self-cohesion is a psychological concept that is difficult to translate into questions that are addressed in a simple, clear, and understandable way in Spanish. Self-cohesion was also the only domain where the inter-rater reliability was relatively low. The items comprising this domain attempt to assess the presence or absence of both dissociative symptoms and tendencies to compartmentalize experience. In Latino culture, it is more common to find somatization and a configuration of symptoms known as *ataques de nervios* (attack of nerves) as a consequence or response following a traumatic experience (Farías, 1991). These symptoms, which are untapped by current MTRR-99 items, are considered problems in self-cohesion or forms of displacement that are more common in certain cultural groups, including Latino culture. Unless asked directly if they had ever experienced "nervios" or "ataques de nervios" or particular physical complaints, it is unlikely that the women would provide the information.

The tendency to compartmentalize is another aspect of self-cohesion that is explored by the MTRR measures. Compartmentalization or having a double life is generally seen as a symptom of poor self-cohesion. However, for some people–particularly people in flight from oppression–compartmentalization may in fact be quite adaptive. For example, undocumented refugees often have maintained double identities in order to get to and survive in new and often unwelcoming new countries.

These findings suggest that it is the area of self-cohesion the MTRR measures should be modified to better address and assess cultural differences in respondents' adaptation to trauma. In general, however, these same findings suggest that the MTRR measures provides a respectful and effective means of assessing a wide array of the traumatic experiences of Central American women refugees of war and other violent events, and highlights the resilient adaptations and expressions of recovery that women in this population may exhibit. The progression of the interview, from questions that invite disclosure of personal experience through those that explore symptomatic and affective responses to those that ask the respondent to consider and reflect upon their ways of making meaning of their experience, also appears to provide respondents a safe and reassuring way of telling and reflecting upon very painful stories.

## Limitations of the Study

The 30 women interviewed in this investigation are women who had successfully fled their homelands and arrived safely in the United States under conditions of enormous duress. While they may be representative of highly resilient (and very fortunate) war survivors, they are not representative of women war survivors in general. Also, because the women interviewed were, in essence, a sample of convenience, we have no information about their psychological functioning prior to flight, and we do not know how they compare with other women in the community who did not know about or chose not to participate in the study.

## Directions for Future Research

Clearly, more research is needed with additional populations of trauma survivors and with non-English language versions of the MTRR measures. Additional examination of the qualitative material yielded by this investigation is also required (and is in progress). Future studies should examine, as well, the cross-cultural applicability and validity of specific MTRR scales and items, and modify these as needed to enhance their cross-cultural utility.

## CONCLUSION

That all women interviewed in this investigation had successfully fled the violence, poverty, and devastation of their countries is testimony to their resilience in the wake of traumatic exposure. For at least some of the women, their new environment and the safety and opportunity it afforded offered conditions conducive to their recovery. For them, life in the United States provided new ways of being in the world, new ways of viewing themselves and others, and a host of opportunities that might not have been accessible to them in their home countries. Thus, their flight from an environment of harm, with all the stresses that such flight entailed, ultimately provided access to an environment of safety and empowerment, yielding new opportunities and enhancing their already considerable internal resources.

## REFERENCES

Allodi, F., & Stiasny, S. (1990). Women as torture victims. *Canadian Journal of Psychiatry, 35*(2), 144-148.

Aron, A., Corne, S., Fursland, A., & Zelwer, B. (1991). The gender-specific terror of El Salvador and Guatemala: Post-traumatic stress disorder in Central American refugee women. *Women's Studies International Forum, 14*(1/2), 37-47.

Becker, D., Lira, E., Castillo, M., Gomez, E., & Kovalskys, J. (1990). Therapy with victims of political repression in Chile: The challenge of social reparation. *Journal of Social Issues, 46*(3), 133-149.

Brautigan, C. A. (1996). Traumatized women: Overcoming victimization through equality and non-discrimination. In Y. Danieli, N. S. Rodley, & L. Weisaeth (Eds.), *International responses to traumatic stress: Humanitarian, human rights, justice, peace and development contributions, collaborative actions and future initiatives* (pp. 347-365). New York: Baywood Publishing Co.

Farías, P. J. (1991). Emotional distress and its socio-political correlates in Salvadoran refugees: Analysis of a clinical sample. *Culture, Medicine and Psychiatry, 15,* 167-192.

Fornazzari, X., & Freire, M. (1990). Women as victims of torture. *Acta Psychiatrica Scandinavica, 82,* 257-260.

Friedman, A. R. (1992). Rape and domestic violence: The experience of refugee women. In E. Cole, O. M. Espin, & E. D. Rothblum (Eds.), *Refugee women and their mental health: Shattered societies, shattered lives* (pp. 65-78). New York: The Haworth Press.

Harvey, M. R. (1996). An ecological view of psychological trauma and trauma recovery. *Journal of Traumatic Stress, 9*(1), 3-23.

Harvey, M. R., Liang, B., Harney, P. A., Koenen, K., Tummala-Narra, P., & Lebowitz, L. (2003). A multidimensional approach to the assessment of trauma impact, recovery and resilience: Initial psychometric findings. *Journal of Aggression, Maltreatment & Trauma, 6*(2), 87-109.

Harvey, M. R., Mishler, E. G., Koenen, K., & Harney, P. A. (2000). In the aftermath of sexual abuse: Making and remaking meaning in narratives of trauma and recovery. *Narrative Inquiry, 10*(2), 291-311.

Harvey, M. R., Westen, D., Lebowitz, L., Saunders, E., Avi-Yonah, O., & Harney, P. A. (1994). *Multidimensional Trauma Recovery and Resiliency Interview.* Unpublished Manuscript, Victims of Violence Program, Cambridge, MA.

Liang, B., Tummala-Narra, P., Bradley, R. & Harvey, M. R. (2007). The multidimensional trauma recovery and resiliency instrument: Preliminary examination of an abridged version. *Journal of Aggression, Maltreatment & Trauma, 14*(1/2), 55-174.

Lykes, M. B., Brabeck, M. M., Ferns, T., & Radan, A. (1993). Human rights and mental health among Latin American women in situations of state-sponsored violence. *Psychology of Women Quarterly, 17,* 525-544.

Martín-Baró, I. (1990, August). *War and the psychosocial trauma of Salvadoran children.* Posthumous presentation at the annual meeting of the American Psychological Association, Boston, MA.

Martín-Baró, I. (1994a). The psychological value of violent political repression. In A. Aron & S. Corne (Eds.), *Writings for a liberation psychology: Ignacio Martín-Baró* (pp. 151-167). Cambridge: Harvard University Press.

Martín-Baró, I. (1994b). War and mental health. In A. Aron & S. Corne (Eds.), *Writings for a liberation psychology: Ignacio Martín-Baró* (pp. 108-121). Cambridge: Harvard University Press.

Martín-Baró, I. (1994c). War and psychosocial trauma of Salvadoran children. In A. Aron & S. Corne (Eds.), *Writings for a liberation psychology: Ignacio Martín-Baró* (pp. 122-135). Cambridge: Harvard University Press.

Mollica, R.F., Caspi-Yavin, Y., Bollini, P., Truong, T., Tor, S. & Lavelle, J. (1991). The Harvard Trauma Questionnaire: Validating a cross-cultural instrument for measuring torture, trauma and posttraumatic stress disorder in Indochinese refugees. *The Journal of Nervous and Mental Disease. 180*(2), 110-115.

Roe, M. (1986). Central American refugees in the United States: Psychosocial adaptation. *Refugee Issues, 3,* 21-30.

Salgado de Snyder, V. N., Cervantes, R. C., & Padilla, A. M. (1990). Gender and ethnic differences in psychosocial and generalized distress among Hispanics. *Sex Role, 22*(7/8), 441-453.

doi:10.1300/J146v14n01_08

# Exploration of Recovery Trajectories in Sexually Abused Adolescents

Isabelle Daigneault
Mireille Cyr
Marc Tourigny

**SUMMARY.** This study documents recovery status and symptom changes in a one-year follow-up of sexually abused adolescent girls in child protection services in the province of Québec, Canada. Sixteen French-speaking participants completed questionnaires assessing symptoms, types of maltreatment endured, and services received and were interviewed using the Multidimensional Trauma Recovery and Resiliency Interview (MTRR-I), which was in turn rated by interviewers using the companion rating scale, the MTRR. Analyses of one-year follow-up data revealed statistically significant changes towards better functioning on multiple domains and less symptomatology for a majority of the girls

Address all correspondence to: Mireille Cyr, PhD, Département de Psychologie, Université de Montréal, C.P. 6128, Succursale Centre-Ville, Montréal, Québec, Canada, H3C 3J7 (E-mail: mireille.cyr@umontreal.ca).

This paper is part of the first author's doctoral dissertation. The authors wish to acknowledge financial support from the *Conseil québécois de la recherche sociale* (CQRS), the *Institut de recherche pour le développement social des jeunes* (IRDS, a research institute for youth's social development) as doctoral Fellowships to the first author, as well as financial support from CRIPCAS.

[Haworth co-indexing entry note]: "Exploration of Recovery Trajectories in Sexually Abused Adolescents." Daigneault, Isabelle, Mireille Cyr, and Marc Tourigny. Co-published simultaneously in *Journal of Aggression, Maltreatment & Trauma* (The Haworth Maltreatment & Trauma Press, an imprint of The Haworth Press, Inc.) Vol. 14, No. 1/2, 2007, pp. 165-184; and: *Sources and Expressions of Resiliency in Trauma Survivors: Ecological Theory, Multicultural Practice* (ed: Mary R. Harvey, and Pratyusha Tummala-Narra) The Haworth Maltreatment & Trauma Press, an imprint of The Haworth Press, Inc., 2007, pp. 165-184. Single or multiple copies of this article are available for a fee from The Haworth Document Delivery Service [1-800-HAWORTH, 9:00 a.m. - 5:00 p.m. (EST). E-mail address: docdelivery@haworthpress.com].

interviewed. The recovery status of a minority of research participants seems to have worsened in the interval. The discussion considers these findings and addresses relevancy of the MTRR measures in cases of sexually abused adolescents. doi:10.1300/J146v14n01_09 *[Article copies available for a fee from The Haworth Document Delivery Service: 1-800-HAWORTH. E-mail address: <docdelivery@haworthpress.com> Website: <http://www.HaworthPress.com> © 2007 by The Haworth Press, Inc. All rights reserved.]*

**KEYWORDS.** Child sexual abuse, adolescence, recovery, resilience, child protective services

In Quebec, the involvement of Child Protective Services (CPS) in cases of child sexual abuse (CSA) includes the application of legal or voluntary measures to protect the child from further abuse. When necessary, psycho-educational or therapeutic services are also offered. Currently, CPS workers face the dual challenge of dealing with the most serious cases of behavioral problems in sexually abused (SA) adolescents and assuring their sustained psychosocial development. However, these adolescents constitute a heterogeneous group who has suffered a wide range of abuses (Putnam, 2003). Because of this diversity, their security and developmental achievements vary considerably when they first come to CPS attention. Thus, their need for services may vary and evolve quite differently from case to case. When planning interventions, CPS workers must take into account many variables, including the adolescent's adaptation in several areas of functioning. Given such heterogeneity, there is a great need for reliable and comprehensive assessment of both complex traumatic adaptations and resilience.

## MENTAL HEALTH IMPACTS OF CSA

As of now, three important conclusions have been drawn from studies on symptoms of SA children and adolescents. First, they show a wide range of symptoms, none of which exemplifies the experience of a majority of victims across ages and genders (Beitchman, Zucker, Hood, DaCosta, & Akman, 1991; Kendall-Tackett, Williams, & Finkelhor, 1993). Second, roughly one-third of child and adolescent survivors present no measurable symptoms (Kendall-Tackett et al., 1993). Third, SA adolescents present with more diagnostic comorbidity than do other adolescents, sometimes more than those in psychiatric care who were not sexually abused (Brand, King, Olson, Ghaziuddin, & Naylor, 1996; Silverman, Reinherz, & Giaconia, 1996). This high level of comorbidity may reflect a "failure of syndromic integrity" rather than truly separate and co-occurring "diseases" (Sroufe, 1997, p. 257). Thus, in the past decade researchers and clinicians have developed new diagnostic categories to describe these complex symptomatic presentations, which are regarded as forms of post-traumatic stress resulting from prolonged and repeated interpersonal violence (Herman, 1992; Roth, Newman, Pelcovitz, van der Kolk, & Mandel, 1997; van der Kolk, 1996). This Complex PTSD syndrome includes alterations in self-regulation, self-concept, and interpersonal functioning (Herman, 1992; Pelcovitz et al., 1997).

Despite considerable advances in the assessment of exposure to CSA and its impact, most measures generally fail to evaluate these complex responses across all areas of functioning. An exception is the Structured Interview for Disorders of Extreme Stress (SIDES), which assesses alterations in regulation of affect, consciousness, self-perception, relationships, somatization, and meaning or sustaining belief system (Pelcovitz et al., 1997; Roth et al., 1997). Despite a paucity of studies, there is some evidence that this syndrome may be present in SA children and adolescents (Hall, 1999; Roth et al., 1997; Tremblay, Hébert, & Piché, 2000) and is a "fit" conceptualization of the impact of CSA (Wolfe & Birt, 1995). Consistent with this point of view, in a previous study we found that the majority of the 30 adolescents assessed were at least partly affected in most of the domains assessed and that the symptomatic profile for many participants was consistent with a diagnosis of Complex PTSD (Daigneault, Cyr, & Tourigny, 2003).

## RESILIENT OR ADAPTIVE OUTCOMES POST TRAUMA

While there is an increasing recognition of the need to develop and use multidimensional and integrated measures to describe the impact of CSA, a growing number of researchers and clinicians underscore the importance of also studying resilience (Gore & Eckenrode, 1994; Luthar & Cicchetti, 2000). This concept has been studied in varied populations. For example, some disadvantaged, homeless, or maltreated children have shown positive adaptations to adversity (Cicchetti & Garmezy, 1993; Garmezy, 1993; Rew, Taylor-Seehafer, Thomas, & Yockey, 2001).

Questions of how to measure and conceptualize resilience have been at the center of interest, and a consensus has yet to be reached. Very few studies report the number of asymptomatic adolescents (Boney-McCoy & Finkelhor, 1996; Morrow, 1991; Naar-King, Silvern, Ryan, & Sebring, 2002), which is often used as a resilience criterion (Dufour, Nadeau, & Bertrand, 2000), and fewer directly assess resilience (Spaccarelli & Kim, 1995). Some researchers suggest considering different sources of evaluation and different definitions of resilience to determine a "true" or global resilience over all areas of functioning (Spaccarelli & Kim, 1995), such as in asymptomatic college students who have managed to overcome adversity (Jumper, 1995). Others propose to examine "relative" resilience in the presence of symptoms or distress (Anderson, 1997; Harvey, 1996; Luthar, 1993; Luthar, Cicchetti & Becker, 2000). Luthar et al. (2000), for instance, recommend assessing positive adaptation in areas of functioning that are theoretically or empirically linked to the adversity or risk factor investigated. However resilience is defined, current instruments used to assess the impact of sexual trauma neglect the phenomenon of resilience and the possibility of adaptive functioning.

## RECOVERY AND ASSOCIATED FACTORS

Longitudinal studies of SA children have found that even without treatment, symptoms significantly abate over time (Bolger & Patterson, 2001; Kendall-Tackett et al., 1993; Oates, O'Toole, Lynch, Stern, & Cooney, 1994). However, between 10% and 33% of SA children appear to develop more symptoms and symptom clusters that become increasingly complex and persist for many years (Briere & Elliott, 1994; Oates et al., 1994). To explain this increase, Downs (1993) proposes that when the impact of trauma is not resolved or treated, the dynamics resulting from CSA may cause a "progressive accumulation" of symptoms, which could explain the complex traumatic adaptations seen in adult survivors (van der Kolk, McFarlane, & Weisaeth, 1996). These findings underscore the importance of protecting children from further abuse and of timely treatment of CSA trauma.

Factors such as participation in psychotherapy have been related to symptom improvement and, more rarely, deterioration in SA children (Bagley & LaChance, 2000; Berliner & Kolko, 2000; Finkelhor & Berliner, 1995; Oates et al., 1994; O'Donohue, 1992; Sinclair et al., 1995; Tourigny, 1997; Tourigny, Péladeau, & Doyon, 1993). Other factors, such as co-occurring physical abuse, have been related to poorer outcomes (Green, Russo, Navratil, & Loeber, 1999; Naar-King et al., 2002; Ruggiero, McLeer, & Dixon, 2000). A significant percentage of children have also suffered additional sexual abuse while in CPS' care, which can affect the course of recovery for children who do and who do not receive treatment (Bagley & LaChance, 2000; Daigneault, Tourigny, & Cyr, 1999; Faller, 1991; Lynn, Jacob, & Pierce, 1988; Messier, 1986).

The current exploratory study aimed to find more comprehensive ways to assess complex traumatic adaptations to CSA and to employ a new measure of trauma impact, recovery, and resiliency with SA youths for CPS in Québec. We also attempted to describe changes in multiple domains of functioning of adolescents in CPS during a one-year interval.

## METHOD

### Procedures

All adolescents between 13 and 17 years with an active case in CPS for confirmed SA were eligible for the study unless they were diagnosed with an active phase psychotic disorder. Caseworkers were asked to solicit eligible adolescents and refer those interested in taking part in the study. The first author then contacted these adolescents to inform them of the content and duration of the interview and to schedule a first meeting. Participants were interviewed individually either at their residence, the Université de Montréal, or CPS offices, according to their preference. All participants provided informed consent, as did a legal guardian in the case of adolescents under 14. They were informed that they could terminate the interview at any time and were asked if they would agree to be contacted for a second interview one year later. In addition to the interview and self-report measures, CPS files of all eligible adolescents were screened and scored for SA characteristics and sociodemographic variables by a trained research assistant.

### Participants

The Time 1 (T1) study sample consisted of 30 French-speaking female adolescents aged 13 to 17 years. During the one-year interval, 29 of the 30 adolescents who agreed to be contacted for a follow-up interview received birthday cards and Christmas cards to maintain contact. However, 13 of them did not participate in the second interview: five refused to participate, one had run away, and seven had moved and were unreachable. Thus, for the present study, 16 adolescents (53%) were interviewed at follow-up. No significant differences were found between the 16 participants and the 14 non-participants in any of the variables studied. Since this study is specifically interested in changes over the one-year period, only data obtained from those adolescents who participated in both interviews were kept for the analyses.

## Measures

All measures were used at T1 and T2, except for CSA characteristics collected from CPS files at T1. Self-report measures were administered in a structured interview format.

*Multidimensional Trauma Recovery and Resiliency: Interview and scale* (MTRR-I and MTRR-99, respectively; Harvey et al., 1994; see Appendix A for MTRR-99 and Appendix B for MTRR-I, both at the end of this volume). The MTRR-I is a semi-structured clinical interview designed to elicit information concerning a trauma survivor's psychological functioning in eight domains of trauma and recovery, namely: authority over memory, integration of memory and affect, affect tolerance and regulation, symptom mastery, self-esteem, self-cohesion, safe attachment, and meaning making (for a detailed description, see Harvey, 1996; Lebowitz, Harvey, & Herman, 1993). All interviews were audiotaped and scored by the first author using the MTRR-99 scale (see Appendix A). The 99 items composing the eight domains of the MTRR-99 were rated on a 5-point Likert scale ranging from 1 (*Not at all descriptive*) to 5 (*Highly descriptive*). An average score was computed for each domain, with higher scores associated with more adaptive functioning in all domains. A study using the MTRR-99 with a sample of 164 incarcerated women found an average internal reliability of the subscales of .85 (ranging from .76 to .89; Liang, Tummala-Narra, Bradley, & Harvey, this volume). These investigators reported adequate inter-rater reliabilities for each subscale using 20 pairs of rated interviews (average of .67). The MTRR measures operationalize a multidimensional definition of trauma recovery and have demonstrated the ability to distinguish between traumatized patients who are "largely to fully recovered," "partially recovered," or "largely unrecovered," and as such provide some evidence for the validity of a three-stage model of recovery from interpersonal trauma (Harvey et al., 2003; Liang et al., this volume). No standard cutoffs have been proposed for this scale and different ones have been used for different reasons. We wanted to distinguish three recovery groups, thus we needed two cutoffs. However, since no participant scored at the extreme ends of the scale (i.e., 1 or 5) on any dimension, save for one, to set cut-offs at equal intervals of the scale would have under-represented those who were both largely unre-covered and largely recovered and over-represented those partially re-covered. In Harvey and colleagues' study (2003), results showed that average scores for each of the three recovery groups tended to center around the mean of the scale for all the domains as well as for the total 99 items (average of 2.71, 2.86, and 3.04 for stages 1, 2 and 3 respec-tively). This prompted us to use the average of the 99 items ($M = 3.0$) and its standard deviation ($SD = 0.5$) to set cutoffs that better reflected clinician-assessed stages of recovery. Thus, for all the domains, stage 1 ("largely unrecovered") was operationally defined by mean item scores below 2.5, stage 2 ("partially recovered") by mean item scores between of 2.5 and 3.5 inclusively, and stage 3 ("largely to fully recovered") by mean item scores above 3.5.

*Trauma Symptoms Checklist for Children* (TSCC; Briere, 1996). Psychological symptoms of depression, anxiety, sexual preoccupations, post-traumatic stress, dissociation, and anger were assessed using the TSCC, a 54-item questionnaire evaluating the degree of distress associ-ated with traumatic events in children 8 to 17 years of age. Clinical norms from American populations were used (Briere, 1996). The facto-rial structure and internal consistency of the French-language transla-tion of the instrument were comparable to those of the original version, with alphas of .70 to .84 (Jouvin, Cyr, Thériault, & Wright, 2001).

*Sexual abuse characteristics.* Physical contact, penetration, fre-quency (at least once a week), duration, age at onset, time elapsed since last abuse, relationship with the principal perpetrator, and total number of perpetrators were assessed from information in CPS files.

*Services.* The time since the case had been opened and if the case had been closed during the one-year interval were documented. Many rea-sons justify closing a case, including the adolescent has moved out of territory, is no longer in need of protection, is 18 years old, etc. In the present study, we could only document if cases were closed because the adolescent was legally an adult and no longer eligible for CPS. Adoles-cents also reported all professional services, including the number of sessions they received in the past year. Services included those given by a psychologist or an educational-therapist (psycho-educational therapy focused on day-to-day living and behavior problems). Adolescents were considered to have received professional services in addition to regular CPS if they reported more than one session a month with either professional.

*Concomitant family violence.* Psychological (belittling, shouting, etc.) and physical violence towards adolescents and between parents were assessed through self-report (Thériault, Cyr, & Wright, 1996). Adolescents reported if each of these events ever happened in their family, and if so, how old they were and how long these events lasted. Each type of violence was scored as present (1) or absent (0) and all were combined to yield a global score of family violence. At follow-up, adolescents reported if they experienced these four types of violence since T1.

## Analyses

*T*-tests were conducted on all scales of the MTRR and the TSCC to verify if scores at T2 significantly differed from those at T1. Because of the low number of participants and the exploratory nature of the study, a significance level of $p < .01$ was used. We also examined effect sizes using Cohen's (1988) $d$ formula for independent groups as suggested by Dunlop, Cortina, Vaslow, and Burke (1996). In addition, since the low number of subjects precluded analyses of factors contributing to change over a year, recovery trajectories were qualitatively analyzed by individuals and by racial identity, services received, and further SA or family violence during the study.

## RESULTS

### Participant Characteristics Across Variables at T1

At T1, adolescents participating in the study averaged 15 years of age. Most were living in out-of-home placements (group home, re-adaptation center, etc.), while two were living with a biological parent (see Table 1). A significant number were of Haitian origin. No significant differences were found between Haitian adolescents and others on any outcome or factor assessed.

Sexual abuses suffered by the research participants were all intrafamilial, with fathers being the principal perpetrator in a majority of cases (see Table 1). On average, the sexual abuses were severe (81%) and frequent (69%), involved more than one perpetrator (50%), and had an early onset in childhood ($M = 7.7$ years, $SD = 3.8$), with abuses continuing through to early adolescence. None of the adolescents reported a

TABLE 1. Description of Demographic Variables, Sexual Abuse (SA), and Family Violence Before the Study as Assessed at Time 1 (*N* = 16)

| Variables | Mean (*SD*) or % |
|---|---|
| Mean age (years) | 15.2 (±1.4) |
| Haitian origin | 38% |
| Place of residence at T1<br>With mother<br>Out-of-home placement (group home, readaptation center, etc.)<br>Other family member (grandparents) | 13%81%6% |
| SA with physical contact | 100% |
| SA with penetration | 81% |
| Principal perpetrator<br>Father<br>Stepfather<br>Brother<br>Uncle or grandfather | 56%13%13%19% |
| Multiple perpetrators | 50% |
| Frequent SA (more than once a week) | 69% |
| Age at onset (years) | 7.7 (±3.8) |
| Duration (years) | 3.3 (±2.6) |
| Time elapsed since last SA (years) at T1 | 3.6 (±1.9) |
| Time in child protective services (years) at T1 | 3.5 (±2.9) |
| Mean number of types of family violence at T1 (lifetime) | 2.4 (±1.5) |
| Physical marital violence | 44% |
| Verbal marital violence | 69% |
| Physical violence towards child | 69% |
| Verbal violence towards child | 63% |

unique event of CSA: 19% reported that SA lasted for less than a year, 19% reported that SA lasted one year, and the majority (62%) reported that SA lasted for more than one year. The last sexual abuse incident had occurred more than three and a half years prior to the study and all adolescents had been in CPS for more than three and a half years at T1.

Concomitant family violence was also frequent, with an average of two out of the four types of violence (Table 1). About two-thirds witnessed psychological partner violence (69%) and experienced physical (69%) and psychological violence (63%) within their family. Forty-four percent experienced both physical and psychological violence towards them, and only two did not experience either types of violence (13%).

## *Events and Services Between T1 and T2*

At T2, three (19%) of the adolescents reported being sexually abused by extra-familial perpetrators during the one-year interval. They also reported an average of 0.9 (*SD* = 1.0) type of concomitant family violence during that period, with psychological violence towards themselves being the most frequently reported (38%), followed by verbal violence between parents (25%), physical violence toward themselves (13%), and physical violence between parents (13%). Seven adolescents experienced neither sexual abuse nor family violence during that period, while nine experienced at least one type of violence.

During the follow-up year, five (31%) adolescents stopped receiving services from CPS, four because they were 18 years old. Three adolescents saw a psychologist in individual therapy more than once a month, seven saw an educational therapist more than once a month, and seven did not receive services from either professional more than once a month over the year.

## Description of Recovery and Symptom Changes Over a Year

All MTRR scale scores were on average higher at T2 than at T1 (Table 2) and four scales showed statistically significant improvements. The group thus showed statistically better integration of memory and affect, self-esteem, safe attachment, and meaning making at follow-up than at T1. In addition, average scores on the self-esteem and self-cohesion scales were at 3.6 or higher, indicating that these specific areas of strength were rated as "largely recovered" at T2. Analyses of effect sizes of MTRR scales are reported in Table 2 and indicate that most effects were moderate (between .39 and .64). However, the self-esteem scale and the integration of memory and affect scale both showed larger effect sizes (.74 and .71, respectively).

Furthermore, as a group, the adolescents studied had lower scores on all symptom scales at follow-up, indicating a general reduction of symptoms and a statistically significant improvement on three of the six TSCC scales. The group thus showed significantly fewer symptoms of depression, PTSD, and anger at follow-up than at T1. Analyses of effect sizes of TSCC scales are also reported in Table 2 and indicate that effects were generally moderate. However, the PTSD scale clearly showed a large effect size (Cohen's $d = 1.11$), while the sexual preoccupations scale had a rather small effect size (Cohen's $d = .33$).

Although as a group the adolescents who participated in the study seemed to moderately improve in half of the domains and symptoms, a look at individual changes on the MTRR scales reveals that although

TABLE 2. Mean Scores at T1 and T2, Paired _t_-Tests, Number of Adolescents in Each Stage of Recovery Per Domain and Number of Adolescents Showing Clinical Symptoms Per Symptom Scale at T2, Number of Clinical and Stage Improvements and Deteriorations Between T1 and T2 ($N = 16$)

| Domains of recovery and symptoms | T1 Mean (SD) | T2 Mean (SD) | Difference | Cohen's _d_ | Number of adolescents in each stage of recovery or number of adolescents with clinical symptoms at T2 | Number of adolescents improved and deteriorated at T2 |
|---|---|---|---|---|---|---|
| | | | | | Stage 1-2-3 | |
| _MTRR scales_ | | | | | | |
| Authority over memory | 3.0 (±.6) | 3.4 (±.8) | .4 | −0.56 | 3- 5-8 | 6-3 |
| Integration of memory and affect | 2.8 (±.8) | 3.3 (±.8) | .5* | −0.71 | 2-8-6 | 6-0 |
| Affect tolerance | 2.9 (±.6) | 3.3 (±.6) | .4 | −0.62 | 2-9-5 | 4-2 |
| Symptom mastery | 3.1 (±.6) | 3.3 (±.5) | .2 | −0.40 | 1-10-5 | 4-2 |
| Self-esteem | 3.5 (±.9) | 4.0 (±.6) | .5* | −0.74 | 0-4-12 | 6-1 |
| Self-cohesion | 3.2 (±1.0) | 3.6 (±.8) | .4 | −0.39 | 2-5-9 | 6-2 |
| Safe attachment | 3.0 (±.7) | 3.4 (±.8) | .4* | −0.56 | 3-4-9 | 7-1 |
| Meaning making | 2.5 (±.7) | 3.0 (±.8) | .5* | −0.64 | 4-7-5 | 9-1 |
| TSCC | | | | | | |
| Anxiety | 11.6 (±4.0) | 9.1 (±3.9) | 2.5 | 0.65 | 2 | 2-1 |
| Depression | 12.1 (±5.0) | 9.3 (±4.0) | 2.8* | 0.61 | 2 | 2-0 |
| PTSD | 14.7 (±4.1) | 10.3 (±3.8) | 4.4* | 1.11 | 0 | 3-0 |
| Sexual preoccupations | 8.6 (±4.1) | 7.3 (±4.3) | 1.3 | 0.33 | 7 | 3-1 |
| Anger | 11.8 (±5.5) | 9.1 (±3.6) | 2.7* | 0.40 | 1 | 1-0 |
| Dissociation | 10.3 (6.0) | 7.9 (5.5) | 2.4 | 0.60 | 0 | 4-0 |

*_t_-test significant at $p < .01$
Effect sizes: .2 = small, .5 = moderate, .8 = large

most improved, up to 19% of them deteriorated (Table 2). Similarly, when using clinical norms as cut-points, results showed that while more adolescents reported symptom improvements from a clinical level to a normal level on all symptom measures, up to 13% of them showed a deterioration in symptoms from a normal level to a clinical level. Furthermore, although four adolescents who had at least one symptom at T1 appeared asymptomatic at follow-up, two of the three initially asymptomatic adolescents had clinical symptoms at follow-up.

In an effort to assess which characteristics or factors contributed to changes over a year, we examined follow-up trajectories of small groups of adolescents. Generally speaking, when looking at scores on MTRR and TSCC scales, we see that three adolescents seemed to deteriorate (i.e., more deteriorations than improvements), three seemed to show no changes (no change or equal deteriorations and improvements), and ten seemed to improve over the year (more improvements than deteriorations; see Table 3).

First, we looked at the characteristics of the three adolescents whom, generally speaking, seemed to deteriorate over the year on both the MTRR and the TSCC. Although all three seemed to do worse at T2 than at T1, they had different trajectories over that year. The first adolescent legally became an adult and her case was closed with CPS within less than two months of T1. She did not receive services during that time and reported continued family violence over the year. At T2, she showed clinical symptoms of anger. The second adolescent also became an adult eight months after T1, at which point her case was closed. She did, however, see an educational therapist weekly during her eight months in CPS. Nonetheless, she reported experiencing further SA and family violence over the year and showed clinical symptoms of sexual preoccupations at T2. The last adolescent who showed a global deterioration was of Haitian descent. Her case was open, but she had received no regular services from a professional over that year and reported continued family violence. She showed clinical symptoms of sexual preoccupations at T2.

Second, adolescents who did not seem to change over the year had similarly different profiles. The first one became an adult and her case was closed within two months of T1. She reported continued family violence but no services during that year. The second adolescent whose profile did not change received services from a psychologist over the year and reported no SA or family violence. Her case remained open throughout the year. Although neither of these two adolescents

TABLE 3. Recovery Trajectories of 16 Adolescents, Follow-Up Clinical Status, and Events Occurring Between T1 and T2

| Case number | Trajectory | No. of clinical symptoms T2 | Case Closed | Educational therapist | Psychologist | Sexual Abuse | Family violence | Haitian descent |
|---|---|---|---|---|---|---|---|---|
| 1. | Deteriorated | 1 | yes | no | no | no | yes | no |
| 2. | Deteriorated | 1 | yes | yes | no | yes | yes | no |
| 3. | Deteriorated | 1 | no | no | no | no | yes | yes |
| 4. | Unchanged | 0 | yes | no | no | no | yes | no |
| 5. | Unchanged | 0 | no | no | yes | no | no | no |
| 6. | Unchanged | 2 | no | yes | yes | no | yes | yes |
| 7. | Improved | 1 | yes | no | no | no | yes | no |
| 8. | Improved | 1 | no | yes | no | no | no | no |
| 9. | Improved | 1 | no | yes | yes | no | no | no |
| 10. | Improved | 1 | no | no | yes | no | no | yes |
| 11. | Improved | 3 | no | yes | no | yes | yes | yes |
| 12. | Improved | 0 | yes[1] | yes | no | no | no | yes |
| 13. | Improved | 0 | no | no | no | no | yes | yes |
| 14. | Improved | 0 | no | no | no | no | no | no |
| 15. | Improved | 0 | no | no | no | yes | no | no |
| 16. | Improved | 0 | no | yes | no | no | no | no |

[1]This adolescent's case was closed although she was not 18 years old.

changed, at T2 they showed no clinical symptoms and their MTRR scores were in the second and mostly third stages of recovery. The third adolescent whose profile did not change was of Haitian descent and her case remained open throughout the year. She reported continued family violence during the year and received services from a psychologist and an educational therapist. She showed clinical symptoms of anxiety and sexual preoccupations at T2.

The trajectories of the ten adolescents whose profiles improved were equally diverse. Half reported receiving services and half did not, while two reported SA and three reported continued family violence over the year. Two of these cases were closed during the year; one of these legally became an adult and was no longer eligible for CPS. Half of those who "improved" showed no clinical symptoms at T2, while the other half still showed between one and three symptoms. Sexual preoccupation was the most common symptom for all adolescents at T2.

## DISCUSSION

Following their exposure to severe and prolonged intra-familial sexual abuse, adolescents interviewed in the present study initially showed evidence of both considerable trauma and substantial resilience. A general decline in symptomatology for the group as a whole was observed at a one-year follow-up, a finding consistent with the results of many studies that have reported symptom abatement over time, with or without treatment (Bolger & Patterson, 2001; Kendall-Tackett et al., 1993; Oates et al., 1994). In addition, TSCC scale scores improved over the year with mainly moderate, and one large, effect sizes. This improvement was statistically significant in half of the TSCC scales.

In addition to symptom abatement, the present study brings to light both group and individual changes on many domains of the MTRR scales. Indeed, this instrument was able to detect improvements in the targeted domains. In this regard, results indicate that concomitant with symptom relief, adolescents were also more able to bring new emotions to bear on their understanding of the past and to find meaning in their lives and in the abuses they had suffered. All MTRR changes showed moderate to large effect sizes and half were statistically significant. The data suggest that, even in severely and chronically abused populations such as this one, improvements can be seen over a relatively short period. These changes are not only seen in symptom abatement but are also seen in improved resilience. The MTRR is a sensitive instrument that was able to detect these changes.

The MTRR data also revealed that these adolescents had particular strengths at T2 in the domains of self-esteem and self-cohesion. However, despite the positive changes achieved by many of these adolescents, another result consistent with many findings is the considerable number who were symptomatic at follow-up (Cohen, Brown, & Smailes, 2001; Leifer & Shapiro, 1995; Oates et al., 1994). Most of these adolescents were still receiving services at the end of the study, suggesting that their need for security was adequately assessed as compromised by CPS. However, among those adolescents who were most symptomatic at follow-up, those whose cases were closed were not better off than those whose cases remained open. In fact, cases were typically closed because the adolescents were 18 years old (four out of five cases) and no longer eligible for CPS, rather than because they were asymptomatic or did not need services. Over half of those whose cases were closed were clinically symptomatic and experiencing family violence. The question remains as to what happens to these young adults. Do they seek other services? Are there resources in the community for them if they do?

While most of the adolescents studied did improve in most MTRR domains and on the self-report scales, some experienced little or no changes and some were worse off. No clear recovery pattern emerged. In fact, recovery seemed possible with or without treatment, as half of the adolescents whose profile improved over the year did not receive services from an educational therapist or a psychologist. In addition, within the smaller groups of adolescents whose profile either deteriorated or was unchanged after a year, some did receive therapy while others did not. Future longitudinal studies need to observe changes over longer periods with larger groups of adolescents in order to describe how life circumstances interact with personal characteristics in the recovery process. Our study looked at a general profile of recovery using a total of 14 scales and in doing so might have oversimplified the recovery process. More specific hypotheses could be made in the exploration of change trajectories (e.g., by observing how the different domains of the MTRR interact with each other or with other factors). It may be that therapy is related to improvement in some domains (e.g., meaning) and not in others, while family violence may be related to deterioration in circumscribed areas of functioning (e.g., safe attachment).

One particularity of this sample needs to be addressed. One in three adolescent was of Haitian descent and they were thus over-represented in this sample compared to the general population in the same area. Although no significant difference was found on any variable studied between Haitian adolescents and the others, some cultural considerations came up during interviews. For example, "white magic" or "spirits" were referred to as a means of coping with or giving meaning to adversity but were sometimes difficult to differentiate from dissociation or psychotic behavior. Caution needs to be applied when administering the MTRR with different cultural groups, especially as it assesses self-perceptions, ways of caring for oneself, or ways of making sense of past trauma. To render the scale more culturally sensitive, for example, it may be suggested that some items addressing very specific and maybe culturally tinted ways of making sense of experience (religious, spiritual, or moral values; social or political activism, etc.) be merged into one general item more readily adapted to different cultures. This is true for Quebecois adolescents in general, as almost none reported using religious beliefs or social/political activism to give meaning to their lives or to past abuses.

Although these results are promising for the future study of resilience and recovery in SA populations, they need to be interpreted with caution because of the small number of participants, their very specific profile of severe intrafamilial sexual abuse, and the fact that all participants were receiving or had received child protection services. In this regard, the cutoff scores used in this study, while useful for interpreting the results, are based on this small sample's results and should not be used for other populations. Further community studies of traumatized adolescents need to be carried out in order to better appreciate how largely unrecovered, partially recovered, and largely recovered participants score on these scales. It might be that some MTRR domains always tend to have lower scores in largely unrecovered participants, which would necessitate different cutoff scores for the eight domains. Nonetheless, the *MTRR* measures offer an interesting alternative and/or addition to self-reported symptom measures in describing recovery profiles in multiple domains of functioning of SA adolescents receiving or not receiving treatment.

# REFERENCES

Anderson. K. M. (1997). Uncovering survival abilities in children who have been sexually abused. *Families in Society, 78*, 592-599.

Bagley. C., & LaChance, M. (2000). Evaluation of a family-based programme for the treatment of child sexual abuse. *Child & Family Social Work, 5*, 205-213.

Beitchman. J. H., Zucker, K. J., Hood, J. E., DaCosta, G. A., & Akman, D. (1991). A review of the short-term effects of child sexual abuse. *Child Abuse & Neglect, 15*, 537-556.

Berliner. L., & Kolko. D. (2000). What works in treatment services for abused children. In M. P. Kluger, G. Alexander, & P. A. Curtis (Eds.), *What works in child welfare* (pp. 97-104). Washington, DC: Child Welfare League of America, Inc.

Bolger. K. E., & Patterson. C. J. (2001). Pathways from child maltreatment to internalizing problems: Perceptions of control as mediators and moderators. *Development & Psychopathology, 13*, 913-940.

Boney-McCoy. S., & Finkelhor, D. (1996). Is youth victimization related to trauma symptoms and depression after controlling for prior symptoms and family relationships? A longitudinal, prospective study. *Journal of Consulting and Clinical Psychology, 64*, 1406-1416.

Brand. E. F., King, C. A., Olson. E., Ghaziuddin, N., & Naylor, M. (1996). Depressed adolescents with a history of sexual abuse: Diagnostic comorbidity and suicidality. *Journal of the American Academy of Child & Adolescent Psychiatry, 35*, 34-41.

Briere, J. (1996). *Trauma Symptom Checklist for Children (TSCC): Professional manual*. Odessa: Psychological Resources, Inc.

Briere, J. N., & Elliot, D. M. (1994). Immediate and long-term impacts of child sexual abuse. *The Future of Children, 4*, 54-69.

Cicchetti, D., & Garmezy, N. (1993). Prospects and promises in the study of resilience. *Development & Psychopathology, 5*, 497-502.

Cohen, J. (1988). *Statistical power analysis for the behavioral sciences* (2nd ed.). Hillsdale, NJ: Lawrence Earlbaum Associates.

Cohen, P., Brown, J., & Smailes, E. (2001). Child abuse and neglect and the development of mental disorders in the general population. *Development & Psychopathology, 13*, 981-999.

Daigneault, I., Cyr, M., & Tourigny, M. (2003). Profil psychologique d'adolescentes agressées sexuellement et prises en charge par les services de protection de la jeunesse [The psychological profile of sexually abused adolescents and admitted to youth protection services]. *Santé mentale au Québec, 28*, 211-232.

Daigneault, I., Tourigny, M., & Cyr, M. (1999). *Rapport d'évaluation de l'implantation et de l'efficacité d'une thérapie de groupe pour adolescentes victimes d'agressions sexuelles et d'une intervention post-dévoilement* [An evaluation of the efficacy of group therapy and a post-disclosure intervention among sexually abused adolescents]. Montréal: Institut de recherche pour le développement social des jeunes.

Daigneault, I., Tourigny, M., & Cyr, M. (2003). *Description of trauma and resilience in sexually abused adolescents: An integrated assessment*. Manuscript submitted for publication.

Downs, W. R. (1993). Developmental considerations for the effects of childhood sexual abuse. *Journal of Interpersonal Violence, 8*, 331-345.

Dufour, M. H., Nadeau, L., & Bertrand, K. (2000). Factors in the resilience of victims of sexual abuse: An update. *Child Abuse & Neglect, 24*, 781-797.

Dunlop, W. P., Cortina, J. M., Vaslow, J. B., & Burke, M. J. (1996). Meta-analysis of experiments with matched groups or repeated measures designs. *Psychological Methods, 1*, 170-177.

Faller, K. C. (1991). What happens to sexually abused children identified by child protective services? *Children & Youth Services Review, 13*, 101-111.

Finkelhor, D., & Berliner, L. (1995). Research on the treatment of sexually abused children: A review and recommendations. *Journal of American Academy of Child & Adolescent Psychiatry, 34*, 1408-1423.

Garmezy, N. (1993). Children in poverty: Resilience despite risk. *Psychiatry, 56*, 127-136.

Gore, S., & Eckenrode, J. (1994). Context and process in research on risk and resilience. In R. J. Haggerty, L. R. Sherrod, N. Garmezy, & M. Rutter (Eds.), *Stress, risk, and resilience in children and adolescents* (pp. 19-63). Cambridge: Cambridge University Press.

Green, S. M., Russo, M. F., Navratil, J. L., & Loeber, R. (1999). Sexual and physical abuse among adolescent girls with disruptive behavior problems. *Journal of Child & Family Studies, 8*, 151-168.

Hall, D. K. (1999). "Complex" posttraumatic stress disorder/disorders of extreme stress (CP/DES) in sexually abused children: An exploratory study. *Journal of Child Sexual Abuse, 8*, 51-71.

Harvey, M. R. (1996). An ecological view of psychological trauma and trauma recovery. *Journal of Traumatic Stress, 9*. 3-23.

Harvey, M. R., Liang. B., Harney, P. A., Koenen, K., Tummala-Narra, P., & Lebowitz, L. (2003). A multidimensional approach to the assessment of trauma impact, recovery. and resiliency: Initial psychometric findings. *Journal of Aggression, Maltreatment & Trauma, 6*, 87-109.

Harvey. M. R.. Westen, D.. Lebowitz, L., Saunders, E., Avi-Yonah, O., & Harney, P. (1994). *Multidimensional Trauma Recovery and Resiliency interview*. Cambridge, MA: The Cambridge Hospital Victims of Violence Program.

Herman. J. L. (1992). *Trauma and recovery*. New York: Basic Books.

Jouvin, É.. Cyr, M., Thériault, C., & Wright, J. (2001). *Study on the psychometric qualities of the French version of the Trauma Symptom Checklist for Children (TSC-C)*. Montreal: Psychology Department. Université de Montréal.

Jumper. S. A. (1995). A meta-analysis of the relationship of child sexual abuse to adult psychological adjustment. *Child Abuse & Neglect, 19*, 715-728.

Kendall-Tackett. K. A., Williams, L. M., & Finkelhor, D. (1993). Impact of sexual abuse on children: A review and synthesis of recent empirical studies. *Psychological Bulletin, 113*. 164-180.

Lebowitz, L., Harvey, M. R., & Herman. J. L. (1993). A stage-by-dimension model of recovery from sexual trauma. *Journal of Interpersonal Violence, 8*, 378-391.

Leifer. M., & Shapiro, J. P. (1995). Longitudinal study of the psychological effects of sexual abuse in African American girls in foster care and those who remain home. *Journal of Child Sexual Abuse, 4*, 27-44.

Liang. B.. Tummala-Narra, P., Bradley, R., & Harvey, M. R. (2007). The Multidimensional Trauma and Resilience instrument: Preliminary examination of an abridged version. *Journal of Aggression, Maltreatment & Trauma, 14*(1/2), 55-74.

Luthar. S. S. (1993). Annotation: Methodological and conceptual issues in research on childhood resilience. *Journal of Child Psychology & Psychiatry, 34*, 441-453.

Luthar, S. S., & Cicchetti, D. (2000). The construct of resilience: Implications for interventions and social policies. *Development & Psychopathology, 12*, 857-885.

Luthar, S. S., Cicchetti, D., & Becker, B. (2000). The construct of resilience: A critical evaluation and guidelines for future work. *Child Development, 71*, 543-562.

Lynn, M.. Jacob, N., & Pierce, L. (1988). Child sexual abuse: A follow-up study of reports to a protective service hotline. *Children & Youth Services Review, 10*, 151-165.

Messier. C. (1986). *Le traitement des cas d'inceste père-fille: une pratique difficile* [Treatment of father-daughter incest: A difficult feat]. Québec: Ministère de la Justice.

Morrow, K. B. (1991). Attributions of female adolescent incest victims regarding their molestation. *Child Abuse & Neglect, 15*, 477-483.

Naar-King, S.. Silvern, L., Ryan, V., & Sebring, D. (2002). Type and severity of abuse as predictors of psychiatric symptoms in adolescence. *Journal of Family Violence, 17*, 133-149.

Oates. R. K.. O'Toole. B. I., Lynch, D. L., Stern, A., & Cooney, G. (1994). Stability and change in outcomes for sexually abused children. *Journal of the American Academy of Child and Adolescent Psychiatry, 33*, 945-953.

O'Donohue, W. (1992). Treatment of the sexually abused child: A review. *Journal of Clinical Child Psychology, 21*, 218-228.

Pelcovitz, D., van der Kolk, B., Roth, S., Mandel, F., Kaplan, S., & Resick, P. (1997). Development of a criteria set and a structured interview for disorders of extreme stress (SIDES). *Journal of Traumatic Stress, 10*, 3-16.

Putnam, F. W. (2003). Ten-year research update review: Child sexual abuse. *Journal of the American Academy of Child & Adolescent Psychiatry, 42*, 269-278.

Rew, L., Taylor-Seehafer, M., Thomas, N. Y., & Yockey, R. D. (2001). Correlates of resilience in homeless adolescents. *Journal of Nursing Scholarship, 33*, 33-40.

Roth, S., Newman, E., Pelcovitz, D., van der Kolk, B., & Mandel, F. S. (1997). Complex PTSD in victims exposed to sexual and physical abuse: Results from the DSM-IV field trials for posttraumatic stress disorder. *Journal of Traumatic Stress, 10*, 539-555.

Ruggiero, K. J., McLeer, S. V., & Dixon, F. J. (2000). Sexual abuse characteristics associated with survivor psychopathology. *Child Abuse & Neglect, 24*, 951-964.

Silverman, A. B., Reinherz, H. Z., & Giaconia, R. M. (1996). The long-term sequelae of child and adolescent abuse: A longitudinal community study. *Child Abuse & Neglect, 20*, 709-723.

Sinclair, J. J., Lazelere, R. E., Paine, M., Jones, P., Graham, K., & Jones, M. (1995). Outcome of group treatment for sexually abused adolescent females living in a group home setting. *Journal of Interpersonal Violence, 10*, 533-542.

Spaccarelli, S., & Kim, S. (1995). Resilience criteria and factors associated with resilience in sexually abused girls. *Child Abuse & Neglect, 19*, 1171-1182.

Sroufe, A. L. (1997). Psychopathology as an outcome of development. *Development & Psychopathology, 9*, 251-268.

Thériault, C., Cyr, M., & Wright, J. (1996). *Questionnaire on events from childhood and adolescence*. Unpublished manuscript, Université de Montréal.

Tourigny, M. (1997). Efficacité des interventions pour enfants abusés sexuellement: une recension des écrits [The efficacy of interventions for sexually abused treatments: A compilation of the literature]. *Revue Canadienne de Psycho-Éducation, 26*, 39-69.

Tourigny, M., Péladeau, N., & Doyon, M. (1993). Évaluation sommative du programme de traitement des enfants abusés sexuellement implanté dans la région de Lanaudière par le centre des services sociaux Laurentides-Lanaudière [The evaluation of a treatment program for sexually abused children in the Lanaudière region, offered by the Laurentides-Lanaudière social services]. Montréal: Laboratoire de Recherche en Écologie Humaine et Sociale. Université du Québec à Montréal.

Tremblay, C., Hébert, M., & Piché, C. (2000). Type I and type II posttraumatic stress disorder in sexually abused children. *Journal of Child Sexual Abuse, 9*, 65-90.

van der Kolk, B. A. (1996). The complexity of adaptation to trauma: Self-regulation, stimulus discrimination, and characterological development. In B. A. van der Kolk, A. C. McFarlane, & L. Weisaeth (Eds.), *Traumatic stress: The effects of overwhelming experience on mind, body, & society* (pp. 182-213). New York: The Guilford Press.

van der Kolk, B. A., McFarlane, A. C., & Weisaeth, L. (1996). *Traumatic stress: The effects of overwhelming experience on mind, body, and society.* New York: The Guilford Press.

Wolfe, V. V., & Birt, J. A. (1995). The psychological sequelae of child sexual abuse. *Advances in Clinical Child Psychology, 17,* 233-263.

doi:10.1300/J146v14n01_09

# Assessing Trauma Impact, Recovery, and Resiliency in Refugees of War

## Nancy Peddle

**SUMMARY.** This paper describes the psychometric properties and process of using the Multidimensional Trauma Recovery and Resiliency Scale (MTRR) with 83 untreated war-affected adolescent and adult refugees of diverse cultures, family of origin, age, gender, and time since the war. The MTRR met reliability, validity, and utility criteria with this convenience sample. This paper discusses modifications made to the MTRR-I format, questions, and prompts to enable work with the wide range of ages and cultures represented in the sample. The results support the MTRR as a tool that may have the ability to capture the complexity of culture as well as measure a variety of trauma responses and work with other measurements. Limitations of the study and avenues of future research are discussed. doi:10.1300/J146v14n01_10 *[Article copies available for a fee from The Haworth Document Delivery Service: 1-800-HAWORTH. E-mail address: <docdelivery@haworthpress.com> Website: <http://www.HaworthPress.com> © 2007 by The Haworth Press, Inc. All rights reserved.]*

---

Address correspondence to: Nancy Peddle, PhD, 1927 North Hudson Avenue, Suite 3, Chicago, IL 60614 (E-mail: nancy@lemonaidfund.org).

[Haworth co-indexing entry note]: "Assessing Trauma Impact, Recovery, and Resiliency in Refugees of War." Peddle, Nancy. Co-published simultaneously in *Journal of Aggression, Maltreatment & Trauma* (The Haworth Maltreatment & Trauma Press, an imprint of The Haworth Press, Inc.) Vol. 14, No. 1/2, 2007, pp. 185-204; and: *Sources and Expressions of Resiliency in Trauma Survivors: Ecological Theory, Multicultural Practice* (ed: Mary R. Harvey, and Pratyusha Tummala-Narra) The Haworth Maltreatment & Trauma Press, an imprint of The Haworth Press, Inc., 2007, pp. 185-204. Single or multiple copies of this article are available for a fee from The Haworth Document Delivery Service [1-800-HAWORTH, 9:00 a.m. - 5:00 p.m. (EST). E-mail address: docdelivery@haworthpress.com].

**KEYWORDS.** Trauma, assessment, recovery, resiliency, MTRR-99, war refugees

Research has shown that the wars of the 21st Century leave civilians as targets, victims, potential perpetrators, expendable persons, part of war strategies, and psychologically injured (Ajdukovic & Ajdukovic, 1998; Dyregrov, Gjestad, & Raundalen, 2002; Levy & Sidel, 1997). Many studies show forced displacement is one of the most stressful human experiences (Danieli, Rodley, & Weisaith, 1996; McCallin, 1991), with the U.S. being the world's largest country of resettlement (Myles, 2000). Refugees, in addition to experiencing forced removal and gross human rights violations, have additional stress factors, including poor housing in strange and possibly hostile places, lack of employment opportunities, unfamiliarity with the host country's language and customs, loss of social networks, and poor nutrition (Cardozo, Kaiser, Gotway, & Agani, 2003; Maass, 1996; Weine, 1999; Westermeyer & Wahmanholm, 1996). In contrast, some research findings suggest that refugee status may mediate the effects of war (Legerski, Layne, Saltzman, Djapo, & Kutlac, 2003).

As research on refugees grows, studies on both the understanding of psychological reactions associated with war and the understanding of ethnocultural differences reveal divergent results (Dubrow, Liwski, Palacios, & Gardinier, 1996; Evans, 1996; Friedman & Marsella, 1996; Marans, Berkman, & Cohen, 1996; Stamm, Stamm IV, Hudnall, & Higson-Smith, 2004). Some studies present evidence that the use of the PTSD diagnosis crosses cultures and gender, decreases with time, and is not inevitable (Arcel, Folnegovic-Smale, Kozaric-Kovacic, & Marusic, 1995; Scott, Knoth, Beltran-Quiones, & Gomez, 2003). Other researchers question the PTSD diagnosis and/or the limitations in the cross-cultural methodology used in the studies to understand ethnocultural differences (Bracken, 1998; Friedman & Marsella, 1996; Green, 1996; Summerfield, 1998). Still other recent studies have yielded mixed findings or lack of results associated with such factors as gender, self-disclosure, and postwar long-term impact (Amir & Lev-Wiesel, 2003; Bolton, Glenn, Orsillo, Roemer, & Litz, 2003; Carlson & Dutton, 2003; Dyregrov et al., 2002; Legerski et al., 2003; Scott et al., 2003).

Not unexpectedly, given the range of research findings and limitations of the cross-cultural methodologies employed, treatments based on research driven protocols are not providing the expected healing to a wide variety of people (Marsella, Bornemann, Ekblad, & Orley, 1994; Nader, Dubrow, & Stamm, 1999; Stamm et al., 2004). This may be related to the assessment tools themselves. Most psychological trauma measures have not been developed and evaluated for their cultural validity with untreated war-affected populations. The long-term consequences related to war, the stress of displacement, and posttrauma adjustment problems underscore the need for accurate assessment of trauma in war-affected populations (Wilson & Keane, 1996). In order to measure the complexity and cultural impact of trauma, recovery, and resiliency, it is important to determine if the measures need modification (i.e., for untreated, culturally different, war-affected refugee groups) and further testing of psychometric properties with a broader selection of traumatized populations (Fairbank, Jordon, & Schlenger, 1996; Green, Chung, Daroowalla, deBenedictis, & Krupnick, 2003; Harvey et al., 2003; Solomon, Keane, Newman, & Kaloupek, 1996).

To examine the complexity of both trauma and culture, some researchers draw on the tenets of ecological theory, which takes the person, event, and environment into account and posits that the influence of each can be understood only in relationship to the other as part of an interrelated system (Cicchetti & Lynch, 1993; Greene & McGuire, 1998; Harvey, 1996; McFarlane & Yehuda, 1996). Harvey's (1996) ecological framework, for example, suggests that trauma impact, recovery, and resiliency are expressed and can be assessed in and across eight domains of psychological functioning. The Multidimensional Trauma Recovery and Resiliency Scale (MTRR) and Interview (MTRR-I) are assessment tools that have been developed to operationalize this framework. Preliminary studies of the MTRR instruments show promising results (Harvey et al., 2003).

Researchers and clinicians have used the MTRR measures with treated and untreated trauma survivors (Bradley & Davino, this volume; Harvey et al., 2003; Liang, Tummala-Narra, Bradley, & Harvey, this volume; Radan, this volume). The MTRR-I interview (Harvey et al., 1994) invites survivors to recall and share salient aspects of their trauma story. Researchers have suggested that the process of telling and retelling their story has a healing effect, enabling survivors to begin integrating their experience into a cohesive narrative and, in doing so, gain new insights and new control over difficult symptomatic responses to traumatic exposure (Foa, Molnar, & Cashman, 1995; Herman, 1992). How one tells one's story (Bolton et al., 2003; Klein & Janoff-Bulman, 1996) and how supportive the interviewer and the environment are can influence recovery (Gasker, 1999; Solomon, 1986). Use of the interview for assessment purposes not only helps clarify posttraumatic responses, but also may have therapeutic benefits for the person telling the story (Bolton et al., 2003; Dubrow & Peddle, 1997; Nader, 1996).

Three early studies provide strong preliminary evidence for the reliability and validity of the MTRR scale, as do more recent studies with untreated Guatemalan refugees of war (Radan, this volume) and with a Chilean sample (Haz, Castillo, & Aracena, 2003). Results of these studies suggest that the MTRR measures can be used to assess trauma impact, recovery, and resiliency with diverse populations. As yet, however, there is limited information on the utility of the measures with male survivors, women and men of diverse cultures, and, with the exception of Radan's (this volume) study of Central American women refugees, those who are untreated survivors of the trauma of war. The current study was designed, in part, to address the need for more information about the cross-cultural utility of the MTRR measures with these groups.

The data reported in this investigation are drawn from a larger dissertation project designed to investigate the relationship, if any, between expressions of recovery and the role of forgiveness among survivors of war trauma (Peddle, 2001). The study made extensive use of the MTRR-I and the MTRR-99 (see Appendices A and B at the end of this volume) and involved adapting the assessment protocol to enable interviews to be conducted either solely with the individual or in the presence of other family members (who were also interviewed). This paper examines and describes the utilization of the MTRR-99 and companion interview (MTRR-I) and the process of collecting data with untreated war-affected refugees of diverse cultures, family of origin, age, gender, religion, and time since the war. It adds to a growing literature on the MTRR as a tool able to assess the complexity of trauma, resiliency, and culture currently neglected by other measures.

## METHODS

### Participants

Administrators and caseworkers at 28 established agencies, organizations, and institutes providing support and assistance in refugee resettlement in the Chicago, Illinois, area were asked for help in recruiting refugees, who: (a) had status as war refugees; (b) were willing and able to participate in a one-on-one interview about their life experience before, during, and after a war; (c) had experienced war-related interpersonal violence; (d) were able to communicate in English, directly or through a family interpreter; and (e) were at least 13 years of age. No limitation was applied on length of time since war exposure. The final convenience sample was composed of 83 refugees from 12 countries ranging in age from 13 to 85 with a median age of 34 (see Table 1).

The majority of participants in the study were female (59%), from former Yugoslavia (71%), and identified as Muslim (73.5%). For the purpose of this study, participants chose either to be interviewed together with other family members (74.7%), in which case individual interviews were conducted sequentially (and in the presence of one another) with all family members or individually. All participants identified at least two current social support systems (i.e., resettlement agency, religious institution, family).

TABLE 1. Demographic Variables for Participants and T-Tests and Analysis of Variance Scores

| Demographic Variables | % | MTRR $M$ | $t$-Tests | Analysis of Variance | DF |
|---|---|---|---|---|---|
| Number of Years Since Experienced War | | | | $F = 5.30^{**}$ | 2 |
|    5 years ago and less | 77.1 | 4.551 | | | |
|    6-16 | 14.5 | 4.666 | | | |
|    Greater than 16 | 8.4 | 4.826 | | | |
| Gender | | | $t = .51$ | | 1 |
|    Female | 59.0 | 4.580 | | | |
|    Male | 41.0 | 4.607 | | | |
| Age | | | | $F = .57$ | 2 |
|    18 and under | 21.7 | 4.639 | | | |
|    19-39 | 49.4 | 4.589 | | | |
|    40-85 | 28.9 | 4.558 | | | |
| Religion | | | $t = -3.18^{**}$ | | 1 |
|    Muslim | 73.5 | 4.543 | | | |
|    Christian | 26.5 | 4.724 | | | |
| Country of Origin | | | | | |
|    Kosovo | 59.0 | 4.524 | | | |
|    Bosnian-Herzegovina | 12.0 | 4.604 | | | |
|    African | 24.1 | 4.716 | | | |
|    Other | 4.9 | 4.751 | | | |

Notes. $N = 83$ for all demographic variables, $n$ varies for subcategories (Female, Male) under demographic variables.
$^{**}p < .01$.

All of the refugees in the study shared the experience of dislocation due to war and the war-related devastation of their homeland. They had faced death and survived. All but one participant self-reported life threatening exposure to violence such as ethnic cleansing, rape, beatings, scalding with burning oil, witnessing the killing of relatives and friends, bombardment, fleeing from burning homes, torture, and other experiences that fulfill Criterion A of the *Diagnostic and Statistical Manual of Mental Disorders-IV* (American Psychiatric Association, 1994) diagnostic criteria for PTSD. Only a few had been treated. Participants were asked to rank the severity of their exposure using a question from the Enright Forgiveness Inventory (EFI) Likert-scale of 1-5. The EFI is a tool tested for its validity and reliability cross culturally (Rique et al., 1999). Most participants (64.6%) ranked the exposure as a 5 (*a great deal of hurt*), with 31.7% giving ranks of 4 (*much hurt*), and only 3.7% a 3 (*some hurt*). The partial account told by "Nessa," age 16 from Kosovo, is typical of the events participants had suffered:

> March 22, seeing people crying, running just like animals. Seeing people shot for nothing. We couldn't do anything about it. [We] couldn't help anybody. With what could you help? All the kids were crying. The old people couldn't walk. Three days later it was our time. . . . While we were eating breakfast, someone knocked on the door and then broke the door and came in. We were shaking like we were so cold. I remember their faces. We stopped eating. My little brother didn't know anything. He said, 'I'm not finished, I want to eat.' They took him and stopped him eating. One said, 'You better get out of here or I'll kill your son.' While we were walking, we had to jump over dead bodies, smell the smell of blood. It was really hard to get to our car. Tried to get to Macedonia. We had to drive on the landmines. We weren't sure of anything. I wanted to be dead. I was crying so much but my eyes were still strong, stronger than ever."

### Instruments

Three data collection instruments were used: (a) a background questionnaire, (b) the MTRR-I (Harvey, Mishler, Koenen, & Harney, 2000; see Appendix B), and (c) companion rating scale, the MTRR-99 (see Appendix A). The background questionnaire sought basic demographic information (e.g., gender, age, country of origin) and information about the treatment experiences of participants, if any.

The MTTR-I consists of 19 open-ended questions to guide the participant through telling his or her story with attention to experiences, images, and feelings related to his or her history, relationships, feelings about self and others, survival coping skills, and the nature of his or her current life. Following administration of the MTRR-I, the MTRR-99 can be used to rate narrative material on each of eight domains of psychological functioning (Appendix A). It yields both a composite recovery/resiliency (r/r) score and eight domain-specific scores.

## Procedures

*Recruiting research participants.* Three of the contacted refugee organizations contacted referred research participants, stating the purpose of the study from the Informed Consent form provided to them. All participants were told that they would participate in an individual interview asking about their life history including traumatic events such as ones they experienced through exposure to war. One referral organization told potential participants that their stories would be written down and included in a book. The principal investigator then called all who were referred to clarify the purpose and schedule interviews. Some participants then referred other friends and family members. Participants were paid $10 for the interviews, which lasted from 1-3 hours depending on the number of family members being interviewed.

*Informed consent.* Prior to conducting any interview, the purpose of the study and the nature of the interview was described, questions regarding the investigation were answered in depth, and informed consent and parental consent (for family members under age 18) was obtained. Informed consent and parental consent was also obtained when family members under 13 years of age translated, interpreted, and or chose to draw a picture of his or her experience. However, children under 13 were not interviewed and did not otherwise participate in the study.

*Modifications in MTRR-I content and process.* In order to better assess trauma impact, recovery, and resilience in this diverse group of refugees, a number of modifications were made to the MTRR-I protocol and to MTRR-99 scoring. In addition to employing designated MTRR-I prompts, participants were also questioned regarding their experience of the interview and their perception of the effects of telling their story. These modifications are described below.

*(1) Creating age-appropriate questions and prompts.* A number of modifications were made to ensure the study was age-appropriate when children and adolescents under the age of 18 were present. Specifically,

some interview questions and prompts were modified to replace an emphasis on sexual or romantic relationships with an emphasis on re-lationships generally. For example, MTRR-99 questions and prompts designed to elicit information concerning sexual relationships and sex-ual promiscuity were eliminated or modified in favor of questions about the nature and quality of relationships generally when interviews were conducted with children under 18 years of age and/or when children un-der 18 served as interpreters or translators. In addition, some children who were not interviewed but were present as translators and interpret-ers asked to be involved in the research. In response to their requests, the interviewer invited them to draw pictures of their experiences, an age appropriate therapeutic technique used with children who have ex-perienced war (Dubrow & Peddle, 1997; Evans, 1996; Suzic, Patel, & Doran, 1995).

*(2) Interviews in individual and family contexts.* Each participant was asked to complete a short background questionnaire and was then inter-viewed, either individually or in the company of other family members based on the choice of each study participant. Participants who chose to be interviewed alone (i.e., not in the presence of other family members) were interviewed using the standard MTRR-I protocol. These partici-pants were designated "Individual" interviewees and spoke English. Modifications in the protocol were required when entire families came together to the interview, requesting that they be interviewed together. Families explained that they experienced the atrocities together and wanted to be together to tell the story. In almost all cases, these families included children of all ages and any extended family members who lived at the same residence. After a number of requests to participate as a family, the interviewer gave all participants the choice to participant as a family. These participants were designated "Family" participants. Typically, they collaborated on the "core" trauma story with other family members, usually selecting a primary narrator with other mem-bers interjecting comments. Individual interviews were then con-ducted sequentially (and in the presence of one another) to elicit individual responses to standard MTRR-I questions (and prompts) with all individuals comprising the family.

## RESULTS

Psychometric results of this investigation are summarized in Tables 1, 2 and 3. Five of the initial 88 interviews were eliminated due to insufficient information. The analyses on the remaining 83 interviews yielded data that permitted ratings on 96 of the MTRR-99 items that were of interest in this study. As indicated, the MTRR met reliability, validity, and utility with the sample of 83 war refugees who then comprised the research participants of this investigation. Pearson bivariate correlations were computed among the MTRR Scale's eight domains and between domains and the total r/r. As indicated in Table 2, correlations among the MTRR Scale's eight domains were substantial and significant (i.e., significance in all domains was $p < .01$ or higher) with the exception of the safe attachment domain, which demonstrated significance ($p < .05$). There were also strong correlations between domains and the total r/r mean score. These findings are consistent with Harvey et al.'s (2003) findings on inter-correlations across all domains. Internal consistency was sound with a coefficient Cronbach's alpha of .88 for the composite score. Individual domain alphas ranged from .41-.78. The alpha among the eight domains and the MTRR total showed strong internal consistency with a Cronbach's alpha of .93.

Inter-rater reliabilities of items within each of the eight MTRR domains in the case of five participants were examined. The measure demonstrated reasonable inter-rater reliability, achieving a .75 level of agreement or higher in all but three items, which were dropped from the analysis: "Is comfortable with her or his sexual orientation" (Domain 5: Self-Esteem), "Has assumed control over dissociate capacities that once compromised psychological status and daily functioning" (Do-

TABLE 2. Correlations Among Subscales and Total Mean of the MTRR Scale

| MTRR Domains | 1 | 2 | 3 | 4 | 5 | 6 | 7 | 8 | 9 |
|---|---|---|---|---|---|---|---|---|---|
| Authority over Memory | | | | | | | | | |
| Integration of Memory & Affect | .603*** | | | | | | | | |
| Affect Tolerance | .701*** | .567*** | | | | | | | |
| Symptom Mastery | .704*** | .488*** | .744*** | | | | | | |
| Self Esteem | .651*** | .419*** | .733*** | .731*** | | | | | |
| Self Cohesion | .782*** | .571*** | .816*** | .711*** | .699*** | | | | |
| Safe Attachment | .222* | .310** | .337** | .434*** | .428*** | .343** | | | |
| Meaning- Making | .621*** | .594*** | .678*** | .605*** | .570*** | .744*** | .248* | | |
| Total MTRR Score | .840*** | .676*** | .913*** | .858*** | .835*** | .890*** | .481*** | .810*** | |

$N = 83$
*$p < .05$. **$p < .01$. ***$p < .001$, two-tailed test of significance.

TABLE 3. Number of Items, Means, and Standard Deviation for Scales of the Modified MTRR

| MTRR Domains | Items | Mean | SD |
|---|---|---|---|
| Authority over Memory | 11 | 4.401 | .393 |
| Integration of Memory & Affect | 5 | 4.559 | .307 |
| Affect Tolerance | 14 | 4.353 | .380 |
| Symptom Mastery | 12 | 4.566 | .357 |
| Self Esteem | 15 | 4.819 | .233 |
| Self Cohesion | 8 | 4.644 | .275 |
| Safe Attachment | 16 | 4.823 | .145 |
| Meaning- Making | 15 | 4.470 | .343 |
| Total MTRR Score | 96 | 4.591 | .241 |

Note. $N = 83$

main 6: Self Cohesion), and "Avoids sexual contact" (Domain 7: Safe Attachment). The final analysis of data used only the ratings from the remaining 96 items.

Table 1 presents demographic variables for participants, *t*-tests, and ANOVA scores. As shown in Table 3 the ANOVA on the Number Of Years Since Experienced War group scores were statistically significant, $F(1, 81) = 5.30, p < .01$, while the ANOVA on the three age groups did not differ significantly. A *t*-test for independent samples showed no statistical significance between the scores of males or females (Gender) on the r/r, $t(81) = .51, p > 0.10$. These results suggest that gender differences were not predictive of differences in MTRR scores. A *t*-test for the variable Religion showed that MTRR scores for Muslim participants' r/r scores differed significantly from those for participants who identified as Christian, with a negative and statistically significant *t*-test on the MTRR, $t(81) = -3.18, p < .01$. Because of variations in sample size, Country of Origin differences were not tested.

Overall, study participants received high ratings on all eight r/r domains and the MTRR overall score (see Table 3). The total mean score on the overall MTRR was 4.59 ($SD = .241$). The range was 3.75 to 5.00, where 3.75 represented low (for this sample) r/r and 5.00 represents high r/r. The Safe Attachment domain showed the least degree of variation across all participants ($SD = .145$) and the highest degree of resilience or recovery of the eight domains.

When asked about the interview process, participants talked about how the self-disclosure of telling their story brought back intense emotions as well as release, a finding that is consistent with the literature that suggests self-disclosure before empathic witnesses is therapeutic (Bolton et al., 2003; Herman, 1992; Weine, 1999). One participant likened telling the story to opening a Coke bottle: "the fizzes come out and it lets a little pressure out. The healing deal." In addition, many participants finished their interviews with a thank-you to the U.S. for support and to the interviewer for making it possible for them to tell their story to someone.

## DISCUSSION

This paper describes the psychometric characteristics of the MTRR assessment tool and results of using the MTRR with predominantly untreated war-affected refugees of diverse cultures, ages, genders, religions, and time since war exposure. It also describes the modifications to MTRR questions, prompts, and interview procedure that were used to gather MTRR data on trauma impact, recovery, and resiliency with this population.

### Psychometric Characteristics

Results of this study showed reasonable reliability and validity with this sample, further supporting the utility of the MTRR in assessing the impact of trauma as well as trauma recovery and resilience with a greater range of traumatized populations (Harvey et al., 2003; Haz et al., 2003). In this study, the MTRR met criteria of reliability, validity, and utility with a mean alpha of .88 and significant correlations among the eight domains and the total r/r score for this sample. Moreover, MTRR interrater reliability results also appeared to be sound, with .75 or higher agreement among ratings on all but three of the 99 items. Given the low standard error of the mean alpha of .88, there are positive implications for comparisons among participants' MTRR scores. Furthermore, results from Pearson's correlations, *t*-tests, and ANOVA's showed significant differences on this group of diverse participants' MTRR mean scores. These results provide evidence that the MTRR may have the ability to capture the complexity of culture as well as measure a variety of trauma responses.

### MTRR Scores of Diverse Participants

Significant differences in participants' MTRR scores were related to two demographic variables: number of years since experienced war and religion. MTRR scores did not differ significantly as a result of either age or gender. These findings provide additional information about the MTRR as a tool able to assess differences of trauma impact, recovery, and resiliency with a wider array of traumatized populations (i.e., a number of different cultures, both genders, and a wide range of ages). While the trauma recovery literature indicates the prominent role of variables such as number years since experienced war (Mullet & Girard, 2000; Solomon, Laor, & McFarlane, 1996), age (Amir & Lev-Wiesel, 2003), gender (Dyregrov et al., 2002; Scott et al., 2003), and religion (Rye et al., 2000; Williams, Zinner, & Ellis, 1999), these findings suggest the need for further exploration of how these variables interact with each other in the recovery process.

In this study, MTRR scores were generally on the high side of the scale, consistent with Radan's (this volume) study of Central American women refugees of war. There are a number of reasons that may account for these high scores, including some of which are related to this study's procedures (i.e., recruitment and modifications).

The three agencies that referred participants did so because they had close relationships with those they referred. All participants had relocated to the U.S. a minimum of six months ($M = 2.8$) prior to the referral and a minimum of one year ($M = 5.9$) had lapsed since any participant had experienced the trauma. During the interviews, the majority of the participants reported that many of the symptoms that they had felt in the immediate post-war period (i.e., nightmares, headaches, heartaches, inability to pay attention, intrusive thoughts and great anxiety) had either gone away or were greatly reduced. There is research that points to the need for the passage of time in order to assess differences in normal versus abnormal adaptation (Yehuda & McFarlane, 1999). Some studies report the development of PTSD among war refugees several years after traumatic exposure (Kinzie, Sack, Angell, & Clarke, 1989). In this study, one participant who had experienced rape and forced displacement four years prior to the interview did report reexperiencing a traumatic event, "like it's happening [now]" in the context of the interview. However, another participant who, in this study, was representative of the majority, described time as a change agent, "I'm much more committed to a spiritual nature in these 16 years since the war, I've changed, I'm more committed to the common good now." These findings and examples suggest that there may be considerable variability in individuals' adjustments over time. Research shows that this is even more likely with children because of developmental issues (Amir & Lev-Wiesel, 2003; Pynoos & Eth, 1999; Yehuda & McFarlane, 1999). In the current study, the differences in MTRR-99 scores as a function of number of years since experienced war suggests that time itself may indeed have a healing effect. However, this study did not examine such factors as age at initial exposure or the impact of prior trauma experiences.

All participants in this study identified a religious affiliation, with a much higher number of Muslim versus Christian participants. The differences in MTRR mean scores for Muslim and Christian participants may be confounded by the number of years since the participants had experienced war. No Muslim participant in this study had experienced war less than eight years prior to the interview. The fact that this study yielded significant differences between the MTRR ratings of Muslim and Christian participants is a topic that merits discussion that is beyond the scope of the current paper. Full consideration of the issue is found in Peddle (2001).

Other mediating psychosocial resilience and protective factors may have contributed to the generally high MTRR ratings in this study. It may be that this particular sample of refugees is, in fact, more resilient (reflecting the protective factors of, e.g., faith and family) and/or more recovered (indicating the positive contribution of social support, especially the refugee agency they were working with during resettlement, and other resources available in the U.S.) than other groups of trauma survivors, particularly those who seek psychotherapy. All participants in this study reported positive social supports, had religious affiliations, and had elected to remain in the U.S., turning down repatriation benefits. All of the adolescents interviewed were attending school; most of the adult participants were employed and/or attending some type of school. All but one participant reported having some family support, with 67% citing extended family. Additional supports identified by participants in this investigation included friends (36.6%), church or mosque (19.5%), schoolmates (28%), and work colleagues (17.1%). All of these are considered key predictor variables for resiliency and may prevent and mitigate long-term impact of a traumatic event (Garmezy & Rutter, 1983; Irving, Telfer, & Blake, 1997; Whittaker & Garbarino, 1983). It is important to emphasize, however, that resiliency is not synonymous with invulnerability; it is not a constant and can vary across time and circumstances (McCallin, 1991).

### *Modifications in MTRR-I Content and Process*

The MTRR-I was selected for this study because of its use of the unstructured interview, one of the most effective ways to gather information on trauma impact and recovery (Carlson & Dutton, 2003) and because it is designed for both clinical and research purposes (Harvey et al., 2003). Yet, modifications to the MTRR-I process and prompts regarding age appropriateness, the presence of family, and family interpreters were also needed to elicit a full response from participants in this study. The modifications appear to have had their intended effect of making research participants more comfortable with the interview process and therefore more able to tell terribly painful stories in a way that enabled (a) the researcher to utilize the MTRR-99 as an assessment tool, and (b) the research participant to experience the process as both helpful and healing. They may also have had unintended effects.

Modifications to the MTRR-I questions and prompts to ensure age appropriateness, for example, may have had the unintended effects of eliminating information about dysfunctions in sexual relationships and thus inadvertently skewed the Safe Attachment domain (4.82, $SD$ = .145) and the Self-Esteem domain (4.82, $SD$ = .233) scores. This adaptation may have also elevated the total MTRR scores, as all domains affect the total MTRR.

This study also employed noteworthy modifications in MTRR interview protocol to accommodate the presence of family members in the interviews and the use of family members as interpreters. These modifications too may have had an effect on this study's findings. All individuals identified as "Family" participants in this study came from countries that cultivate a collective identity unlike the United States, which tends to celebrate individual experience and accomplishment. They assumed they would be interviewed together and, in almost all cases, wanted to tell their story collectively. Most of these families had experienced the same traumatic events together, although there were a number of women who had experienced rape and wanted their husbands to be present while they told their stories. Participants then answered the prompts individually and, in most cases, in the presence of all other family members. In many cases when one family member did not share some information, another member would. Family interpreters also prompted individual members to remember additional information that helped them to answer questions more completely. These answers, in turn, allowed for a more accurate scoring of the MTRR-99. Based on the outcomes of this study, it is recommended that when future researchers working with participants from countries that cultivate a collective existence, the "family interview" methodology be explored as a choice.

The extent to which the refugees who participated in this investigation experienced both family and community support to openly discuss the trauma (as evidenced by their willingness, e.g., to grant newspaper interviews, give school presentations, agree to be interviewed for this research, and refer others to be interviewed) may also have contributed to their recovery and resiliency. These results are consistent with research showing that self-disclosure or screening interviews can be therapeutic (Bolton et al., 2003; Green & Wessells, 1997; Nader, 1996; Pynoos & Eth, 1999; Scott et al., 2003) and with trauma recovery programs that use telling as a therapeutic tool (Dubrow & Peddle, 1997; Evans, 1996; Friedlander, 1993; Garbarino, Kostelny, & Dubrow, 1991; Green & Wessells, 1997; Peddle, Monteiro, Guluma, & Macaulay, 1999; Suzic et al., 1995).

Finally, those who were working with participants in this study may have perceived them as more recovered and/or resilient. Many professionals who work with war-affected people are trained to avoid pathologizing them. In this context, refugees' reactions are seen as normal for those who have experienced the horrors of war and terror and the stresses associated with relocation (Arcel et al., 1995). This is the orientation of the principal investigator (and interviewer) and of the individual who scored the MTRR for inter-rater reliability purposes. This orientation may underlie a research bias, which in turn may inflate MTRR scoring relative to scores assigned by mental health professionals who are more likely to use the language of psychopathology in describing pain.

## *Limitations and Future Directions*

A number of limitations of this study should be taken into consideration. One of the limitations relevant to internal and external validity of this study was the convenience sampling and the possible bias inherent in convenience sampling. Moreover, only refugees who could speak English or who had someone in the household who could speak English could be referred to this investigation. This restriction excluded many non-English speaking individual refugees and refugee families that may otherwise have been included and whose MTRR profiles might have looked quite different from those of the English-speaking sample. Further, MTRR research with non-English speaking populations is needed to confirm the cross-cultural utility of these measures. Because a standardized translation of the MTRR was not available for each language spoken as a native tongue by the participants in this investigation, the interviewer had to rely on someone in the family to both translate the questions and interpret the story being told. Clearly, this process could have led to misunderstanding and misinformation. However, using a family interview methodology also helped mitigate misunderstandings as stories were shared and information was added or clarified by individual family members. Further studies could consider the ways in which this methodology may have contributed to or inhibited the disclosure of information.

While the factors described in the scope of this study limit generalization of the sample to the greater population of refugees, the study results nevertheless contributed to understanding trauma impact, recovery, and resiliency and add to the growing evidence of the effectiveness of using the MTRR with war-affected refugees across cultures, religions, genders, age groups, and throughout a person's life.

## REFERENCES

Ajdukovic, M., & Ajdukovic, D. (1998). Impact of displacement on the psychological well-being of refugee children. *International Review of Psychiatry, 10*(3), 186-195.

American Psychiatric Association. (1994). *Diagnostic and statistical manual of mental disorders* (4th ed.). Washington, DC: Author.

Amir, M., & Lev-Wiesel, R. (2003). Time does not heal all wounds: Quality of life and psychological distress of people who survived the Holocaust as children 55 years later. *Journal of Traumatic Stress, 16*(3), 295-299.

Arcel, L. T., Folnegovic-Smale, V., Kozaric-Kovacic, D., & Marusic, A. (1995). *Psycho-social help to war victims: Women refugees and their families.* Copenhagen: International Rehabilitation Council for Torture Victims.

Bolton, E. E., Glenn, M. D., Orsillo, S., Roemer, L., & Litz, B. T. (2003). The relationship between self-disclosure and symptoms of posttraumatic stress disorder in peacekeepers deployed to Somalia. *Journal of Traumatic Stress, 16*(3), 203-210.

Bracken, P. J. (1998). Hidden agendas: Deconstructing post traumatic stress disorder. In P. J. Bracken & C. Petty (Eds.), *Rethinking the trauma of war* (pp. 38-59). London: Free Association Books.

Bradley, R., & Davino, K. (2007). Interpersonal violence, recovery and resilience in incarcerated women. *Journal of Aggression, Maltreatment & Trauma, 14*(1/2), 123-146.

Cardozo, B. L., Kaiser, R., Gotway, C. A., & Agani, F. (2003). Mental health, social functioning, and feelings of hatred and revenge of Kosovar Albanians one year after the war in Kosovo. *Journal of Traumatic Stress, 16*(4), 351-360.

Carlson, E. B., & Dutton, M. A. (2003). Assessing experiences and responses of crime victims. *Journal of Traumatic Stress, 16*(2), 133-148.

Cicchetti, D., & Lynch, M. (1993). Toward an ecological/transactional model of community violence and child maltreatment: Consequences for children's development. In D. Reiss, J. E. Richters, M. Radke-Yarrow, & D. Scharff (Eds.), *Children and violence* (pp. 96-118). New York: Guilford Press.

Dubrow, N., Liwski, N. I., Palacios, C., & Gardinier, M. (1996). Traumatized children: Helping child victims of violence. In Y. Danieli, N. Rodley, & L. Weisaith (Eds.), *International responses to traumatic stress* (pp. 327-346). Amityville, NY: Baywood Publishing Company, Inc.

Dubrow, N., & Peddle, N. (1997). *Trauma healing and peace education training manual* (2nd ed.). Chicago, IL: Taylor Institute.

Dyregrov, A., Gjestad, R., & Raundalen, M. (2002). Children exposed to warfare: A longitudinal study. *Journal of Traumatic Stress, 15*(1), 59-68.

Evans, J. L. (1996). Children as zones of peace: Working with young children affected by armed violence. *Coordinators' Notebook: An International Resource for Early Childhood Development, 19*, 1-26.

Fairbank, J. A., Jordon, B. K., & Schlenger, W. E. (1996). Designing and implementing epidemiologic studies. In E. B. Carlson (Ed.), *Trauma research methodology* (pp. 105-125). Lutherville, MD: Sidran.

Foa, E. B., Molnar, C., & Cashman, L. (1995). Change in rape narratives during exposure therapy for posttraumatic stress disorder. *Journal of Traumatic Stress, 8*(4), 675-690.

Friedlander, B. Z. (1993). Community violence, children's development, and mass media: In pursuit of new insights, new goals, and new strategies. In D. Reiss, J. E. Richters, M. Radke-Yarrow, & D. Scharff (Eds.), *Children and violence* (pp. 66-81). New York: Guilford Press.

Friedman, M. J., & Marsella, A. J. (1996). Posttraumatic stress disorder: An overview of the concept. In A. J. Marsella, M. J. Friedman, E. T. Gerrity, & R. M. Scurfield (Eds.), *Ethnocultural aspects of posttraumatic stress disorder: Issues, research, and clinical applications* (pp. 11-32). Washington DC: American Psychological Association.

Garbarino, J., Kostelny, K., & Dubrow, N. (1991). What children can tell us about living in danger. *American Psychologist, 46*(4), 376-383.

Garmezy, N., & Rutter, M. (Eds.). (1983). *Stress, coping, and development in children.* New York: McGraw-Hill Book Company.

Gasker, J. A. (1999). *"I never told anyone this before": Managing the initial disclosure of sexual abuse re-collections.* New York: The Haworth Press, Inc.

Green, B. L. (1996). Cross-national and ethnocultural issues in disaster research. In A. J. Marsella, M. J. Friedman, E. T. Gerrity, & R. M. Scurfield (Eds.), *Ethnocultural aspects of posttraumatic stress disorder: Issues, research, and clinical applications* (pp. 341-361s). Washington DC: American Psychological Association.

Green, B. L., Chung, J. Y., Daroowalla, A., deBenedictis, C., & Krupnick, J. (2003). *Evaluating the cultural validity of a trauma history measure (SLESQ).* Washington DC: Georgetown University Medical School.

Green, E., & Wessells, M. (1997). *Mid-term evaluation of the province-based war trauma team project: Meeting the psychosocial needs of children in Angola* (Evaluation report). Richmond, VA: Christian Children's Fund.

Greene, R. R., & McGuire, L. (1998). Ecological perspective meeting the challenge of practice with diverse populations. In R. R. Greene & M. Watkins (Eds.), *Serving di-*

*verse constituencies: Applying the ecological perspective* (pp. 1-27). New York: Aldine de Gruyter.

Harvey, M. R. (1996). An ecological view of psychological trauma recovery. *Journal of Traumatic Stress, 9*(1), 3-24.

Harvey, M. R., Liang, B., Harney, P. A., Koenen, K., Tummala-Narra, P., & Lebowitz, L. (2003). A multidimensional approach to the assessment of trauma impact, recovery and resilience: Initial psychometric findings. *Journal of Aggression, Maltreatment & Trauma, 6*(2), 87-109.

Harvey, M. R., Mishler, E. G., Koenen, K. C., & Harney, P. A. (2000). In the aftermath of sexual abuse: Making and remaking meaning in narratives of trauma and recovery. *Narrative Inquiry, 10*(2), 291-311.

Harvey, M. R., Westen, D., Lebowitz, L., Sanders, E., Avi-Yonah, O., & Harney, P.A. (1994). *Multidimensional trauma recovery and resiliency assessment manual.* Unpublished manuscript. The Cambridge Hospital Victims of Violence Program.

Haz, A. M., Castillo, R., & Aracena, M. (2003). Adaptacion preliminar del instrumento multidimensional trauma recovery and resilience (MTRR) en una muestra de madres maltratadoras fisicas con historia de maltrato fisico y madres no maltratadoras con historia de maltrato fisico. *Child Abuse & Neglect, 27*(7), 807-820.

Herman, J. (1992). *Trauma and recovery.* New York: BasicBooks.

Irving, L. M., Telfer, L., & Blake, D. D. (1997). Hope, coping, and social support in combat-related posttraumatic stress disorder. *Journal of Traumatic Stress, 10*(3), 465-480.

Kinzie, J. D., Sack, W., Angell, R., & Clarke, G. (1989). A 3 year follow-up of Cambodian young people traumatized as children. *Journal of American Academy of Child & Adolescent Psychiatry, 28*, 501-504.

Klein, I., & Janoff-Bulman, R. (1996). Trauma history and personal narratives: Some clues to coping among survivors of child abuse. *Child Abuse & Neglect, 20*(1), 45-54.

Legerski, J.-P., Layne, C. M., Saltzman, W., Djapo, N., & Kutlac, M. (2003). *Post-war adjustment in war-exposed Bosnian youths: An SEM analysis.* Paper presented at the International Society for Traumatic Stress Studies 9th annual Meeting, Chicago, IL.

Levy, B. S., & Sidel, V. W. (1997). The impact of military activities on civilian populations. In B. S. Levy & V. W. Sidel (Eds.). *War and public health* (pp. 149-167). New York: Oxford University Press.

Liang, B., Tummala-Narra, P., Bradley, R. & Harvey, M. R. (2007). The multidimensional trauma recovery and resiliency instrument: Preliminary examination of an abridged version. *Journal of Aggression, Maltreatment & Trauma, 14*(1/2), 55-74.

Maass, P. (1996). *Love thy neighbor: A story of war.* New York: Alfred A. Knopf.

Marans, S., Berkman, M., & Cohen, D. (1996). Child development and adaptation to catastrophic circumstances. In R. J. Apfel & B. Simon (Eds.), *Minefields in their hearts: The mental health of children in war and communal violence* (pp. 104-127). New Haven, CT: Yale University Press.

Marsella, A. J., Bornemann, T., Ekblad, S., & Orley, J. (Eds.). (1994). *Amidst peril and pain: The mental health and well-being of the world's refugees.* Washington DC: American Psychological Association.

McCallin, M. (Ed.). (1991). *The psychological well-being of refugee children: Research, practice and policy issues.* Geneva: International Catholic Child Bureau.

McFarlane, A. C., & Yehuda, R. (1996). Resilience, vulnerability, and the course of posttraumatic reactions. In B. A. van der Kolk, A. C. McFarlane, & L. Weisaeth (Eds.), *Traumatic stress: The effects of overwhelming experience on mind, body, and society* (pp. 155-181). New York: The Guilford Press.

Mullet, E., & Girard, M. (2000). Developmental and cognitive points of view on forgiveness. In M. E. McCullough, K. I. Pargament, & C. E. Thoresen (Eds.), *Forgiveness: Theory, research, and practice* (pp. 111-132). New York: The Guilford Press.

Myles, I. (2000, October 12). Numb2000.pdf [Internet]. UNHCR. Retrieved December 13, 2000 from, http:www.unhcr.ch/un&ref/numbers/numb2000.pdf

Nader, K., Dubrow, N., & Stamm, B. H. (Eds.). (1999). *Honoring differences: Cultural issues in the treatment of trauma and loss.* Philadelphia, PA.: Brunner/Mazel.

Nader, K. O. (1996). Assessing traumatic experiences in children. In J. P. Wilson & T. M. Keane (Eds.), *Assessing psychological trauma and PTSD* (pp. 291-348). New York: Guilford Press.

Peddle, N. (2001). *Forgiveness in recovery/resiliency from the trauma of war among a selected group of adolescents and adult refugees.* Unpublished dissertation, The Fielding Institute, Santa Barbara, CA.

Peddle, N., Monteiro, C., Guluma, V., & Macaulay, T. E. A. (1999). Trauma, loss and resilience in Africa: A psychosocial community based approach to culturally sensitive healing. In K. Nader, N. Dubrow, & B. H. Stamm (Eds.), *Honoring differences: Cultural issues in the treatment of trauma and loss* (pp. 121-149). Philadelphia, PA: Brunner/Mazel.

Pynoos, R. S., & Eth, S. (1999). Witness to violence: The child interview. In M. J. Horowitz (Ed.), *Essential papers on posttraumatic stress disorder* (pp. 360-386). New York: New York University Press.

Radan, A. (2007). Exposure to violence and expressions of resilience in Central American women survivors of war. *Journal of Aggression, Maltreatment & Trauma, 14*(1/2), 147-164.

Rique, J., Waltman, M., Sarinopoulos, S., Wee, D., Engstrand, E. A., & Enright, R. (1999). *The tools of forgiveness education: Validity studies of the Enright forgiveness inventory.* Paper presented at the Moral Development of Forgiveness: Research and Education, Minneapolis, MN.

Rye, M. S., Pargament, K. I., Ali, M. A., Beck, G. L., Dorff, E. N., Hallisey, C., et al. (2000). Religious perspectives on forgiveness. In M. E. McCullough & K. I. Pargament & C. E. Thoresen (Eds.), *Forgiveness: Theory, research, and practice* (pp. 17-40). New York: The Guilford Press.

Scott, R. L., Knoth, R. L., Beltran-Quiones, M., & Gomez, N. (2003). Assessment of psychological functioning in Adolescent earthquake victims in Colombia using the MMPI-A. *Journal of Traumatic Stress, 16*(1), 49-57.

Solomon, S. D. (1986). Mobilizing social support networks in times of disaster. In C. R. Figley (Ed.), *Trauma and its wake, volume II: Traumatic stress theory, research, and intervention* (pp. 232-263). New York: Brunner/Mazel.

Solomon, S. D., Keane, T. M., Newman, E., & Kaloupek, D. G. (1996). Choosing self-report measures and structured interviews. In E. B. Carlson (Ed.), *Trauma research methodology* (pp. 56-81). Lutherville, MD: Sidran.

Solomon, Z., Laor, N., & McFarlane, A. C. (1996). Acute posttraumatic reactions in soldiers and civilians. In B. A. van der Kolk & A. C. McFarlane & L. Weisaeth (Eds.), *Traumatic stress: The effects of overwhelming experience on mind, body, and society* (pp. 102-114). New York: The Guilford Press.

Stamm, B. H., Stamm IV, H. E., Hudnall, A. C., & Higson-Smith, C. (2004). Considering a theory of cultural trauma and loss. *Journal of Trauma & Loss, 9*(1), 89-111.

Summerfield, D. (1998). The social experience of war and some issues for the humanitarian field. In P. J. Bracken & C. Petty (Eds.), *Rethinking the trauma of war* (pp. 9-37). London: Free Association Books.

Suzic, D., Patel, M., & Doran, C. (1995). *An evaluative review of psychosocial programme studies and documents (Evaluation Review of psychosocial programmes in ESA region)*. Nairobi: UNICEF ESARO.

Weine, S. M. (1999). *When history is a nightmare: Lives and memories of ethnic cleansing in Bosnia-Herzegovina*. New Brunswick, NJ: Rutgers University Press.

Westermeyer, J., & Wahmanholm, K. (1996). Refugee children. In R. J. Apfel & B. Simon (Eds.), *Minefields in their hearts: The mental health of children in war and communal violence* (pp. 75-103). New Haven, CT: Yale University Press.

Whittaker, J. K., & Garbarino, J. (Eds.). (1983). *Social support networks: Informal helping in the human services*. New York: Aldine de Gruyter.

Williams, M. B., Zinner, E. S., & Ellis, R. R. (1999). The connection between grief and trauma: An overview. In E. S. Zinner & M. B. Williams (Eds.), *When a community weeps: Case studies in group survivorship* (pp. 3-17). Philadelphia, PA: Brunner/Mazel.

Wilson, J. P., & Keane, T. M. (Eds.). (1996). *Assessing psychological trauma and PTSD*. New York: Guilford Press.

Yehuda, R., & McFarlane, A. C. (1999). Conflict between current knowledge about posttraumatic stress disorder and its original conceptual basis. In M. J. Horowitz (Ed.), *Essential papers on posttraumatic stress disorder* (pp. 41-60). New York: New York University Press.

doi:10.1300/J146v14n01_10

# SECTON FOUR: ECOLOGICALLY INFORMED INTERVENTION

# Trauma and Resilience: A Case of Individual Psychotherapy in a Multicultural Context

Pratyusha Tummala-Narra

**SUMMARY.** The decision to seek professional help and the efficacy of such help are influenced by several factors, including individual and cultural definitions of trauma, access to services, and social support. This paper is focused on psychotherapy as one avenue of recovery for trauma survivors. A case of a biracial woman coping with a history of traumatic experience, working in the context of weekly individual psychotherapy

Address correspondence to: Pratyusha Tummala-Narra (E-mail: ushatummala@ yahoo.com).

[Haworth co-indexing entry note]: "Trauma and Resilience: A Case of Individual Psychotherapy in a Multicultural Context." Tummala-Narra, Pratyusha. Co-published simultaneously in *Journal of Aggression, Maltreatment & Trauma* (The Haworth Maltreatment & Trauma Press, an imprint of The Haworth Press, Inc.) Vol. 14, No. 1/2, 2007, pp. 205-225; and: *Sources and Expressions of Resiliency in Trauma Survivors: Ecological Theory, Multicultural Practice* (ed: Mary R. Harvey, and Pratyusha Tummala-Narra) The Haworth Maltreatment & Trauma Press, an imprint of The Haworth Press, Inc., 2007, pp. 205-225. Single or multiple copies of this article are available for a fee from The Haworth Document Delivery Service [1-800-HAWORTH, 9:00 a.m. - 5:00 p.m. (EST). E-mail address: docdelivery@haworthpress.com].

is presented. The case is conceptualized from a culturally informed, ecological perspective that considers the relevance of individual, interpersonal, and cultural factors in determining the trajectory of trauma
recovery. The psychotherapeutic relationship is seen as a significant
force in helping the client to mobilize and make use of her resilient capacities.

doi:10.1300/J146v14n01_10 *[Article copies available for a fee from The Haworth
Document Delivery Service: 1-800-HAWORTH. E-mail address: <docdelivery@
haworthpress.com> Website: <http://www.HaworthPress. com> © 2007 by The
Haworth Press, Inc. All rights reserved.]*

**KEYWORDS.** Trauma recovery, resilience, ecological theory, culturally informed psychotherapy, race and psychotherapy, transference

Individuals and communities heal from traumatic experiences in
multiple ways. Supportive family relationships and friendships, psychotherapy, group intervention, and social movements are examples of
contexts through which healing occurs. It is well established in the research and clinical literature that recovery from trauma encompasses a
multidimensional and dynamic process (Harvey, 1996; Herman, 1992).
Research on help-seeking behavior among trauma survivors indicates
that both formal (i.e., police, legal advocates, psychotherapists) and informal (i.e., family, friends, clergy) supports are critical to the recovery
process (Goodkind, Gillum, Bybee, & Sullivan, 2003; Goodman, Dutton,
Weinfurt, & Cook, 2003). The decision to seek professional help (i.e.,
crisis intervention, psychotherapy, legal advocacy), often pivotal in the
recovery from trauma, is influenced by several factors, including individual and cultural definitions of trauma, access to services, and social
support (Bui, 2003; Harvey, 1996; Liang, Goodman, Tummala-Narra, &
Weintraub, 2005). These same factors almost certainly help to determine the relevance and the efficacy of professional interventions post-
trauma (Harvey, 1996, this volume; Koss & Harvey, 1991; Mollica &
Son, 1989).

This paper is focused on psychotherapeutic intervention as one avenue of recovery for trauma survivors. Specifically, the author presents a
case of a biracial woman coping with a history of traumatic experience
with whom she has worked in individual psychotherapy. The case is
conceptualized from an ecological perspective that considers the relevance of individual, interpersonal, and cultural factors in determining
the trajectory of trauma recovery. This case highlights the psychothera-

peutic relationship as a context for recovery and a force capable of mobilizing resilience in the lives of trauma survivors.

## A THEORETICAL FRAMEWORK FOR PSYCHOTHERAPY WITH TRAUMA SURVIVORS

Several perspectives in the treatment of trauma have been discussed extensively in the psychotherapy literature. These approaches focus on biological, intrapsychic, interpersonal, and community influences in individual responses to traumatic experience (Davies & Frawley, 1994; van der Kolk, McFarlane, & Weisaeth, 1996). While each of these perspectives addresses important aspects of trauma recovery, none provides an integrated understanding of individual, community, and cultural factors affecting recovery (Harvey, 1996). Furthermore, traditional approaches to psychotherapy, which emphasize values of individual achievement and autonomy and are based on European and North American white middle class contexts without consideration for one's racial, ethnic, and socioeconomic history, can exacerbate the effects of traumatic experience. For instance, many ethnic minority individuals who cope with the intergenerational effects of historical trauma (i.e., slavery, genocide) are vulnerable to further violation of their sense of dignity in a treatment setting that minimizes a connection to social and historical context (Daniel, 2000; Tummala-Narra, this volume; Whitbeck, Adams, Hoyt, & Chen, 2004). If they are to be helpful and effective, psychotherapeutic approaches need to consider the cultural, economic, and sociopolitical realities that traumatized individuals often face on an ongoing basis. In light of the impact of one's cultural context on the individual's processing of and healing from trauma, it is critical that therapists address both internal (i.e., intrapsychic) experience and external (i.e., family, community) ramifications of individual and collective traumatic experience.

Herman (1992) has defined trauma recovery as a process occurring across three stages, including establishment of safety, remembrance and mourning, and reconnection. According to this model, a central goal of trauma recovery is "the empowerment of the survivor and the creation of new connections" (p. 133), a recovery goal that occurs in the context of relationships. This view of trauma recovery emphasizes the impact of the relational context on the individual's understanding of and recovery from traumatic experience.

The integration of individual and contextual elements in the treatment of trauma is further elaborated by the ecological perspective. An ecological approach to trauma recovery attempts to bridge some of the gaps between traditional psychotherapy with its focus on intrapsychic processes with awareness of the larger ecosystem of the individual (Harvey, 1996). A central feature of the ecological framework is its emphasis on the resilient capacities of individuals and communities (Harney, in press; Harvey, this volume). An individual's sources of resilience are considered to be critical in determining the nature and helpfulness of clinical interventions, in the individual's search for understanding and in her/his reframing the experiences of trauma across life transitions (Harvey, this volume; Harvey, Mishler, Koenen, & Harney, 2000).

Harvey (1996) outlined eight different dimensions or outcome criteria, including authority over the remembering process, integration of memory and affect, affect tolerance, symptom mastery, self-esteem, self-cohesion, safe attachment, and meaning-making, which encompass recovery from trauma. According to Harvey, each of these criteria reflects a specific domain of functioning that may be impacted by one or more traumatic events. The utility of this multidimensional approach to assessing trauma recovery, as defined by these eight domains of functioning, has been documented in psychometric studies of the Multidimensional Trauma Recovery and Resiliency Scale (i.e., the MTRR-135 and the MTRR-99; Bradley & Davino, this volume; Harvey, Liang, Tummala-Narra, Harney, & Lebowitz, 2003; Liang, Tummala-Narra, Bradley, & Harvey, this volume). These measures have also been used to study recovery and resiliency in culturally diverse populations of trauma survivors. A number of these studies are included in this volume (see, e.g., Bradley & Davino, this issue; Daigneault, Cyr, & Tourigny, this volume; Lynch, Keasler, Reaves, Channer, & Bukowski, this volume; Peddle, this volume; Radan, this volume, and Sorsoli, this volume).

In recent years, various researchers and clinicians have confirmed the value of the ecological perspective by exploring the experience of trauma in diverse contexts. Specifically, the question of how cultural and racial context shape one's psychological life has been explored in the psychotherapy literature (Akhtar, 1999; Foster, 1996; Roland, 1996). Other authors have focused on the effects of racial trauma, political trauma, and ethnic strife (Aron & Corne, 1994; Daniel, 2000; Keinan-Kon, 1998; Radan, this volume; Peddle, this volume). There has also been an increasing interest in the role of racial, ethnic, and socioeconomic factors in the client-therapist relationship (Altman, 1995; Leary, 2000).

While there is empirical evidence for the effectiveness of several psychotherapeutic approaches for certain psychological problems, such as phobias and depression, empirical evidence that any of these is effective with ethnic minority populations is sorely lacking (Alvidrez, Azocar, & Miranda, 1996; Hall, 2001). This is in sharp contrast with the reality of the increasing demand for psychotherapy services that are culturally sensitive. Several culturally sensitive theoretical models of psychotherapy have been developed for specific ethnic minority groups, some of which emphasize worldview differences between ethnic groups, and some that emphasize racial identity development (Hall, 2001; Helms & Cook, 1999; Sue et al., 1998). Hall (2001), for example, identified three major constructs including interdependence, spirituality, and discrimination that broadly differentiate ethnic minority from majority individuals in the U.S. in these cross-cultural models. The three constructs define areas of central value to ethnic minority groups (African American, American Indian, Asian American, and Latino American), which may help guide treatment planning. For instance, several cross-cultural researchers and clinicians, noting the centrality of group identity and interdependence in the lives of ethnic minorities, suggest the use of family and interpersonal therapies for ethnic minorities (Leyendecker & Lamb, 1999; Romero, Cuellar, & Roberts, 2000; Rosello & Bernal, 1999). While cross-cultural models provide a useful framework for understanding broad differences among different racial and cultural groups, it is important that psychotherapy with ethnic minorities also involve a fine tuned approach attending to the heterogeneity among individuals within each ethnic group.

As an elaboration of the ecological perspective of trauma recovery, this paper uses a single case study to illustrate and explore the impact of racial, cultural, and economic contexts on the experience of and recovery from trauma. The treatment with trauma survivors from a culturally informed, ecological perspective begins with the assessment of several factors, in addition to individual psychopathology, including cultural definitions of recovery and resilience, culturally salient expressions of resilience, and cultural and racial identity. Each of these aspects of experience has significant impact on resiliency and impairment in the eight domains of functioning described by Harvey (1996). The case discussion highlights the interplay of cultural context and individual psychology in a survivor's recovery from trauma along these eight domains.

## THE CASE OF LISA

The following case illustration involves my work with Lisa who sought treatment with the encouragement from a friend. I worked with her for 10 months in weekly individual psychotherapy.[1]

### Presenting Problem

Lisa is a 30-year-old biracial (African American and white) woman who complained of headaches and anxiety. She sought treatment after being physically assaulted by a female stranger at a local night club. Lisa left the club with bruises on her arms and chest, and stayed at her friend's home. Her friends discouraged her from seeking help from the police, and told her that the incident would be dismissed as a "brawl between black people." After several days, Lisa sought medical help from her primary care provider who questioned her about why she had not come in sooner for treatment. Lisa told her physician that she worried that the incident would be reported to the police, whom she did not trust. In her follow up visit with this physician, Lisa told her that she had trouble sleeping and seemed to be "hyper-aware" of her surroundings. Her physician suggested that she meet with a psychotherapist to discuss her condition. Initially, Lisa responded with some suspicion and trepidation about the idea of talking with a therapist. After four months of coping with frequent nightmares, however, she confided in a colleague at work, who also suggested that Lisa consider psychotherapy. Reluctantly, she made the decision to meet with a therapist and received a referral from her physician.

### History and Background

Lisa was born and raised in an urban, working class neighborhood in the northeastern part of the United States. Her mother and father both died in a car accident when she was seven years old, after which she lived with her younger sister and her maternal aunt and uncle. Her father was white and her mother was African American, as were her maternal aunt and uncle. Lisa reported having had a close relationship with her mother and that she felt devastated when her mother died. Although she had felt more distant from her father, who had spent less time with her in her childhood, she had missed his presence, too, following his death.

After her parents' deaths, Lisa had a difficult time readjusting to school and interacting with her friends. She described her childhood as "lonely and depressing." She also recalled that she would pray everyday for her parents to heal her sadness. While she loved her sister, she also felt that she carried a great deal of responsibility for taking care of her, as her aunt and uncle worked long hours in their business. She also remembered that her aunt and uncle had not encouraged either Lisa or her sister to talk about their parents.

Lisa reported that she had been sexually abused from ages 8 to 10 by her uncle's brother, who periodically visited their home during this time. He had stopped molesting her when he moved to another state. Lisa recalled that she did not reveal the abuse to her aunt and uncle because she feared that they would not believe her and that she and her sister would lose yet another set of parents. Following the physical assault that predated her entry into therapy with me, she had begun to have increasingly intrusive memories of her sexual abuse.

During her elementary and high school years, Lisa had pursued her interest in art and music. She also had developed a few close friendships through her church, which she attended regularly. She felt that these friends had helped her to gain "an inner strength" to cope with her emotional pain. She also reported that her high school experiences had been mostly positive, with the exception of a group of white kids who had teased her for being biracial. Although she does not recall specific instances of racism at her primarily African American church, she mentioned that she always "felt different" there. After high school graduation, she lost contact with most of her friends as they moved to different parts of the state. In college, she studied graphic design, and after graduating, she obtained a job in a large company where she still works.

Today, Lisa maintains infrequent contact with her sister and with her aunt and uncle, and she has a small group of African American friends most of whom she knows from her workplace. She stated that she confides in her friends about her childhood history, including the sexual abuse. She described her friends as "stable and supportive." Lisa attends her church every Sunday, and reported that prayer gives her a "sense of peace." When she began therapy, she had been dating a man whom she met through a friend for approximately four years, and was considering ending the relationship. She described her boyfriend as a "self-pitying black man who is silently controlling." Lisa had difficulty being sexually intimate with him, and felt used by him whenever they had sex. She increasingly found herself withdrawing from him, although she felt extremely lonely in his absence.

## Course of Treatment

Lisa began individual psychotherapy a week before the anniversary of her parents' deaths. In our initial session, Lisa expressed her reluctance to work with a therapist. When I questioned her about what she hoped to gain in psychotherapy, she stated that she felt that she had "no choice at this point," as she had been unable to cope with her nightmares and traumatic memories. Lisa stated that her goals for her treatment involved reducing her anxiety and becoming more effective in coping with her traumatic experiences. She had discussed her sexual abuse with her friends, but worried that she would "burden them" with her problems. She reported that she had been assaulted and that she had a history of sexual abuse, but she did so with little emotion connected with her words.

Lisa also stated that she wanted the therapy to last no more than a couple of months. She stated, "I don't want to delve into all of my past. I need solutions for dealing with what happened to me. It's weird for me to be doing this, being black. We're not supposed to go to therapy when we have these kinds of problems." Lisa explained that seeking therapy, particularly in light of her religious beliefs, felt alien to her. From the church's perspective, the conventional approach to dealing with psychological distress was to seek counseling from members of the clergy. Although her relationship with the church had helped her in grieving the loss of her parents, she felt that her church ignored issues of trauma, particularly the sexual violation of girls and women. Lisa felt that she would not be able to discuss her sexual abuse with the clergy, and worried that she would be blamed for the abuse.

In the initial three months of treatment, Lisa focused on practicing some relaxation techniques (i.e., breathing, listening to music) at home, particularly before sleeping at night. She also talked in therapy about her relationship with her boyfriend. She stated that he was indifferent to her assault and that he cared only for himself. Lisa had refused his offer to move in with him, after which he had verbally abused her and threatened to end their relationship. She expressed feeling confused about why she continued dating him, despite her unhappiness.

In our eighth session, she stated, "I don't know if I can delve further with you . . . I mean it's helping to talk about Jim (boyfriend), but I don't know if I can get into all of my problems." I responded, "I wonder what might be making it difficult for you to tell me more." Lisa then discussed how hard it was for her to talk about the fear of losing people in her life. This issue, interestingly, arose in the context of my impending two-week long vacation. We discussed her continuing to use relaxation techniques to help reduce her anxiety and improve her sleep during our separation.

After my return from vacation, Lisa expressed her curiosity about me. She stated, "Are you from India? I feel like I need to know something about you to feel more comfortable in here." I replied, "Yes, I am originally from India. I am wondering how knowing more about me would help you feel more comfortable." She revealed that she held an image of therapists as people who "just repeat what you say," and she worried that I would evaluate her negatively or not understand her African American background. She also mentioned that it was difficult for her to have such a long break from therapy.

Her transference to me reflected her fear of attaching to someone and then losing him/her, as she found it difficult to express any anger toward me or toward other significant people in her life (i.e., her boyfriend) for not fulfilling her need for emotional closeness. In an attempt to protect herself from further loss, she also treaded carefully in therapy and tried not to "delve" too much into her past. My countertransference involved both curiosity and some anxiety about learning more about the deaths of Lisa's parents and her sexual abuse. I was concerned with helping her to maintain her progress in stabilizing her sleep and ameliorating her anxiety, while helping her to better understand her long-standing relational conflicts.

As we continued to discuss her fear of separation and loss from others, she began to talk about her feelings of shame and anger about being assaulted, and how this had shattered her self-image as a strong and self-reliant woman. In Lisa's view, being strong and self-reliant was related to her racial identity. In one session, she stated, "I am a strong African American woman, and I don't get seen that way." She explained that her aunt, uncle, and peers at school had treated Lisa differently than they had treated her sister. Lisa has a light skin complexion and light brown hair, while her sister has darker skin and darker hair. Growing up, Lisa was frequently identified as a white person, which she saw as an invalidation of her true racial identity as a black woman. She felt as though her family had treated her as a more sensitive and needy child than her sister and she thought the difference was connected to her "whiteness." She also attributed to her "whiteness" her inability to ward off her uncle's brother, who "chose" her as his victim. She also believed that being seen as white had led to the conflict with the woman who had assaulted her.

In the fourth month of treatment, Lisa began to talk more about her uncle's brother. She talked about how she had initially admired and trusted him, and then feared him and felt disgusted by his molestation of her. During this phase of our work, she frequently interrupted our discussion of her abuse, indicating to me that it felt too overwhelming, but at later points in the session, would resume our discussion. She noted that she had more difficulty with sleeping at night following these sessions. Our focus would then turn to practical strategies to cope with her anxiety, including some breathing exercises in session.

In one session, Lisa mentioned that she hated her perpetrator's light skin, and that she wished that she had dark skin like her sister, imagining that he would not have hurt her had she not been "so white." Lisa also stated, "I wish my skin was as dark as yours. I bet nobody ever thinks you are anything other than what you are. You probably know what it's like to be discriminated against." I stated, "You are still working on figuring out all of the things that make you who you are. Being black is one of them, and so is being white." Lisa then expressed, "I know I am part white, but I always felt closer to my mother than to anyone else, and she is who I want to be like. . . . I wish that my mother was there. She would have protected me. I loved the way she took care of us. She knew who I really was and how I really felt."

With respect to our relationship, Lisa's perceptions of me involved both a sense of connection and disconnection. While she felt that she could identify with me as an ethnic minority and as a potential dark skinned mother figure, she also felt as though I would not be able to identify with her conflicts about being biracial. As an Indian-American, I empathized with her attempt to make sense of two different cultural contexts, and at the same time, I felt anxious about not being able to identify with her conflict with her black and white racial identities. I also realized that her racial identity conflicts reflected her sense of deep loss and her struggle with defining herself as a whole person. Her sexual abuse had further broken her trust in the ability of parental figures to take care of her, and her racial identifications became symbolic of the "good" and "bad" people in her life, as well as the parts of herself that felt competent or inadequate. These identifications also shaped the way she saw herself as "weak" for having been victimized, first by her uncle's brother and later by the stranger who assaulted her.

In the following weeks, Lisa was able to speak about her sexual abuse in more detail and with fewer disruptions to her sleep and less anxiety.

This eventually led to more discussion about her feelings of sadness about losing her parents, and her longing to connect with someone she could trust. She also contemplated how to approach her relationship with her boyfriend. She decided to "take a break" from him and asked him not to call her for a few weeks, so that she could think further about her decision. She eventually ended the relationship, and spent more time with friends from her workplace and her church where she felt supported and accepted.

Toward the end of the eighth month of treatment, Lisa decided to accept a position in a company in a different part of the state. As we prepared to end the treatment, Lisa expressed her ambivalence about ending therapy and feeling "on my own again." We discussed ways in which she could continue to maintain her safety in her relationships, and to feel more connected to her feelings about herself and others in her life. In the last month of our work together, she had begun to draw pictures of herself and her family. She planned to continue creating her art, which also helped her to connect with her feelings about different events in her life. She also met with a priest in a church that was more racially diverse (i.e., white, black, Latino) near her new home. She hoped to someday be able to talk with the priest about the church's perspective on sexual abuse. Lisa also stated that therapy, in a different way than being at church or talking with friends, had given her a place to connect with her innermost thoughts and feelings. In our last few sessions, she expressed that she would miss me, and also that she would consider working in therapy in the future.

## CASE DISCUSSION

Lisa's ability to cope with her traumatic experiences and her decision to seek psychotherapy were shaped by individual, family, and cultural factors, and her treatment was guided by a culturally informed approach that examined these factors. While the goals of her treatment focused on reducing her trauma-related stress, an ecological perspective allowed for a more expansive understanding of her cultural and religious contexts, which influenced her recovery. For instance, Lisa's changing connection with her church played a significant role in her healing from trauma, as did her decision to seek psychotherapy. Her recovery involved the examination of and resolution of psychological distress (i.e., nightmares, anxiety, depression) as well as the mobilization of multiple sources of resilience (i.e., friendships, creativity).

## *Eight Domains of Functioning*

Harvey's (1996) ecological model of trauma recovery and resilience provides a useful framework in which the various aspects of Lisa's traumatic history and her current functioning can be conceptualized. This case illustrates Lisa's resilience as well as her impairment in eight domains of functioning identified in this model. In considering the first three domains (i.e., authority over the remembering process, integration of memory and affect, and affect tolerance and regulation), for example, it is worth noting Lisa's ability to remember the circumstances around the death of her parents and her history of childhood sexual abuse with clarity and detail. She recounted the sadness of her parents' death and her feelings of fear and disgust when she was abused by her uncle's brother. However, when she first entered treatment, she had a difficult time with connecting any emotions with her factual report of these events.

One of the initial goals of individual psychotherapy with Lisa involved creating a safe space for her to discuss not only her history but also her emotional life. As she felt increasingly safe in our relationship, she began to take more risks by revealing her feelings about her abuse. For instance, when she stated that she wished that her mother was there to protect her, she was able to connect her loss with the abuse in the present tense. In other words, she was no longer recounting a past longing for her mother, but felt her loss in the moment as she described the abuse in our session. In a similar vein, as Lisa experimented with expressing her emotions in session, her ability to tolerate her sometimes intense affect improved over time. Outside of therapy, with her friends at work she became less defensive in guarding her emotional pain.

The fourth domain of functioning, symptom mastery, refers to one's mastery over certain symptoms related to or produced by traumatic experience. Relaxation techniques were used as a therapeutic mechanism for reducing stress, anxiety, and nightmares. Lisa continued to struggle with sleep throughout our work together, and as she practiced her stress management techniques more regularly, she felt more relieved. Her openness to creating artwork in the context of healing from trauma further served a purpose of relieving stress and anxiety.

With respect to the impact of trauma on her self-esteem and self-cohesion, Lisa experienced significant shifts in her sense of competence, self-reliance, and her racial identity. Her experience of being assaulted triggered her long-standing fear of being "weak" and of not being seen as a strong African American woman. She felt shamed by the assault as she had by her sexual abuse. Her negative view of herself was apparent in her relationship with her boyfriend, in which she felt emotionally and sexually unsafe. Her understanding of the effects of her abuse and the loss of her parents on her sense of self was critical to her decision to establish safety in her intimate relationships. Furthermore, her therapeutic work aimed to help her to mobilize existing resources, such as her friends and her church, in order to gain a more realistic, positive view of herself. Her friends were instrumental in helping her to connect with her strengths and abilities and in accepting her vulnerability. They verbally praised her ability to survive terrible loss and encouraged her to consider seeking help from a therapist when she felt overwhelmed by her traumatic memories.

The seventh domain of recovery has to do with building safe attachments with others. The process of building safe, intimate relationships requires the grieving of loss (Harvey, 1996; Herman, 1992). As she discussed the loss of her parents and the fragmentation of her family, Lisa became increasingly aware of her feelings toward significant others. Lisa had struggled with her feelings of isolation since the time of her parents' deaths. Her sense of loneliness coupled with her fear of losing significant people in her life pervaded her choices regarding intimate relationships. She did enjoy memories of being close with her mother and had positive experiences with friends from her church as an adolescent, and carried these feelings with her as an adult. She was able to form close friendships with her colleagues at work. Her ambivalence about emotional intimacy was explored in the context of the psychotherapeutic relationship, and Lisa's gains in the therapy eventually made possible her decision to end a relationship that felt unsafe and to strengthen her positive relationships with friends.

The last domain of recovery involves a process whereby a survivor gives new meaning to her traumatic experiences. While this is a highly personal and complicated task, often evolving over a long period of time, it was clear as Lisa prepared to leave psychotherapy that she had begun to question her conceptualization of what her trauma meant in her life. For instance, when she first entered therapy, she was convinced that a "strong black woman" should not "delve into" or reveal her vulnerabilities. By actually sharing her experiences with a therapist, she began to move toward a different perspective on what had happened to her. Specifically, Lisa wondered about what might have been different if her mother had been alive at the time of her abuse. She also thought about whether or not she would have been sexually abused if she had had darker skin color. Outside of therapy, Lisa had begun to explore these questions in the context of her religious beliefs. She considered talking to a priest about why terrible things like sexual abuse happen, the nature of accountability of the perpetrator, and the process of healing. Another way in which she tried to form meaning of her experiences was to bring together her artistic and relational worlds. These types of inquiry were critical to Lisa's understanding of what had happened in her life, and to determining the course of her recovery.

## Cultural Definition of Trauma Recovery and Resilience

The ecological perspective emphasizes that recovery from trauma and expressions of resilience are multidetermined, influenced by various individual, interpersonal, and cultural factors (Harvey, 1996, this volume; Tummala-Narrra, this volume). It is also important to note that resiliency is a dynamic process with effects that vary with changing circumstances and developmental transitions (Ashford, Le-Croy, & Lortie, 2001; Harney, in press). The contextual nature of resilience is evident in Lisa's recovery process. Lisa expressed her unfamiliarity with psychotherapy in light of her background as an African American woman raised in a working class environment. The effects of culture and context can be profound in the help-seeking process, from the challenge of defining an experience as traumatic to that of choosing a provider (Cauce et al., 2002; Haeri, this volume; Liang et al., 2005). Initially, Lisa viewed psychotherapy as an "alien" resource for dealing with stress. Her reluctance to reveal her personal experiences to individuals outside of her community was reinforced by some of her African American friends, who cautioned her against reporting the assault to the police or any other white people. She was concerned that she would either be dismissed or pathologized by a therapist, feelings that are not uncommon among African Americans who seek mental health services (Daniel, 2000; Jordan, Bogat, & Smith, 2001).

Several studies emphasize the role of social support from friends, clergy, and community members in coping with trauma within African American communities (Fraser, McNutt, Clark, Williams-Muhammed, & Lee, 2002; Snowden, 2001). Lisa had survived significant loss and both child and adult trauma prior to seeking psychotherapy. Her connection with her church, her friends, and her art were important sources of resilience congruent with her cultural and religious contexts. It is clear that Lisa's recovery from trauma began long before she sought psychotherapy. Harvey et al. (2000) discuss the importance of "turning points" that allow for new ways of understanding and coping with past traumas. The decision to seek psychotherapy was one such turning point for Lisa, providing her with a new and unfamiliar means of connecting with her fears, her vulnerabilities, and her strengths. Critical features of the psychotherapeutic process were (a) that it provided Lisa with new resources for coping with her post-traumatic stress, and (b) that it simultaneously sought to strengthen her sense of connection to her community. In this way, Lisa was able to access not only increased support, but more options for defining herself and making sense of her experiences.

## Racial and Cultural Context and the Psychotherapeutic Relationship

Lisa's case highlights several aspects of the client's transference and the therapist's countertransference that can help guide a culturally informed, ecological approach to the treatment of trauma. Herman (1992) discussed the relevance of "traumatic transference," where the client's responses to the therapist are shaped at least in part by his/her experience of terror, and "traumatic countertransference," which includes the therapist's reactions both to the traumatized client and to the traumatic event itself. In this case, both Lisa and I experienced some degree of helplessness in the face of a complex and long-standing history of trauma. When we felt ourselves locked into this position, it became more difficult to identify those sources of resilience that could prove critical to her confronting her trauma and moving beyond with her life. Therefore, it was necessary to attend both to the areas of difficulty that Lisa experienced and to her strengths.

The therapeutic dyad reflects larger societal structuring of socioeconomic class, race, culture, gender, and sexual orientation. A critical component of Lisa's identity involved race. Her strong sense of identification as an African American woman influenced her view of her traumatic experience and the recovery process. It also shaped the nature of our therapeutic relationship. Her fear of being pathologized by a therapist was evident in her transference. Lisa indicated that it was important for her to know something more personal about me. Several researchers and clinicians have noted the ability of therapists to take risks in race-related disclosures as helpful in creating a trusting interpersonal space when working with ethnic minority clients (Constantine & Kwan, 2003; Helms & Cook, 1999; Sue & Sue, 2003). One reason for why this may be particularly salient to the establishment of safety and trust is that some race-related disclosure by the therapist is affirming of the interdependent context valued by many ethnic minorities. For Lisa, my attempt to engage her around our cultural differences and similarities was also essential to communicating my openness to the discussion of racism and conflicts with racial identity.

In the transferential relationship, Lisa and I experienced ourselves as both similar and different from each other. While she viewed me as a fellow member of a minority group, she expressed her concern about me not fully understanding or appreciating black and white racial conflicts. From her perspective, I was in a position of power as a therapist, and as an immigrant, less prone to discrimination than she or other African American and biracial people. With respect to my countertransference, I felt anxious, at times, with her seemingly conflicted choice of denouncing her white racial identity, and wondered about how she felt about her father, of whom she spoke only rarely during our work together. I also wondered if she spoke less about the parts of her that are more identified with being white, because she feared that this identification would diminish our shared connection as ethnic minorities. Our discussion of racial identity led to these questions about her relational life that were left unexplored in the treatment. I hoped that Lisa would have the opportunity to address these questions in another context of healing.

An area that is often overlooked in addressing culture and race in clients' lives involves the heterogeneity in the experiences of individuals within a particular ethnic group. Stereotyping derived from distorted images of individuals from diverse contexts can contribute to the therapist's countertransference, typically in the direction of the therapist viewing the client as less able or at "higher risk" for maladjustment due to his/her minority status. In these instances, the therapist may approach a client with excessive curiosity about his/her culture as the sole force in shaping the client's traumatic experience and subsequent recovery. At other moments, the therapist and the client may avoid the discussion of race and culture altogether in the attempt to take a universalistic approach to the impact of trauma on the client's life, by focusing solely on behavioral symptoms without considering the client's relationships with his/her family and/or cultural contexts (Gorkin, 1996). The paucity of public images of ethnic minorities as both vulnerable and resilient can exacerbate the therapist's misnomers about the client's full range of emotional experiences. Contradictory messages about ethnic minorities, such as the ones implied in television images of African Americans as competent, successful musicians and athletes, and other images as intellectually inferior and disadvantaged, create confusion and misconstruals of any individual African American's experience (Daniel, 2000).

These images internalized by both therapist and patient, if left unexamined, can create obstructions in building a genuine and effective therapeutic relationship.

While race and culture shape individual development and traumatic experience, it is also true that within all racial, cultural, and ethnic groups there is significant variation among individuals in how trauma is processed. Within given racial, ethnic, and cultural groups, individual recovery trajectories are influenced by those cultural and religious beliefs the individual adheres to, the nature and quality of relationships with family members, and the quality of his/her interactions with various elements of mainstream U.S. society. In Lisa's treatment, she expressed her concern about being seen as a white instead of as an African American woman. Her connection with her African American community was a central source of strength in her life, but at the same time, she was aware of her "feeling different" within the African American community because of her biracial status. The psychotherapy process needed to respect her unique path to recovery, in light of her different racial identifications. One way in which this was made possible was through an active and non-evaluative discussion of what dark and light skin meant to her (i.e., good vs. bad), where she maintained her sense of control in defining herself. This was particularly important in light of her past abusive interactions with her perpetrator, and her current relationship with her boyfriend, both in which she felt controlled and helpless.

## CONCLUSION

Psychotherapy is a powerful means of helping trauma survivors mobilize their resilient capacities and secure recovery from trauma. An ecological perspective that attends to cultural differences in defining recovery and resilience, cultural and racial identity, and the impact of social context on the psychotherapeutic relationship is critical in providing psychotherapy that is effective across diverse contexts. In particular, the therapist's recognition of culturally congruent sources of resilience lays the foundation for a therapeutic process that respects the unique recovery pathway of the individual client.

As the applications of ecological and multicultural perspectives continue to expand into the treatment of trauma, several lines of inquiry are worth exploring in the future. First, psychotherapy outcome research with ethnic minorities coping with traumatic experience is imperative in order to better understand the unique trajectories of survivors from various backgrounds. Second, the attention to within group differences (i.e., heterogeneity within ethnic groups) with respect to the experience of trauma and expressions of resilience needs to be further explored. Finally, it would be interesting to study aspects of the therapeutic relationship (i.e., transference, countertransference), and specifically intercultural dynamics, that contribute to the recovery process. These areas of inquiry would help establish a better understanding of the nuances of the trauma recovery process and expressions of resilience across diverse racial, cultural, and economic contexts.

## NOTES

1. Lisa gave her consent to the author to include relevant information from her treatment.

## REFERENCES

Akhtar, S. (1999). *Immigration and identity: Turmoil, treatment, and transformation.* Northvale, NJ: Jason Aronson, Inc.

Altman, N. (1995). *The analyst in the inner city: Race, class, and culture through a psychoanalytic lens.* Hillsdale, NJ: The Analytic Press.

Alvidrez, J., Azocar, F., & Miranda, J. (1996). Demystifying the concept of ethnicity for psychotherapy researchers. *Journal of Consulting and Clinical Psychology, 64*(5), 903-908.

Aron, A., & Corne, S. (Eds.). (1994). *Writings for a liberation psychology. Ignacio Martín-Baró.* Cambridge, MA: Harvard University Press.

Ashford, J. B., LeCroy, C. W., Lortie, K. L. (2001). *Human behavior in the social environment: A multidimensional perspective* (2nd ed.). Belmont: Brooks/Cole Thomson Learing.

Bradley, R., & Davino, K. (2007). Interpersonal violence, recovery, and resilience in incarcerated women. *Journal of Aggression, Maltreatment & Trauma, 14*(1/2), 123-146.

Bui, H. N. (2003). Help-seeking behavior among abused immigrant women: A case of Vietnamese American women. *Violence Against Women, 9*(2), 207-239.

Cauce, A., Domenech-Rodríguez, M., Paradise, M., Cochran, B., Shea, J. M., Srebnik, D., et al. (2002). Cultural and contextual influences in mental health help seeking: A focus on ethnic minority youth. *Journal of Consulting and Clinical Psychology, 70*, 44-55.

Constantine, M. G., & Kwan, K. (2003). Cross-cultural considerations of therapist self-disclosure. *Journal of Clinical Psychology, 59*(5), 581-588.

Daigneault, I., Cyr, M., & Tourigny, M. (2007). Exploration of recovery trajectories in sexually abused adolescents. *Journal of Aggression, Maltreatment & Trauma, 14*(1/2), 165-184.

Daniel, J. H. (2000). The courage to hear: African American women's memories of racial trauma. In L. C. Jackson & B. Greene (Eds.), *Psychotherapy with African American women: Innovations in psychodynamic perspectives and practice* (pp. 126-144). New York: The Guilford Press.

Davies, J. M., & Frawley, M. G. (1994). *Treating the adult survivor of childhood sexual abuse: A psychoanalytic perspective.* New York: Basic Books.

Foster, R. P. (1996). Assessing the psychodynamic function of language in the bilingual patient. In R. P. Foster, M. Moskowitz, & R. A. Javier (Eds.), *Reaching across boundaries of culture and class* (pp. 243-263). Northvale, NJ: Jason Aronson, Inc.

Fraser, I. M., McNutt, L., Clark, C., Williams-Muhammed, D., & Lee, R. (2002). Social support choices for help with abusive relationships: Perceptions of African American women. *Journal of Family Violence, 17*(4), 363-375.

Goodkind, J. R., Gillum, T. L., Bybee, D. I., & Sullivan, C. M. (2003). The impact of family and friends' reactions on the well-being of women with abusive partners. *Violence Against Women, 9*(3), 347-373.

Goodman, L. A., Dutton, M. A., Weinfurt, K., & Cook, S. (2003). The Intimate Partner Violence Strategies Index: Development and application. *Violence Against Women, 9*(2), 163-186.

Gorkin, M. (1996). Countertransference in cross-cultural psychotherapy. In R. Perez-Foster, M. Moskowitz, & R. A. Javier (Eds.), *Reaching across boundaries of culture and class: Widening the scope of psychotherapy* (pp. 159-176). Northvale, NJ: Jason Aronson.

Haeri, S. (2007). Resilience and posttraumatic recovery in cultural and political context: Two Pakistani women's strategies for survival. *Journal of Aggression, Maltreatment & Trauma, 14*(1/2), 287-304.

Hall, G. C. N. (2001). Psychotherapy research with ethnic minorities: Empirical, ethical, and conceptual issues. *Journal of Consulting and Clinical Psychology, 69*(3), 502-510.

Harney, P. A. (in press). Resilience processes in context: Literature review and implications for intervention. *Journal of Aggression, Maltreatment & Trauma.*

Harvey, M. R. (1996). An ecological view of psychological trauma and trauma recovery. *Journal of Traumatic Stress, 9*(1), 3-23.

Harvey, M. R. (2007). Towards an ecological understanding of resilience in trauma survivors: Implications for theory, research, and practice. *Journal of Aggression, Maltreatment & Trauma, 14*(1/2), 9-32.

Harvey, M., Liang, B., Harney, P., Koenan, K., Tummala-Narra, P., & Lebowitz, L. (2003). A multidimensional approach to the assessment of trauma impact, recovery and resiliency: Initial psychometric findings. *Journal of Aggression, Maltreatment & Trauma, 6*(2) 87-109.

Harvey, M. R., Mishler, E. G., Koenen, K., Harney, P. A. (2000). In the aftermath of sexual abuse: Making and remaking meaning in narratives of trauma and recovery. *Narrative Inquiry, 10*(2), 291-311.

Helms, J. E., & Cook, D. A. (1999). *Using race and culture in counseling and psychotherapy: Theory and process.* Boston, MA: Allyn & Bacon.

Herman, J. L. (1992). *Trauma and recovery.* New York: Basic Books.

Jordan, L. C., Bogat, G. A., & Smith, G. (2001). Collaborating for social change: The Black psychologist and the Black community. *American Journal of Community Psychology, 29*(4), 599-620.

Keinan-Kon, N. (1998). Internal reality, external reality, and denial in the gulf war. *Journal of the American Academy of Psychoanalysis, 26*(3), 417-442.

Koss, M., & Harvey, M. (1991). *The rape victim: Clinical and community interventions* (2nd ed.). Newbury Park, CA: Sage.

Leary, K. (2000). Racial enactments in dynamic treatment. *Psychoanalytic Dialogues, 10,* 639-653

Leyendecker, B., & Lamb, M. E. (1999). Latino families. In M. E. Lamb (Ed.), *Parenting and child development in "nontraditional" families* (pp. 247-262). Mahwah, NJ: Erlbaum.

Liang, B., Goodman, L., Tummala-Narra, P., & Weintraub, S. (2005). A theoretical framework for understanding help-seeking processes among survivors of intimate partner violence. *American Journal of Community Psychology, 36*(1/2), 71-84.

Liang, B., Tummala-Narra, P., Bradley, R., & Harvey, M. R. (2007). The Multidimensional Trauma Recovery and Resiliency Instrument: Preliminary examination of an abridged version. *Journal of Aggression, Maltreatment & Trauma, 14*(1/2), 55-74.

Lynch, S. M., Keasler, A. L., Reaves, R. C., Channer, E. G., & Bukowski, L. T. (2007). The story of my strength: An exploration of resilience in the narratives of trauma survivors early in recovery. *Journal of Aggression, Maltreatment & Trauma, 14*(1/2), 75-97.

Mollica, R. F., & Son, L. (1989). Cultural dimensions in the evaluation and treatment of sexual trauma: An overview. *Psychiatric Clinics of North America, 12*(2), 363-379.

Peddle, N. (2007). Assessing trauma impact, recovery and resiliency in refugees of war. *Journal of Aggression, Maltreatment & Trauma, 14*(1/2), 185-204.

Radan, A. (2007). Exposure to violence and expressions of resilience in Central American women survivors of war. *Journal of Aggression, Maltreatment & Trauma, 14*(1/2), 147-164.

Roland, A. (1996). *Cultural pluralism and psychoanalysis: The Asian and North American experience.* New York: Routledge.

Romero, A. J., Cuellar, I., & Roberts, R. E. (2000). Ethnocultural variables and attitudes toward cultural socialization of children. *Journal of Community Psychology, 28,* 79-89.

Rossello, J., & Bernal, G. (1999). The efficacy of cognitive-behavioral and interpersonal treatments for depression in Puerto Rican adolescents. *Journal of Consulting and Clinical Psychology, 67,* 734-745.

Snowden, L. R. (2001). Social embeddedness and psychological well-being among African Americans and Whites. *American Journal of Community Psychology, 29*(4), 519-536.

Sorsoli, L. (2007). Where the whole thing fell apart: Race, resilience, and the complexity of trauma. *Journal of Aggression, Maltreatment & Trauma, 14*(1/2), 99-121.

Sue, D. W., Carter, R. T., Casas, J. M., Fouad, N. A., Ivey, A. E., Jensen, M. et al. (1998). *Multicultural counseling competencies: Individual and organizational development.* Thousand Oaks, CA: Sage.

Sue, D. W., & Sue, D. (2003). *Counseling the culturally diverse: Theory and practice* (4th ed.). Hoboken, NJ: John Wiley & Sons, Inc.

Tummala-Narra, P. (2007). Conceptualizing trauma and resilience across diverse contexts: A multicultural perspective. *Journal of Aggression, Maltreatment & Trauma, 14*(1/2), 33-53.

van der Kolk, B. A., McFarlane, A. C., & Weisaeth, L. (Eds.). (1996). *Traumatic stress: The effects of overwhelming experience on mind, body, and society.* New York: The Guilford Press.

Whitbeck, L. B., Adams, G. W., Hoyt, D. R., & Chen, X. (2004). Conceptualizing and measuring historical trauma among American Indian people. *American Journal of Community Psychology, 33*(3/4), 119-130.

doi:10.1300/J146v14n01_11

# Group Therapy as an Ecological Bridge to New Community for Trauma Survivors

Michaela Mendelsohn
Robin S. Zachary
Patricia A. Harney

**SUMMARY.** Group therapy counteracts the isolating effects of interpersonal trauma and enables survivors to connect with sources of resilience within themselves and others. By providing an alternative relational experience in which the survivor and her safety are valued, groups empower members to establish self-affirming and supportive relationships in their outside lives. The current paper reviews the psychological impact of chronic interpersonal violence and the relevant literature regarding group therapy for trauma survivors. We describe an approach to group treatment for complexly traumatized patients developed at the Victims of Violence Program, and through a clinical vignette, illustrate some of the ways in which group therapy can expand the relational world of survivors. doi:10.1300/J146v14n01_12 *[Article copies available for a fee from The Haworth Document Delivery Service: 1-800-HAWORTH. E-mail address: <docdelivery@haworthpress.com> Website: <http://www.HaworthPress.com> © 2007 by The Haworth Press, Inc. All rights reserved.]*

---

Address correspondence to: Michaela Mendelsohn, PhD, Victims of Violence Program, The Cambridge Health Alliance, 26 Central Street, Somerville, MA 02143 (E-mail: m.mendelsohn@rcn.com).

[Haworth co-indexing entry note]: "Group Therapy as an Ecological Bridge to New Community for Trauma Survivors." Mendelsohn, Michaela, Robin S. Zachary, and Patricia A. Harney. Co-published simultaneously in *Journal of Aggression, Maltreatment & Trauma* (The Haworth Maltreatment & Trauma Press, an imprint of The Haworth Press, Inc.) Vol. 14, No. 1/2, 2007, pp. 227-243; and: *Sources and Expressions of Resiliency in Trauma Survivors: Ecological Theory, Multicultural Practice* (ed: Mary R. Harvey, and Pratyusha Tummala-Narra) The Haworth Maltreatment & Trauma Press, an imprint of The Haworth Press, Inc., 2007, pp. 227-243. Single or multiple copies of this article are available for a fee from The Haworth Document Delivery Service [1-800-HAWORTH, 9:00 a.m. - 5:00 p.m. (EST). E-mail address: docdelivery@haworthpress.com].

doi:10.1300/J146v14n01_12

**KEYWORDS.** Group therapy, interpersonal trauma, abuse, posttraumatic stress

Interpersonal trauma violates one's sense of safety in the social world. Profound isolation results from ruptured trust, shame, fear of future violence, and the wide range of protective or defensive measures that victims develop in the wake of trauma, particularly under conditions of chronic exposure. In isolation, victims are prevented from functioning to their fullest capacities. Their personal power and competence are diminished by post-traumatic symptoms, a shattered sense of meaning, and disrupted self-cohesion. Additionally, in the context of abusive relationships characterized by domination and subordination, survivors are taught to devalue themselves and their physical and emotional safety, frequently placing them at risk for further trauma.

We conceive of individual and group psychotherapy for trauma survivors as transitional spaces within which they can restore foundations of safety within themselves and with others. Individual therapy offers survivors an opportunity to develop trust and experience the possibility of a safe hierarchical relationship. Groups provide survivors with experiences of community that counteract their isolation and enable them to connect with sources of resilience within themselves and others. Importantly, groups also offer a model of reciprocal relationships marked by caring and compassion. They serve as a microcosm in which survivors can rework problems associated with their traumatic past within a safe and structured relational network. The norms of the group stand in sharp contrast to those of the original abusive relationships, and provide a framework within which survivors can learn to value themselves and their safety. They are empowered to seek out affirming and compassionate relationships in their lives outside of group; it is in this way that groups serve as an ecological bridge to new community.

In this article, we briefly review the effects of interpersonal trauma and the empirical evidence regarding group treatment efficacy. We describe a model of group treatment designed to meet various clinical needs and recognize the resilience of survivors of complex trauma at different phases of recovery. Using a clinical example, we demonstrate some of the ways in which group treatment can serve as an "ecological bridge" (Harvey, this volume); in other words, the ways in which it can facilitate transition from positions of helpless isolation, distrust, and withdrawal to positions of engagement within intimate, social, and community relationships.

## EFFECTS OF CHRONIC INTERPERSONAL TRAUMA

The psychiatric sequelae of chronic interpersonal trauma such as childhood abuse and domestic violence are considerably more diverse, numerous, and pervasive than would be suggested by the diagnosis of uncomplicated posttraumatic stress disorder (PTSD; American Psychiatric Association, 1994) that is frequently associated with single-incident or circumscribed trauma. In addition to PTSD, survivors of chronic interpersonal trauma often report symptoms of other anxiety disorders, major depression, dissociative disorders, conversion disorders and somatization, personality disorders, eating disorders, and substance abuse (Dube et al., 2001; Edwards, Holden, Felitti, & Anda, 2003; Felitti et al., 1998; Herman, Perry, & van der Kolk, 1989; Loewenstein, 1990). Adult survivors of childhood abuse are at increased risk for self-destructive behavior and suicide attempts (Boudewyn & Liem, 1995; van der Kolk, Perry, & Herman, 1991). Childhood sexual abuse is a strong predictor for revictimization in adulthood (Coid et al., 2001). Survivors of chronic interpersonal trauma are also more vulnerable to a variety of physical health problems (Drossman et al., 1990; Wurtele, Kaplan, & Keairnes, 1990).

Herman (1992a) formulated the concept of complex PTSD to describe characteristics of survivors of prolonged and repeated trauma commonly reported in the literature and observed in clinical practice but not adequately captured by the narrow diagnostic criteria of simple PTSD. Complex PTSD involves three broad areas of disturbance: (a) a complicated and tenacious symptoms picture with multiple complaints, including somatization, dissociation, and affective dysregulation; (b) characteristic personality changes, including relational difficulties and dis- turbances of identity; and (c) vulnerability to repeated harm, either self- inflicted or perpetrated by others. The DSM-IV field trials (van der Kolk et al., 1996) confirmed that PTSD, dissociation, somatization, and affect dysregulation were highly interrelated, and that these problems co-occurred most frequently among survivors of early onset interpersonal trauma. Furthermore, a considerable proportion of participants who no longer met criteria for PTSD continued to suffer from high levels of these other symptoms.

## GROUP THERAPY FOR SURVIVORS
## OF INTERPERSONAL TRAUMA

Group therapy has a number of unique advantages for survivors of complex trauma. Social disruption is frequently a primary effect of traumatic events (Sewell & Willliams, 2001). It is thus not surprising that the power of group interventions lies in their potential to restore and rebuild social connections. Herman (1992b) identifies the experience of commonality as a central curative component of group therapy for trauma survivors. Joining with others who have experienced similar traumas creates a sense of belonging, reduces feelings of isolation and alienation, and provides support and understanding not available elsewhere. Groups are especially helpful in combating the sense of secrecy, shame, and stigma that characterize the experience of survivors of child abuse (Herman & Schatzow, 1984), rape (Koss & Harvey, 1991), or combat (Lifton, 1973). Groups provide an opportunity for previously unrecognized resilience among group members to be noticed and utilized. They promote empowerment by offering group members the opportunity to share coping skills and help one another. They foster self-esteem as the survivor learns to value herself through establishing connections with valued others and experiencing their acceptance (Harney & Harvey, 1999). Allen and Bloom (1994) note that by virtue of its social and interpersonal nature, group therapy provides an excellent environment for repairing the cognitive schemas for safety, trust/ dependency, independence, power, self-esteem, and intimacy that are often disrupted by psychological trauma.

Based on a comprehensive review of empirical studies of group psychotherapy for adult trauma survivors, Foy et al. (2000) found that regardless of approach, group psychotherapy was associated with favorable outcomes in a range of symptom domains. Abatement of PTSD and depression were the most commonly included outcomes, but efficacy was also demonstrated for other symptoms, including dissociation, self-esteem, anxiety, fear, and global distress. Beneficial effects have also been found in studies focusing specifically on victims of complex trauma (primarily adult survivors of childhood sexual abuse) and including a wide variety of group treatment approaches such as problem-solving (Richter, Snider, & Gorey, 1997), affect management (Zlotnick et al., 1997), psychoeducation (Lubin, Loris, Burt, & Johnson, 1998), body-oriented interventions (Westbury & Tutty, 1999), trauma-focused therapy (Classen, Koopman, Nevill-Manning, & Speigel, 2001; Saxe & Johnson, 1999), and process groups (Carver, Stalker,

Stewart, & Abraham, 1989; Hazzard, Rogers, & Angert, 1993). Commonly reported improvements involve reductions in PTSD symptoms (e.g., Lubin et al., 1998), depression (e.g., Richter et al., 1997), and dissociation (e.g., Zlotnick et al., 1997), as well as increases in self-esteem and locus of control (e.g., Hazzard et al., 1993).

## GROUP TREATMENT
## AT THE VICTIMS OF VIOLENCE PROGRAM

The Victims of Violence Program (VOV) is an outpatient clinic of the Department of Psychiatry at the Cambridge Hospital, a public-sector hospital affiliated with Harvard Medical School, which serves an economically disadvantaged, multi-racial, and multi-cultural population. VOV provides victims of crime and violence with a range of clinical and community services, among which the group therapy program is a central component. Most VOV patients are survivors of prolonged and repeated interpersonal violence. Many are victims of chronic childhood abuse who have also experienced multiple traumas during their adult lives. Patients seeking services at VOV typically have a very complicated clinical presentation consistent with complex PTSD, as well as a variety of other stressors, such as unemployment, housing difficulties, and health concerns. Their comorbidity, multiple risk factors, and adverse life circumstances would frequently serve as exclusion criteria for many other types of group treatment.

The VOV approach to group therapy has several distinguishing features. It is informed by an explicit theoretical framework for trauma recovery, and uses this theory as a basis for focusing treatment, identifying existing sources of strength, and matching patients to appropriate groups. Group guidelines and support are used to provide a framework for the development of individualized treatment goals. The connections among group members are mobilized to rebuild relational capacities damaged by trauma. Co-leadership by therapists is intentionally designed to provide an alternative relational model. All VOV groups "model" the norms and values of safe and supportive community ecosystems.

### Stages-by-Dimensions Approach

The VOV utilizes a model for trauma recovery that integrates (a) an ecological view of trauma (Harvey, 1996); (b) recognition that recovery from trauma unfolds in a progressive, identifiable series of stages (Herman, 1992b); and (c) a multifaceted definition of what constitutes recovery and resilience (Harvey, 1996). The ecological framework (Harvey, 1996, this volume) draws upon the theoretical premise of community psychology to emphasize the complex interactions of individuals and their environments (Kelly, 1968, 1986; Moos, 2002), the reality of varied–even resilient and agentic–adaptations to conditions of extreme adversity (Riger, 2001; Sandler, 2001), and the viability of both clinical and community interventions (Cowen, 1994; Koss & Harvey, 1991). Within this framework, individual variations in traumatic response are attributed to a complex interplay of person, event, and environmental factors. These factors interact dynamically to produce individual difference in posttraumatic response and recovery. Thus, to be effective, interventions must be attuned to and achieve "ecological fit" with the survivor's unique personal, interpersonal, environmental, and socio-cultural circumstances. The ecological perspective provides an overall framework for assessing the symptoms and strengths and formulating the care of patients seeking treatment at the VOV (Lebowitz, Harvey, & Herman, 1993).

The stage model of trauma recovery developed by Herman (1992b) is based on the assumption that helplessness, meaningless, and disconnection from oneself and others are central components of the experience of interpersonal trauma. Empowerment and the creation of new meanings and connections are thus key aspects of the recovery process, which unfolds over three stages. The initial treatment goal and first stage of recovery involves the establishment of safety. This focus may begin with the body (e.g., regulation of basic functions such as sleep and eating; management of intrusive PTSD symptoms; control over self-destructive behaviors) and proceed outwards to the environment (e.g., establishment of a safe and stable living situation; attention to issues such as work and money). Only once safety is established can recovery move to the next stage where the focus is remembrance, integration, and mourning. The therapeutic work of the second stage involves carefully paced in-depth exploration of the traumatic experience(s), with the goal of integrating memory, affect, and cognition, rather than simply facilitating catharsis. This stage inevitably involves a period of intense grief and mourning, during which the victim is sustained by his or her connections to the therapist and peers, the hope of building new, more adaptive relationships, and the creation of new meaning in the traumatic experiences. The third stage of recovery involves reconnecting with others through the process of establishing mutual, non-exploitative relationships. The survivor may have to renegotiate the boundaries and limits of longstanding relationships, particularly those that have been abusive (Herman, 1992b; Lebowitz et al., 1993). The value of a phase-oriented approach to working with trauma survivors has been recognized across theoretical orientations and is now a core feature of many treatment models (Ford, Courtois, Steele, van der Hart, & Nijenhuis, 2005).

The VOV uses criteria developed by Harvey (1996) for assessing resilience and conceptualizing recovery in eight interrelated domains. These include (a) authority over memory: the process by which survivors experience a sense of choice and control over the remembering process; (b) integration of memory and affect: the extent to which survivors experience their memories as interwoven with feeling, including new feelings born of remembering and reflecting on the past; (c) affect tolerance: the degree to which survivors can bear painful feelings and experience their emotions in a differentiated way; (d) symptom mastery and positive coping: the extent to which survivors can anticipate, manage, contain, or prevent the cognitive and emotional disruption that arises from posttraumatic arousal; (e) self-esteem (self-care and self-regard): the degree to which survivors experience themselves as worthy of care and behave in ways that promote their best interest; (f) self-cohesion: the extent to which survivors can experience themselves as integrated or fragmented in regard to cognition, affect, or behavior; (g) safe attachment: the survivor's ability to negotiate and maintain personal safety within relational contexts and to develop feelings of trust, safety, and enduring connections with others; and (h) meaning-making: the process by which the survivor assigns new meaning to the trauma, to the self as survivor, and to the world in which the trauma occurred (Harney & Harvey, 1999; Harvey, 1996).

The stage model and the recovery criteria reviewed above can be integrated by using the eight criteria as dimensions of psychological functioning to be examined across each of the three stages of recovery. We call this a "stages-by-dimensions" analysis. This approach produces a matrix that can be used to identify the central tasks and sources of resilience within each dimension at each stage, thus providing a well-defined focus for treatment as well as explicit recognition of the specific strengths that the survivor brings to the recovery process. It is important to note that this model does not imply an invariant progression from one stage to the next in all domains. Rather, recovery is conceptualized as a dynamic process in which the individual may be more recovered and resilient on some domains than in others. He or she may move back and forth between stages based on the nature of the traumatic material encountered at the time, current life stressors, and the total resources of the individual. Survivors will also not typically be at one stage on all dimensions at one time. As treatment progresses, however, a consolidation of gains is expected, reflected in increased coping skills, increased integration of traumatic memory, and a more balanced perception of self and the world (Harvey et al., 2003; Lebowitz et al., 1993).

## Stage-Based Matching of Patients to Treatment

A major contribution of the VOV group treatment approach is its well-developed rationale for how to match patients to appropriate group treatments based on their stage of trauma recovery and the domains in which they experience greatest difficulty. Stage 1 groups are offered to patients whose primary needs involve the establishment of safety, stability, and self-care. These groups have a didactic format with an emphasis on helping participants develop behavioral, cognitive, and psychosocial skills for managing their symptoms and caring for themselves appropriately. They are present-focused and actively discourage significant disclosure of trauma histories to protect group members from becoming overwhelmed (Harney & Harvey, 1999). The VOV program currently offers three Stage 1 (safety and stabilization) groups: (a) Trauma Information Group, a manualized psycho-educational group where participants learn about the effects of trauma (Glass, Hamm, & Koenen, 1998); (b) Stress Management Group, a group aimed at helping participants achieve mastery over posttraumatic symptoms (Flannery, Perry, & Harvey, 1993); and (c) Safety and Self-Care Group (SSC), a group for participants who actively harm themselves or care for themselves in otherwise inadequate or self-destructive ways (Harney & Harvey, 1999). Survivors are ready for a Stage 2 group when safety and self-care are reasonably established, symptoms are under a comfortable degree of control, social supports are reliable, and life circumstances permit engagement in the demanding endeavor of trauma-focused work (Herman, 1992b). The VOV program offers separate Stage 2 groups for women and men, as well a co-ed group. These groups have as their focus the integration of the traumatic past with patients' present lives. A new group called Passageways was recently created to bridge the first and second stages of recovery, using expressive techniques. Stage 3 groups are not usually offered within VOV, partly due to the nature of the patient population served by the program and partly because heterogeneous psychotherapy groups that focus more generally on interpersonal issues are often more appropriate for individuals in this advanced stage of recovery than groups that revolve around their identity as trauma survivor.

### Focus on Individual Goals

During the screening process and early group sessions, members are helped to formulate specific individual goals attainable within the lifespan of the group that organize and focus their group work. The type of goals set for Stage 1 versus Stage 2 groups will clearly vary; patients in Stage 1 groups will work on goals related to safety, stabilization, and self-care, whereas the goals of patients in Stage 2 groups will focus on the integration of past trauma within their current lives. The stages-by-dimensions approach provides a helpful framework for identifying appropriate treatment goals.

### Relational Focus

A fundamental characteristic of the VOV treatment groups is the utilization of the connections that develop among group members as a central vehicle for change, with the underlying idea that the damage created by interpersonal trauma can only be corrected in a safe relationship. Although the interpersonal process among group members is not the focus of these groups, they rely heavily on the interpersonal context to facilitate the progress of individual group members. For example, a key aspect of these groups involves giving and receiving empathic feedback, and time is specifically allotted for this purpose after each member shares his or her goal-related work. Group leaders model the empathic feedback process and help members do the same. This feedback process is distinct from the process of "trading stories," and provides members with a reparative experience of mutuality and equality that counteracts the experiences of humiliation and subordination so familiar to the patients we treat. The group is also used as a powerful context in which survivors can rework maladaptive attributions about themselves and their experiences in the here-and-now. Negative and self-blaming self-statements that impede recovery are actively confronted by others who have had similar experiences. The direct use of the relational context of the group to facilitate healing distinguishes VOV group treatments from approaches that seek to effect change primarily by psychoeducation (e.g., Lubin et al., 1998), exposure and cognitive restructuring (e.g., Schnicke & Resick, 1993), skills training (e.g., Linehan, 1993), or other means.

## Co-Leadership

Co-leadership is a central feature of the VOV group program (Koss & Harvey, 1991). For the group members, co-leadership sets an example of a relationship of mutuality and collaboration in contrast to the relationships of domination and subordination that characterize the histories of so many patients. It provides an alternative experience of adult care taking, and models a cooperative and collective approach to solving problems and handling differences. It minimizes attributions of power and control to a single group leader. It also communicates the notion that one person cannot "do it all" without support. Co-leadership also has a number of important benefits for the group leaders. Most importantly, it provides therapists with the peer support and feedback that is essential in preventing vicarious traumatization and burnout (Yassen, 1995). In this way, co-leadership keeps the leaders safe so that they can extend safety to the group.

Having reviewed the literature on group therapy for interpersonal trauma and described the VOV approach to group treatment, we now present a vignette reflecting some of the ways in which groups can mobilize the resilience of individual members and function as a bridge to new community at different stages of recovery. Identifying details have been changed to protect patient confidentiality.

## CLINICAL VIGNETTE: LISA

Lisa was a participant in the Women's Time-Limited (WTL) group, a prototypical Stage 2 group for patients who have achieved sufficient safety and stability to look more directly at their traumatic experiences and their impact. This group involves active exploration of survivors' trauma histories with the overall aim of integrating memories and feelings about their past into their present lives. Participants included in such groups are typically doing reasonably well in their life, have several supportive relationships and a steady, strong individual therapy that addresses the impact of their trauma history, are involved in some consistent work or study, and have been free of any self-harming behaviors for at least one year. The specific domains of trauma recovery targeted by the WTL group include authority over memory, integration of memory with affect, self-esteem, safe attachment, and meaning making.

The clinical example of Lisa illustrates the ways in which the secrecy that fostered divisions within this patient's family, and then within herself, was replaced over the course of the group with a sense of choice about her ability to remain private or disclose her thoughts, feelings, and experiences. Increased abilities to integrate memory with emotion led Lisa to a stronger sense of self, which in turn, enabled her to widen her social support network significantly.

After six years of individual therapy, Lisa felt ready to join a psychotherapy group for female trauma survivors. Her therapist had suggested group treatment through the years, but Lisa's anxiety and fears about possible condemnation from a group made this a dim possibility until this point. Lisa had assembled a life of which she was quite proud, given the tumult of her earlier years. She had a solid relationship with her partner, and was the parent of a daughter, now four years old. She was a conscientious professional, respected for her careful work yet unknown to any social degree by her colleagues. She had a few good friends, but was always aware of an inner pressure to be pleasant and keep herself tucked away. Her partner was her steady confidante. To Lisa's own amazement, she widened her support by establishing an intimate rapport with her therapist.

Shame and self-blame were central themes early in her individual therapy. She had been abused by her father, a man beloved in the community for his humor and helpfulness. He had begun sexually abusing her when she was about four years old and continued until she reached puberty. Its end was marked by a bitter confrontation. Lisa's rage stood in stark contrast to the dissociative demeanor that she usually assumed when her father was near. Lisa suspected that her mother always knew about the abuse. She never addressed this issue with her directly, out of a desire to avoid feelings associated with this profound betrayal. She had one sister; the abuse by her father had created a deep sense of division between the two. Initially, she felt that she protected her sister by enduring the abuse. Later, she yearned to confide in her sister, but feared that she would not be believed or that she would taint her sister's seemingly close relationship with their father. Now in her adulthood, Lisa rarely saw other members of her family, all of whom resided in another state.

Disclosing the abuse to her sister was Lisa's primary goal as she interviewed for the WTL group at the VOV. She was apprehensive, though reachable, during the interview. She called to cancel her interest in the group not long after this first meeting. She stated that she did not know how she would mesh with the other members, and feared that her account would not be taken seriously. These fears were normalized for Lisa. Joining a new community, particularly one of abuse survivors, was understandably fraught with fear and anxiety for her. She had learned in the proverbial first group–namely, her family of origin–that betrayal was insured and isolation was her only protection. This lesson had now outlived its usefulness, however, and she acknowledged her restlessness to shed what had become a stifling armor. Rather than abandon her fears, she agreed simply to see if her worries would be confirmed. She closed this conversation with a renewed zest to begin group.

In the first few weeks of the WTL group, as expected, Lisa felt extremely shy and anxious. She fought the urge to dissociate, and would speak in a quiet, wavering voice, barely able to make eye contact with the other members. Her goal to disclose to her sister was broken down and it was recommended that she initially aim to speak about some aspect of her experience within group, with affective presence. Breaking the silence with a group of peers would be the first step toward breaking the silence with her sister.

Concurrently, Lisa witnessed the work of others in the group. The members felt her presence when they spoke. She gave thoughtful, heartfelt comments in response, and earned their respect and compassion. She was remarkably able to discuss the aftermath of revealing more of herself in group. She would refer to feeling anxious or dissociated, or signal that her fears of being disbelieved or disliked were activated. These statements served as an invitation for the other group members to help her alter the internal script that she would be betrayed if seen. They affirmed what she had shared and let her know how they experienced it, contradicting the toxic response that she expected. They would help her ground herself if needed, and praise her for the risks she was taking. As the group progressed and this graduated exposure to her past continued, Lisa appeared more embodied. She laughed more often, indulged in sarcasm, and shared poignant memories.

By the time the group moved toward its final five weeks, Lisa decided to forego her initial goal and not disclose to her sister. She felt it would be too rushed. She realized that the important preparation she needed–rehearsing the disclosure, exploring her hopes, assessing likely outcomes–would require much more time. At this point, the group and the group leaders could see the growing impact of her work as Lisa became more confident in evaluating her needs and in considering what was important to her in this process. She expressed contentment in her therapeutic work, and gradually wanted to disclose more until the close of the group. Her use of the relational connections in the group impacted her authority over memory. Memories that at one point had seemed terrifying to share she was now able to approach incrementally. Lisa's memories were varied and contextual. There was a sense of release when she would speak to her childhood experience, as if the lens was finally sharpening. Armed with the validation of attentive group members, her experience began to take a narrative shape, told in a somber, adult voice.

Lisa also utilized her experiences in the group to rework her sense of relationship with other people in her life. Faced with an upcoming family event, she used the group to strengthen her ability to let her sister know that she would bypass that gathering but wanted to make alternative plans for their own individual families to get together. This was something she had not dared do in the past. Similarly, she considered approaching her mother for some private time, something her mother historically was loath to do for fear of alienating her husband. She rehearsed what she might say, surprising herself with the sudden grief she felt at how much had been lost between the two of them.

Lisa was as reluctant to end group as she had been to begin. She laughed heartily about this at the end of the group. She planned to participate in another such group at some point in the future, after having fully digested this experience. Her accomplishments were evident to herself as well as to the other group members. Not only did Lisa have a more authentic relationship with her family, but she had shed her reflexive secret stance and became more open with others about her present life. A few months after the group's end, for example, she hosted a party at her home for her colleagues for the first time. The group provided a crucial template of acceptance that she could now transfer to another social setting.

## CONCLUSION

The groups described in this paper were developed to address different therapeutic goals depending on a survivor's stage of recovery and dimensions of psychological functioning most affected by trauma. They have in common an underlying ecological perspective that focuses attention on the group member's relationship with her environment at each stage of recovery. Thus, early in recovery when the goal of treatment is the establishment of safety and self-care, the group focuses not only on assisting the individual stabilize her symptomatic response, but also on helping her secure physical and emotional safety in the larger world. Later in recovery when reviewing the past becomes the focus of treatment, the group work draws attention to the ways in which the member's larger world may have kept her from seeking safety or caused her devalue herself. Consideration is then given to qualities of the larger environment that signal safety, support, and validation (replicated in group rules, values, and boundaries).

In the clinical vignette, we see an example of how group treatment, through its provision of an alternative relational experience, offers survivors the opportunity to rebuild the sense of belonging, connection, and community that trauma destroys. A commonality among the groups described here is the belief that a safe, structured network of relationships among peers and authority figures creates a crucible within which the isolation and alienation felt by trauma survivors can be reduced, their self-worth can be strengthened, and their values and expectations regarding interpersonal relationships can be reworked. In the clinical example, we see both the terrible legacy and enduring resilience that Lisa brought to the experience of group treatment. We see, too, evidence of how the group mobilizes the resilience of the individual member and how the anchoring of self to safe others in the treatment setting creates a bridge to new outside relationships. Lisa's ability to talk about her abuse in the group and thereby receive the support, empathy, and respect accorded to her was a veritable antidote to the years of invisibility and silence that she endured. As a result, she reclaimed parts of herself that had been shut down, and then reclaimed aspects of the relationships with her sister and mother that had not seemed possible previously. She was also more able to engage socially with her colleagues and integrate different aspects of her life. Lisa used group therapy in a way that fundamentally shifted her experience of herself and her relationships in her life beyond the group. In this way, groups function as bridges out of worlds in which violence and abuse, shame, and secrecy are familiar realities to new worlds in which survivors are able to seek and find membership in communities that reject violence, offer safe haven, and affirm the value of intimate, caring, and compassionate relationships.

## REFERENCES

Allen, S. N., & Bloom, S. L. (1994). Group and family treatment of post-traumatic stress disorder. *Psychiatric Clinics of North America, 17*, 425-437.

American Psychiatric Association. (1994). *Diagnostic and statistical manual of mental disorders* (4th ed.). Washington, DC: Author.

Boudewyn, A. C., & Liem, J. H. (1995). Childhood sexual abuse as a precursor to depression and self-destructive behavior in adulthood. *Journal of Traumatic Stress, 8,* 445-459.

Carver, C. M., Stalker, C. A., Stewart, E., & Abraham, B. (1989). The impact of group therapy for adult survivors of childhood sexual abuse. *Canadian Journal of Psychiatry, 34,* 753-758.

Classen, C. C., Koopman, C., Nevill-Manning, K., & Speigel, D. (2001). A preliminary report comparing trauma-focused and present-focused group therapy against a wait-listed control condition among childhood sexual abuse survivors with PTSD. *Journal of Aggression, Maltreatment & Trauma, 4,* 265-288.

Coid, J., Petruckevitch, A., Feder, G., Chung, W. S., Richardson, J., & Mooney, S. (2001). Relation between childhood sexual and physical abuse and risk of revictimisation in women: A cross-sectional survey. *The Lancet, 358,* 450-454.

Cowen, E. L. (1994). The enhancement of psychological wellness: Challenges and opportunities. *American Journal of Community Psychology, 22,* 140-179.

Drossman, D. A., Leserman, J., Nachman, G., Zhiming, L., Gluck, H., Toomey, T. C., et al. (1990). Sexual and physical abuse in women with functional and organic gastrointestinal disorders. *Annals of Internal Medicine, 113,* 828-833.

Dube, S. R., Anda, R. F., Felitti, V. J., Chapman D. P., Williamson, D. F., & Giles, W. H. (2001). Childhood abuse, household dysfunction, and the risk of attempted suicide throughout the lifespan: Findings from the Adverse Childhood Experiences study. *Journal of the American Medical Association, 286,* 3089-3096.

Edwards, V. J., Holden G. W., Felitti, V. J., & Anda, R. F. (2003). Relationship between multiple forms of childhood maltreatment and adult mental health in community respondents: Results from the Adverse Childhood Experiences study. *American Journal of Psychiatry, 160,* 1453-1460.

Felitti, V. J., Anda, R. F., Nordenberg, D., Williamson, D. F., Spitz, A. M., Ewards, V., et al. (1998). Relationship of childhood abuse and household dysfunction to many of the leading causes of death in adults: The Adverse Childhood Experiences (ACE) study. *American Journal of Preventive Medicine, 14,* 245-258.

Flannery, R., Perry, J. D., & Harvey, M. R. (1993). A structured stress-reduction approach modified for victims of psychological trauma. *Psychotherapy, 30,* 646-650.

Ford, J. D., Courtois, C. A., Steele, K., van der Hart, O., & Nijenhuis, E. R. S. (2005). Treatment of complex posttraumatic self-dysregulation. *Journal of Traumatic Stress, 18,* 437-447.

Foy, D. W., Glynn, S. M., Schnurr, P. P., Jankowski, M. K., Wattenberg, M. S., Weiss, D. S., et al. (2000). Group therapy. In E. B. Foa, T. M. Keane, & M. J. Friedman (Eds.), *Effective treatments for PTSD* (pp. 155-175). New York: The Guilford Press.

Glass, L., Hamm, B., & Koenen, K. (1998). *Trauma information group manual.* Unpublished manuscript.

Harney, P. A., & Harvey, M. R. (1999). Group psychotherapy: An overview. In B. H. Young & D. D. Blake (Eds.), *Group treatments for post-traumatic stress disorder* (pp. 1-13). New York: Brunner/Mazel.

Harvey, M. R. (1996). An ecological view of psychological trauma and trauma recovery. *Journal of Traumatic Stress, 9,* 3-23.

Harvey, M. R., Liang, B., Harney, P. A., Koenen, K., Tummala-Narra, P., & Lebowitz, L. (2003). A multidimensional approach to the assessment of trauma impact, recovery and resiliency: Initial psychometric findings. *Journal of Aggression, Maltreatment & Trauma, 6,* 87-109.

Harvey, M. R. (2007). Towards an ecological understanding of resilience in trauma survivors: Implications for theory, research, and practice. *Journal of Aggression, Maltreatment & Trauma, 14*(1/2), 9-32.

Hazzard, A., Rogers, J. H., & Angert, L. (1993). Factors affecting group therapy outcome for adult sexual abuse survivors. *International Journal of Group Psychotherapy, 43,* 453-468.

Herman, J. L. (1992a). Complex PTSD: A syndrome in survivors of prolonged and repeated trauma. *Journal of Traumatic Stress, 3,* 377-391.

Herman, J. L. (1992b). *Trauma and recovery.* New York: Basic Books.

Herman, J. L., Perry J. C., & van der Kolk, B. A. (1989). Childhood trauma in borderline personality disorder. *American Journal of Psychiatry, 146,* 490-495.

Herman, J., & Schatzow, E. (1984). Time-limited group therapy for women with a history of incest. *International Journal of Group Psychotherapy, 34,* 605-615.

Kelly, J. G. (1968). Toward an ecological conception of preventive intervention. In J. W. Carter, Jr. (Ed.), *Research contributions from psychology to community mental health* (pp. 75-99). New York: Behavioral Publications.

Kelly, J. G. (1986). Content and process: An ecological view of the interdependence of practice and research. *American Journal of Community Psychology, 14,* 581-589.

Koss, M. P., & Harvey, M. R. (1991). *The rape victim: Clinical and community interventions* (2nd ed.). Thousand Oaks, CA: Sage.

Lebowitz, L., Harvey, M. R., & Herman, J. L. (1993). A stage-by-dimension model of recovery from sexual trauma. *Journal of Interpersonal Violence, 8,* 378-391.

Lifton, R. J. (1973). *Home from the war: Vietnam veterans: Neither victims nor executioners.* New York: Simon & Schuster.

Linehan, M. M. (1993). *Cognitive-behavioral treatment of borderline personality disorder.* New York: Guilford Press.

Loewenstein R. J (1990). Somatoform disorders in victims of incest and child abuse. In R. Kluft, (Ed.), *Incest related syndromes of adult psychopathology* (pp. 75-112). Washington, DC: American Psychiatric Press.

Lubin, H., Loris, M., Burt, J., & Johnson, D. R. (1998). Efficacy of psychoeducational group therapy in reducing symptoms of posttraumatic stress disorder among multiply traumatized women. *American Journal of Psychiatry, 155,* 1172-1177.

Moos, R. (2002). The mystery of human context and coping: an unraveling of clues. *American Journal of Community Psychology, 30,* 67-88.

Richter, N. L., Snider, E., & Gorey, K. M. (1997). Group work intervention with female survivors of childhood sexual abuse. *Research on Social Work Practice, 7,* 53-69.

Riger, S. (2003). Transforming community psychology. *American Journal of Community Psychology, 29,* 62-81.

Sandler, I. (2003). Quality and ecology of adversity as common mechanisms of risk and resilience. *American Journal of Community Psychology, 29,* 19-61.

Saxe, B. J., & Johnson, S. M. (1999). An empirical investigation of group treatment for a clinical population of adult female incest survivors. *Journal of Child Sexual Abuse, 8*, 67-88.

Schnicke, M., & Resick, P. (1993). *Cognitive processing therapy for rape victims.* Thousand Oaks, CA: Sage.

Sewell, K. W., & Williams, A. M. (2001). Construing stress: A constructivist therapeutic approach to posttraumatic stress reactions. In R. A. Niemeyer (Ed.), *Meaning reconstruction and the experience of loss* (pp. 293-310). Washington, DC: American Psychological Association.

van der Kolk B. A., Pelcovitz, D., Roth, S., Mandel, F., McFarlane, A., & Herman J. L. (1996). Dissociation, affect dysregulation and somatization: The complexity of adaptation to trauma. *American Journal of Psychiatry, 153*(Festschrift Supplement), 83-93.

van der Kolk, B. A., Perry, J. C., & Herman, J. L.(1991). Childhood origins of self-destructive behavior. *American Journal of Psychiatry, 148*, 1665-1671.

Westbury, E., & Tutty, L. M. (1999). The efficacy of group treatment for survivors of childhood abuse. *Child Abuse and Neglect, 23*, 31-44.

Wurtele, S. K., Kaplan, G. M., & Keairnes, M. (1990). Childhood sexual abuse among chronic pain patients. *Clinical Journal of Pain, 6*, 110-113.

Yassen, J. (1995). Preventing secondary traumatic stress disorder. In C. Figley (Ed.), *Compassion fatigue: Coping with secondary traumatic stress disorder in those who treat the traumatized* (pp. 178-208). New York: Brunner/Mazel.

Zlotnick, C., Shea, M. T., Rosen, K. H., Simpson, E., Mulrenin, K., Begin, A. et al. (1997). An affect-management group for women with posttraumatic stress disorder and histories of childhood sexual abuse. *Journal of Traumatic Stress, 10*, 425-436.

doi:10.1300/J146v14n01_12

# Revolutionizing the Clinical Frame: Individual and Social Advocacy Practice on Behalf of Trauma Survivors

Carol Gomez

Janet Yassen

**SUMMARY.** In this article, we discuss the role of individual and social advocacy as practices that promote resilience and enhance the ecological relationship between trauma survivors and their communities. Issues of access, comprehension, linguistic and social isolation, cultural disorientation and displacement, and feelings of powerlessness within governmental and non-governmental systems encompass common challenges that trauma survivors experience. We discuss two composite cases that explore what individual advocacy and social action entail, how these activities can change a victim's relationship with, inform and mobilize health-promoting competencies within the larger community that assist in the healing from trauma. Included in the article are guidelines and handouts intended to be useful for service providers who are interested in incorporating advocacy into their work settings. doi:10.1300/J146v14n01_13 *[Article copies available for a fee from The Haworth Document Delivery Service: 1-800-HAWORTH. E-mail address: <docdelivery@haworthpress.com> Website: <http://www.HaworthPress.com> © 2007 by The Haworth Press, Inc. All rights reserved.]*

---

Address correspondence to: Carol Gomez, Victims of Violence Program, 26 Central Street, Somerville, MA 02143 (E-mail: caroljg@gmail.com).

[Haworth co-indexing entry note]: "Revolutionizing the Clinical Frame: Individual and Social Advocacy Practice on Behalf of Trauma Survivors." Gomez, Carol, and Janet Yassen. Co-published simultaneously in *Journal of Aggression, Maltreatment & Trauma* (The Haworth Maltreatment & Trauma Press, an imprint of The Haworth Press, Inc.) Vol. 14, No. 1/2, 2007, pp. 245-263; and: *Sources and Expressions of Resiliency in Trauma Survivors: Ecological Theory, Multicultural Practice* (ed: Mary R. Harvey, and Pratyusha Tummala-Narra) The Haworth Maltreatment & Trauma Press, an imprint of The Haworth Press, Inc., 2007, pp. 245-263. Single or multiple copies of this article are available for a fee from The Haworth Document Delivery Service [1-800-HAWORTH, 9:00 a.m. - 5:00 p.m. (EST). E-mail address: docdelivery@haworthpress.com].

**KEYWORDS.** Advocacy, trauma, resilience, social action

This article considers innovative advocacy practices based on an out-patient trauma clinic that incorporates a sociopolitical understanding of interpersonal violence and an approach to clinical care that is informed by an ecological understanding of psychological trauma (Harvey, 1996). The Victims of Violence Program (VOV) at the Cambridge Health Alliance (CHA), a teaching hospital of the Harvard Medical School, integrates mental health care with individual and social advocacy on behalf of victims. The program draws guidance and direction from a community and political perspective that is rooted in the ecological theory of community psychology and a feminist analysis of violence and abuse (Harvey, 1996; Harvey, this volume). Clinical and community services of the program are based on an ecological view of trauma and recovery from trauma, and are grounded in social movements that stress social justice. In 2000, with Victims of Crime Act (1984) funds administered by the Massachusetts Office of Victim Assistance, VOV expanded to include the Victim Advocacy and Support Team (VAST). VAST was developed as an expression of the value that VOV places on the aim of fostering both individual and community resilience through the medium of empowering interventions.

VAST was established on July 1, 2000 with the goal of developing advocacy services for crime victims throughout the multi-site public healthcare system of the CHA. The first 18 months of the program concentrated on intensive outreach to the various departments within the hospital setting. Today, VAST advocates assess client needs, assess the risk and safety of clients, offer supportive counseling, link clients to community resources, provide consultation to hospital staff and community settings to ensure appropriate care to clients in crisis, and initiate systemic and community change and interventions to improve the quality of care for survivors of violence. Now in its fourth year, VAST is a recognized and heavily utilized service. During the period July 1, 2003 until June 30, 2004, for example, VAST advocates served 116 crime victims, referred by six major service units within the hospital. Events precipitating these referrals included patient disclosures of contemporary or past partner or family violence, sexual assault, stranger assault, stalking, bias crime, workplace harassment, trafficking and labor exploitation, and torture and trauma experienced in home countries. Services rendered included centralized case coordination, safety planning, court accompaniment, legal advocacy (including probate, child custody and support, restraining order applications, immigration, and criminal court issues), emergency funds for food, clothing, and transportation, and housing and shelter advocacy.

This paper describes the VAST concept of advocacy; how it functions; how it provides individual, systemic, and community advocacy; and how it addresses barriers to collaboration. Incorporated into the text are guidelines designed to assist other settings as they incorporate advocacy into their service delivery system.

## ADVOCACY AS INDIVIDUAL AND SOCIAL JUSTICE

*Ad-vo-cate\n. 1. One that pleads the cause of another before a tribunal or judicial court \v. to plead in favor of, support* (Merriam Webster's Collegiate Dictionary, 1994)

The term advocacy is used throughout this article. What is meant by the role and practice of advocacy in working with victims of violence and trauma survivors in a mental health and healthcare setting? It is important to emphasize that the practice of advocacy in a mental health setting may be undertaken by clinicians, social workers, nurses, victim service professionals, psychiatrists and other physicians, health educators, medical interpreters, and hospital administrators; it may also be performed by those whose professional identity is that of Advocate. The work of advocacy constantly moves between the ecological realms of micro and macro, individual and sociopolitical, intra-psychic and relational. Examples of macro-level or systems-based advocacy include creating hospital policy that requires domestic violence screening by all physicians; educating child protective services workers about the complexities facing a mother escaping domestic abuse; and advocating for the state legislature to reinstate funding for rape crisis centers. These advocacy efforts are interrelated and interdependent. Advocates provide care in the contexts of community and institutional cultures. They identify and recognize gaps or obstacles in the provision of services.

## ADVOCACY IN THE AFTERMATH OF VIOLENCE:
## A CLIENT EXAMPLE
### (Based on a Composite of VAST Clients)

*Christina is a 36-year-old woman who was referred to VAST by her primary care physician at the hospital. Christina's husband had been abusive to her throughout their ten year marriage. In the last three years, the violence had escalated. Ray had hit her numerous times and demanded sex from her regardless of her consent. Eight months ago, Christina fled to a battered women's shelter but returned home after two weeks, hoping that things at home would improve. However, nothing changed. In fact, even though the physical violence decreased, her husband's emotional and psychological abuse of her worsened. Christina had not been sleeping well for months, was depressed, anxious, and easily startled. She complained of debilitating headaches. Christina confided in her doctor about the stresses in her relationship, when the doctor provided routine screening for domestic violence. She disclosed that Ray had raped her the night before. In addition to her physical care, which included a Sexual Assault Nurse Examine (SANE), her physician encouraged her to seek counseling and advocacy at VAST to help her deal with her situation, plan for her safety, and make decisions about criminal prosecution.*

In order to help clients effectively, mental health care providers must understand the complex interactions of clients with their social environments and consider how to facilitate client access services that are appropriate for them within these environments. VAST worked with Christina to help her assess her needs and her safety, and to sort through her ambivalence about leaving her husband. Christina did not accept the abuse or believe that she deserved such treatment. She did, however, hold on to the hope that her husband would change and would begin to respect her as an equal and to treat her with kindness and dignity. As a result of the years of abuse, and of at times being embarrassed and humiliated in public, Christina was socially isolated. Her self-esteem and social confidence had eroded. She never felt comfortable or safe making connections that her husband was certain to sabotage. Christina worked a minimum wage job as a sales assistant. She and Ray jointly owned their home. She contemplated separation, but felt terrified about how could support herself or continue the mortgage payments.

Christina's greatest source of anxiety, however, was that she was a dependant spouse of a United States citizen. She holds a passport from a country in South Asia, and Ray must sponsor her application for legal permanent residency (also commonly referred to as a "green card"). Since their relocation to the U.S., Ray had been tardy in completing the application papers. He constantly reminded Christina that her only hope of remaining in this country legally was through him and he used this reminder as a means to secure her compliance and her silence. When he finally did file her papers, which allowed her conditional residency and employment authorization, he undermined the process by writing a letter to immigration authorities withdrawing his support.

Advocacy with Christina included supportive, non-judgmental counseling aimed at empowering her to make decisions for herself and regain control over her life while supporting her choices and helping her move forward at a pace that was comfortable to her. The VAST advocate helped Christina continuously assess her risk and safety, validated her perceptions and instincts, and most importantly, offered her clear, accurate information about her options and the protections available to her as a victim of domestic violence. VAST advocacy helped Christina forge connections with a network of supportive resources, including a probate attorney, an immigration attorney familiar with domestic violence case law, and court-based victim witness advocates in case she decided to obtain a restraining order and file criminal charges against Ray. Christina also joined a community-based support group for battered women that helped her realize that she was not alone in her situation, and to receive positive validation, gain confidence, connect socially with others, and believe in her own worth and potential.

A year and a half after coming to VAST, Christina made the difficult decision to obtain a restraining order and remove her abusive husband from her home. Christina has rented the extra room in her house in order to secure additional income to support her mortgage payments. She is also embarking on two new business ventures in catering and as a cosmetologist, aside from her regular job, which both supplements her income and allows her to make use of her creative talents and of her natural social inclinations. She is beginning to organize women in her community to support each other and break their isolation. While her life is still intertwined with Ray because of various court actions still in process, and although she still fears him, she is able to face court appearances with more confidence, feels entitled to live her life free from abuse, has expanded her social network, and enjoys her liberation from a life of daily terror.

Clients who are referred to VAST often experience factors in their lives that increase their vulnerability, limit their access to more traditional services, and need to be taken into consideration when developing a comprehensive treatment plan. The tools of advocacy need to be expanded to incorporate these added vulnerabilities. For instance, if Christina had been a part of a same-sex couple, safety planning and intervention would need to consider the dynamics and realities of the gay, lesbian, bisexual, transgender, and queer (GLBTQ) communities they may belong to. Screening for abuse, particularly emotional and psychological violence, with same-sex couples can be complex and perhaps less evident, given a presumed parity of gender roles. In addition, since services specific to GLBTQ communities are limited within any service region, it may be common for both parties to be seeking services and utilizing the same limited resources. If Christina had been a woman who spoke little or no English or was hearing impaired, intervention might have looked a little different from what was offered to her by VAST. The advocate would have had to work closely with an interpreter or find a service provider with specialized expertise who might be able to offer her advocacy and counseling in her own language. If there were no service providers in the local area who might be able to work directly with her, then the advocate would offer to work in close consultation and collaboration with service providers and specialized services from outside the region to ensure Christina's safety.

### *ADVOCACY PRACTICE: SAFETY PLANNING, RISK ASSESSMENT, AND NEEDS ASSESSMENTS*

Many victims of crime or violence do not need in-depth therapy to begin reconstructing life after victimization. Effective intervention, building links with appropriate resources, and education about rights and reassurance that what they are feeling and experiencing in the aftermath is normal can be equally important resources toward restoring equilibrium and promoting resilient response to violent and abusive circumstances. Essential components of crisis intervention and advocacy include client needs assessment, continuous safety planning, and risk assessment. Three main areas of safety that require assessment are: (a) safety from perpetrators of violence; (b) safety from re-traumatization and adverse consequences of being involved in community systems, such as the criminal justice system, shelter, child protective services; and (c) availability of resources to meet basic needs such as sustenance, shelter, clothing, medical and mental health care, income/ employment, mobility/transportation, immigration status, ability to communicate/linguistic, and able-ness access.

Once these areas are identified, it is important to empower the client to take steps to reclaim and resume control of her life. Education about rights, legal information, strategy, and linkages to appropriate resources are tools for empowering clients and helping them to achieve safety, control, and self-confidence. It is important to make clients aware of all options and information available, and with input, to fully allow the client to make decisions about her strategy herself.

## *IT TAKES A VILLAGE . . . CREATING A COORDINATED COMMUNITY RESPONSE*
### *(Created from Composite Referrals)*

*Anita was a 29-year-old computer engineer. She had recently gone out on a date with a young man she had met over the Internet. The date was uneventful and Anita did not feel any strong connection to this person. However, over the next five months, Anita was stalked by this individual. He had tracked down her home address, her sister's home address, constantly left messages on her voicemail, and sent her barrages of unwanted email messages, some of which were sexually threatening and explicit. He implied that since he knew where her sister and her family lived he would be paying them a visit soon if she did not return his overtures. She made phone contact with him a few times in an attempt to set boundaries and politely reject his unwanted advances, but he persisted. She found notes on her car, flowers sent to her home, phone calls to her workplace. Her life was altered and she was living in constant fear. She believed his threat to harm her family, which paralyzed her. She was too afraid to call the police and worried that they would not take her seriously. Moreover, she did not understand that what was happening to her was a criminal act. She came in for counseling and advocacy. She was pale, drawn, anxious, and had lost a great deal of weight due to the stress.*

The VAST advocate offered Anita supportive counseling and spent time strategizing with her how to keep herself safe and also what legal and civil recourse she might have available to her. Over the next few weeks, she made some small but practical changes, such as deciding to change her cell phone number and email account. With the advocate's support, Anita decided that she needed to get her workplace involved in her safety plan, since she was getting both unwanted calls and emails from him at the office. She met with her manager, with the support of her advocate who provided consultation to the process. Together, Anita, her manager, and the advocate developed a plan for ensuring her safety at work. This included having the receptionist screen all calls coming into her line and having her computer support department place a block on incoming emails from the stalker's address.

Anita also chose to make use of the criminal justice system. With her permission, the advocate contacted the detective in her neighborhood to explain Anita's plight. The advocate and the detective spent time thinking of workable safety strategies. One strategy was to put Anita in touch with her local neighborhood watch, with detailed information about the stalker. The detective then reached out to Anita, by offering to meet with her and her sister at their homes in order to develop a detailed safety plan and provide them with extra security patrols in their respective neighborhoods. Anita was not comfortable about pressing charges against the stalker, but just wanted the behavior to stop. The detective also directly confronted the stalker and issued him a severe warning about his conduct. Anita also expressed an interest in getting trained in self-defense. She joined a self-defense course that helped her gain confidence.

The result of these varied efforts was a multifaceted safety strategy that entailed close coordination of safety planning by the advocate, Anita, the detective, her parents, her workplace supervisor and staff, the neighborhood watch crew and the self-defense instructors. It was a tailor-made intervention strategy that eventually ended the perpetrator's behavior and resulted in Anita feeling safe, well cared for, and secure with the intervention and with the response of her community. She became less anxious, her appetite resumed, and she slowly began to resume normal function. Once safe, Anita began the journey of acknowledging the emotional and physical fear that she lived under at that time and the effects on future relationships.

## *BEYOND CLINICAL WALLS*

The World Health Organization defines health as "a state of physical, mental and social well being, not just the absence of disease or ailment."[1] This includes emotional, social, and physical welfare and is determined not only by biology, but also by social, political, and economic welfare. In her recommendations for advocacy practice within healthcare settings, labor rights activist and researcher Lora Jo Foo relates best practices in achieving health to the "public health" model (Foo, 2002). Health providers and their patients work in partnership to move patients from "communities of recovery" to "communities of resistance"; to become empowered and knowledgeable; and to recognize and, when safe and possible, to resist systemic and individual oppression, as survivors, activists, mothers, sisters, brothers, and/or healers in our communities (Foo, 2002).

Despite theoretical and social awareness, clients who are trauma survivors often find it difficult to find adequate care. There are very few programs that understand the need for both individual care and an ecological approach to providing care. On the contrary, there is evidence of considerable tension between community-oriented groups and mental health providers. For instance, a survey conducted in 1994 by the National Resource Center on Domestic Violence indicated that over half (53%) of statewide domestic violence coalitions did not feel that mental health professionals understood the dynamics of battering and/or how to assist in safety planning for women and children (Gondolf, 1997). Despite pockets of better working relationships, this mistrust continues today, with reports of mental health providers not valuing or respecting the experience of community advocates. Philosophical and practical differences can be experienced as obstacles to care and confusing for victims of violence, who may be caught in differences of value systems.

The setting and mission in which mental health services are delivered shape the response and services that victims of violence receive. It is, therefore, important to understand some of the challenges that impede the delivery of comprehensive services within a mental health setting and to consider recommendations or opportunities for enhancing your effectiveness as a clinician and advocate. Advocacy involves taking care of clients beyond the confines of the clinical hour and the location of the therapeutic environment. It requires taking an active stand against violence and voicing that premise with your client.

## INSIDER, OUTSIDER

The role of advocacy is determined and affected by the context in which it occurs. Over the last 30 years, advocates for crime victims and battered women have expanded beyond domestic violence shelter programs and rape crisis centers and are now located within court systems, police departments, housing developments, children's services, and healthcare settings. Different contexts provide diverse theoretical approaches and multiple and sometimes conflicting goals for advocacy (Davies, 1998). Victim advocates housed within established institutional structures are in a unique position of being both part of the system and being critical toward and challenging that same system, when necessary.

Clinical practice and advocacy practice are interdependent. The inter-relationship of each discipline can assist in accountability to the inherent goal of being client and community centered. Both lend equal value to the other through the expansion of context for providing holistic and client centered care.

## IMPLICATIONS FOR PRACTICE: GUIDELINES FOR EFFECTIVE ADVOCACY

What can you do to become an effective advocate in your clinical work? Ten attributes are described in the following section as underpinnings of effective clinical advocacy practice.

### 1. Become Knowledgeable About the Systems with Which Victims of Violence May Interface

*Why it is important.* Your anticipation of the strengths and barriers of the system can help you help your client maneuver within the system smoothly and can prepare the client to face those systems effectively. Preparing your client for potential barriers within systems can be useful in preventing and reducing secondary victimization and can help her make more informed choices about steps she can take to keep safe. This systems knowledge will also help you gain understanding and empathy for your client's struggles with the system. When we consider Christina and Anita's cases, a lack of awareness of resources, legal information, or how to utilize systems effectively can create additional difficulties for them both. For instance, if clinicians or medical care providers are not aware that most states have specialized Sexual Assault Nurse Examiners, who are trained to conduct comprehensive medical and forensic examinations for sexual assault survivors, then critical evidence to a criminal case against an offender may be lost. Being an undocumented immigrant, homeless, and/or without health insurance creates additional complications for any client and compromises their emotional functioning.

Clinicians should take the time to become aware of local resources to help clients with these survival needs. In rural areas, you may be less likely to be able to locate the services that someone like Christina might need. Therefore, it may be necessary to lobby for more state funds to enter your area for services and to develop relationships with social services and informal community network in your area for consultation, information, and resource sharing.

*What you can do.*

- Educate yourself about relevant systems. Build alliances with other providers in your own agency or system, and familiarize yourself with in-house resources.
- Build alliances in the community (e.g., with immigration attorneys, probation departments).
- Contact probate lawyers, child protective services workers, domestic violence detectives in local precincts, and victim witness advocates in local prosecutors offices. Offer cross training to each other's staffs. Participate in or initiate community-wide efforts to develop new services, resources, or prevention initiatives. Resource development can diminish the powerlessness that clinicians can feel in the face of inadequate support for their clients.
- Accompany your client to their appointments in court or with their divorce/probate attorney or to the welfare office when possible and appropriate. This helps you to learn first hand what it takes for you and your client to interface with often complicated agencies. Consult the Internet, as many community agencies now have their resources posted and can help familiarize you with local services.
- Include resources packets in all training and orientation materials.

## 2. Advocate for Your Clients in Community Settings

*Why this is important.* Pro-active outreach on the part of a provider to a collateral system provider can go a long way in creating a respectful connection and safe pathway for your client to the referral agency. This particularly rings true in environments, such as police departments, emergency rooms, or child protective services, where crime victims are easily overlooked, lost, or misunderstood. Take this opportunity to educate providers in other systems about the impact of trauma on a crime victim, in order that they are sensitized to the common reactions to trauma that a client may be experiencing.

*What you can do.* A simple call ahead from you as an advocate or representative of healthcare agency fulfills several functions. Accompanying your client to daunting institutions can offer a great deal of

emotional relief and give courage to your client in that situation. This
can be an opportunity to forge a trusting relationship with the providers
on the other side, not only for your client, but also for future clients who
may need their services.

### 3. Facilitate Collaboration, Communication, and Coordinated Response

*Why this is important.* Teamwork and a coordinated community response create a strong safety net for our clients and for future clients.
The relationship built with another provider can enhance creative
problem solving. Coordinated teamwork will also help build confidence of the client and reduce the likelihood of oversights, errors, and
miscommunication being made within the system.

*What you can do.* Keep communication lines among clients and providers open (within the requirements of client and professional confidentiality). Try to resolve interpersonal disputes or disagreements with
colleagues outside of the professional setting, so that these will not in-
terfere with the care of the client. Take time to communicate clearly
with one another about differing perspectives of intervention and care
of the client. Do not hold the individual provider in each system at fault
for institutional policies over which they have no control. Realize that
together we have the power to effect change and paradoxically to transform our own powerlessness within the system.

### 4. Provide and Get Support from Other Providers

*Why this is important.* Providing services to crime victims and abuse
survivors often involves complicated negotiations and can produce a
great deal of anxiety, stress, and compassion fatigue in a caregiver, particularly if a client is still living in an unsafe situation. Positive working
relationships with all providers from the various systems involved with
the trauma survivor can help lessen the stress and burden of responsibility for the safety of our clients. The support given and received can help
reduce secondary trauma for providers.

*What you can do.* Genuinely support each other. Check in periodically,
if only to leave a quick message or email note validating one another's
work, venting constructively about systemic glitches, and acknowledging
how scared, frustrated, or pleased we are about the case.

## 5. Expand and Enhance Your Training and Education Curriculum

*Why this is important.* Mental health providers often do not receive training in their professional education regarding assessment of violence-related factors affecting mental health outcomes. Although many professional schools do offer a trauma-related curriculum, it is often not a requirement. Given our growing awareness of the prevalence of violence in the general population, it is important that mental health training include attention to the social realities of client's lives and to the role of other community-based resources in improving mental health. It is crucial, too, that mental health education and training include attention to cultural forces and offer the clinician opportunities to explore one's own racial, class, and ethnic identity, sexual orientation, and blind spots, which influence how and by whom services are delivered.

*What can you do.*

- Evaluate the professional training curriculum available to you and develop onsite training that includes universal screening for violence and abuse.
- Participate in community-based task forces that inform members about the resources of their own community agencies.
- Develop protocols to assess and provide services for victims of violence that are systemically available and user friendly.
- Assess your setting's multi-cultural curriculum, being sure that it includes opportunities for self-evaluation and growth in order to manage possible unintentional clinical failures and counter-transference traps.

## 6. Actively Learn About and Integrate Different Theoretical Approaches

*Why this is important.* Most mental health clinicians are trained in medical model approaches to providing treatment, which emphasize individual pathology, family dysfunction, and early development. Within this model, there is less awareness of the mental health consequences of violence and abuse. Consequently, medical model approaches to evaluation, diagnosis, and treatment of survivors of violence can constrain or even be harmful to survivors seeking treatment. For instance, if the clinician who first met with Christina had emphasized Christina's early relationships with her family in her initial evaluation, Christina's ability to access much-needed assistance in the here and now could be compromised. Christina may also have been reluctant to talk openly with an evaluator for fear of deportation or to protect those who may have helped her to gain entry to this country illegally. She may also have been reluctant to accept medication to relieve some of her symptoms; for fear that she would be less able to be hypervigilant in order to protect herself. Without this contextual understanding of Christina's presentation and circumstance, the evaluator may have assessed her mental status as "guarded, mistrusting, withholding, non-engaging," or even "treatment resistant."

In addition, treatment evaluation in and of itself might be so foreign to some patients that they need an initial orientation session in order to be able to fully participate in the process. People who come from situations of prolonged and/or chronic trauma or from non-Western countries may have a mistrust or fear of authority or confusion about the therapeutic process, despite our own good will and intentions. Different theoretical orientations can inadvertently lead to inappropriate treatment. For instance, if you are trained in family systems theory, you might suggest that couples treatment is appropriate as a part of a plan for batterer intervention. However, this viewpoint is not applicable when abuse is present. While abuse is still occurring, couples treatment can actually be harmful until the abuser receives specialized treatment.

*What you can do.*

- Invite adherents of diverse perspectives and intervention strategies to participate in onsite training, and facilitate ongoing relationships.
- Create a value system that emphasizes an ecological perspective, one that understands and appreciates the significance of the clients own environment as well as the environment in which care is delivered.
- Include diverse theoretical views as part of core curriculum and concepts.
- Develop supervision guidelines that include the expectation of exploration of personal, professional, and client cultural, racial, ethnic, and sexual orientation as part of sound clinical practice.
- Speak up when you hear misinformation, distortions, lack of awareness, or narrow mindedness in your own settings, educational insti-

tutions, or public forums. Silence perpetuates inadequate care and social injustice.
- Find peer support.

## 7. Advocate for Systemic Change: Time and Productivity Challenges

*Why this is important.* Assisting victims of violence with their various needs often involves collateral contacts, which exceed the traditional 45-50 minute therapeutic hour. This is rarely built into mental health clinical time. Additionally, clients' life situations may require them to attend court appearances, other medical appointments, housing or job interviews, and the like. Therefore, they may need to cancel their therapy appointments, which affect the clinician's productivity–a strong requirement in managed care environments and in light of the many economic pressures facing healthcare institutions. Maintaining flexibility for maximum client care can paradoxically place the clinician in a difficult position, adding new stressors to the stress of attending to the multiple needs of victims of violence.

*What you can do.*

- Develop a positive working environment that appreciates rather than questions the clients' multiplicity of life demands and the demands that these may places on care providers, including the hours of collateral time which may go undocumented and unvalued in a traditional mental health setting.
- Seek sources of outside funding to minimize reliance on health insurance as the sole source of reimbursement for clinical services.
- Create a crisis/walk-in service that could assist in providing non-scheduled appointments for clients who are unable to attend regularly scheduled appointments.
- Develop relationships with community-based resources that might assist in escorting clients to their appointments.
- Participate in legislative policy reforms to ensure that healthcare and mental health care funding is not further reduced in state and federal budgets. Contact your legislators. Inform your clients about they can be involved, if they choose.
- Unionize workers to collectively empower your professional group to have more bargaining power to ensure that practice expectations are productive to clients' health and safety as well as to providers' ability to provide quality care for clients.

## 8. Address the Historic Mistrust Between Mental Health Clinicians and Community-Based Advocates

In the 1994 survey of state domestic violence coalitions conducted by the National Resources Center on Domestic Violence, respondents to the survey felt that "mental health professionals do not respect the work of battered women's advocates and that clinicians considered advocates to be of lower status" (Gondolf, 1997, p. 6). This view is reinforced when professional organizations are reluctant to grant continuing educational credits to conference presenters who do not have professional degrees. Community advocates are mistrustful of mental health professionals who do not understand how do write evaluations or document mental health visits that do not compromise a woman's safety or who discharge a patient to the street without adequate safety planning or linkages to needed resources.

*What you can do.* Develop mutual relationships and mutual training opportunities to learn from each other. Plan a conference together, which brings multiple perspectives and equal participation as presenters.

## 9. Move Beyond Clinical Walls

*Why this is important.* Most clinical work occurs in clinical offices. When it is difficult for clients to leave their homes due to poor health, lack of childcare, no transportation, disability, emotional crises, and other circumstances, clinicians are often unable to make home visits due to constraints of time or limits on insurance coverage. This situation can unintentionally withhold services from clients who need the care. In addition, some clients have a mistrust of institutional care. They may have had bad experiences in the past or come from a country where the state has used social institutions as a weapon of harm.

*What you can do.* Develop creative ways to secure coverage for off site visits (including alternative funding sources). Work collaboratively with community agencies that have more flexibility and mobility in their provision of services.

## 10. Evaluate Your Program

In order to remain truthful to the mission and philosophy of your advocacy program, it is crucial to conduct periodic evaluations to determine if the direction and evolution of your advocacy practice is in synchrony with the changing needs and realities of the communities you serve. The political climate, changing demographics, social and economic welfare policies, immigration policies, and legal reform can directly impact your clients' lives. The complexity of global trauma requires new services to meet new demands.

*What you can do.* Engage in a regular evaluation process that includes assessing your current program, existing systems, and changing community needs. This evaluation process should ensure that the care that we offer our trauma survivors maintains its integrity.

## CONCLUSION:
## SURVIVAL AND HEALING AS A REVOLUTIONARY ACT

It is a revolutionary human act to survive, recognize, and continuously heal from the wounds of gross human and civil rights violations; to overcome emotional, psychic, and psychological scars; to recover from physical bruises; to struggle with sexuality and intimacy issues; to regain control over mind, body, and spirit where control was taken away or never afforded; and to confront and survive within oppressive systems, familial or institutional.

Individual and social advocacy practices in the care of trauma survivors rely on the principle of empowerment, and they engage us as allies with our clients and our communities to foster the healing and restoration necessary to the nurturing of spirit, mind, and body. Offering advocacy and care from a social justice framework also acknowledges our collective vulnerability to violence, oppression, and trauma at any point in our lives, regardless of class, race, education status, nationality, sexual orientation, political affiliation, and medical or mental health status.

Brazilian educator Freire (1994) describes the process of liberation of mind, spirit and physical being as consisting of action and reflection–a praxis that then leads to the transformation of the world. He discusses this human activity as theory and practice, reflection and action. He calls for the revolutionary effort to radically transform oppressive structures (individual or state perpetrators of violence) not by the designation of its leaders as its thinkers and the oppressed (trauma survivors) as mere doers, but for the authentic empowerment of the oppressed from within to lead the path to their own liberation. The healing, survival, caretaking, and care giving of client, community, and advocates is a practice of empowerment, mutual respect, struggle, and perpetual hope in the restoration of justice, dignity, self worth, and a future that values and is free of the pain of violence and oppression.

## NOTE

1. Preamble to the Constitution of the World Health Organization as adopted by the International Health Conference, New York, 19-22 June, 1946; signed on 22 July 1946 by the representatives of 61 States (Official Records of the World Health Organization, no. 2, p. 100) and entered into force on 7 April 1948.

## REFERENCES

Davies, J. (1998). *Safety planning for battered women: Complex lives, difficult choices.* Thousand Oaks: Sage.

Foo, L. (2002). *Asian American women: Issues, concerns, and responsive human and civil rights advocacy.* New York: Ford Foundation.

Freire, P. (1994). *Pedagogy of the oppressed.* New York: Continuum Publishing Co.

Gondolf, E. (Ed) (1997). *Assessing woman battering in mental health services.* Thousand Oaks: Sage.

Harvey, M. R. (1996). An ecological view of psychological trauma and trauma recovery. *Journal of Traumatic Stress,* 9(1), 3-23.

Harvey, M. R. (2007). Towards an ecological understanding of resilience in trauma survivors: Implications for theory, research, and practice. *Journal of Aggression, Maltreatment & Trauma, 14*(1/2), 9-32.

*Merriam Webster's Collegiate Dictionary* (10th ed.). (1994). Springfield, MA: Merriam-Webster.

Victims of Crime Act of 1984, 42 U.S.C.A. §10601 *et seq.*

## RECOMMENDED READING

Abraham, M. (2000). *Speaking the unspeakable: Marital violence among South Asian immigrants in the United States.* New Brunswick, NJ: Rutgers University Press.

de Becker, G. (1997). *The gift of fear: Survival signals that protect us from violence.* Toronto, Canada: Little Brown & Co.

Fortune, M. (1987). *Keeping the faith.* Australia: Harper Collins Publishers.

Gilligan, J. (1996). *Violence: Reflections on a national epidemic.* New York: Vintage Books.

Herman, J. (1992). *Trauma and recovery.* New York: Basic Books.

Hathaway, J., Willis, G., & Zimmer, B. (2002). Listening to survivors' voices: Addressing partner abuse in the health care setting. *Violence Against Women,* 8(6), 687-719.

Koss, M., & Harvey, M. R. (1991). *The rape victim: Clinical and community interventions.* Thousand Oaks, CA: Sage.

Lobel, K. (1986). *Naming the violence: Speaking out about lesbian battering.* Seattle, WA: The Seal Press.

Marcella, A. J., Friedman, M. J., & Gerrity, E. T. (1966) *Ethnocultural aspects of posttraumatic stress disorder: Issues, research and clinical applications.* Washington, DC: American Psychological Association.

Martin-Baro, I. (1994). *Writings from liberation psychology.* Cambridge, MA: Harvard University Press.

Schechter, S., & Jones, A. (1992). *When love goes wrong: What to do when you can't do anything right.* New York: Harper Perennial.

Slater, L., Daniel, J. H., & Banks, A. E. (2003). *The complete guide to mental health for women.* Boston, MA: Beacon Press.

Volpp, L., & Marin, L., (1995). *Working with battered immigrant women: A handbook to make services accessible.* San Francisco, CA: Family Violence Prevention Fund.

Yassen, J. (1995) Preventing secondary traumatic stress disorder. In C. Figley (Ed.), *Compassion fatigue: Coping with secondary traumatic stress in those who treat the traumatized* (pp. 178-208). New York: Brunner/Mazel.

Yassen, J., & Harvey, M. (1998). Crisis assessment and interventions with victims of violence. In P. M. Kleespies (Ed.), *Emergencies in mental health practice: evaluation and management* (pp. 117-144). New York: The Guilford Press.

Zhan, L. (Ed.) (1999). *Asian voices: Asian and Asian American health educators speak out.* Sudbury, MA: Jones and Bartlett Publishing.

doi:10.1300/J146v14n01_13

# Fostering Resilience
# in Traumatized Communities:
# A Community Empowerment Model
# of Intervention

Mary R. Harvey
Anne V. Mondesir
Holly Aldrich

**SUMMARY.** This paper describes the history, composition, and community intervention activities of the Community Crisis Response Team (CCRT) of the Victims of Violence Program and the community empowerment model of intervention that guides its work. The paper uses a single case study to illustrate the nature of community-wide trauma, the core attributes of ecologically informed and effective community intervention, and the intervention design, implementation, and evaluation processes that are embedded in the community empowerment model. The paper includes a description of the CCRT's approach to the conduct

---

Address correspondence to: Mary R. Harvey, 26 Central Street, Somerville, MA 02143.

[Haworth co-indexing entry note]: "Fostering Resilience in Traumatized Communities: A Community Empowerment Model of Intervention." Harvey, Mary R., Anne V. Mondesir, and Holly Aldrich. Co-published simultaneously in *Journal of Aggression, Maltreatment & Trauma* (The Haworth Maltreatment & Trauma Press, an imprint of The Haworth Press, Inc.) Vol. 14, No. 1/2, 2007, pp. 265-285; and: *Sources and Expressions of Resiliency in Trauma Survivors: Ecological Theory, Multicultural Practice* (ed: Mary R. Harvey, and Pratyusha Tummala-Narra) The Haworth Maltreatment & Trauma Press, an imprint of The Haworth Press, Inc., 2007, pp. 265-285. Single or multiple copies of this article are available for a fee from The Haworth Document Delivery Service [1-800-HAWORTH, 9:00 a.m. - 5:00 p.m. (EST). E-mail address: docdelivery@haworthpress.com].

of traumatic stress debriefings and a discussion of the practical and theoretical implications of the CCRT. doi:10.1300/J146v14n01_14 *[Article copies available for a fee from The Haworth Document Delivery Service: 1-800-HAWORTH. E-mail address: <docdelivery@haworthpress.com> Website: <http://www.HaworthPress.com> © 2007 by The Haworth Press, Inc. All rights reserved.]*

**KEYWORDS.** Community intervention, crisis response, trauma, traumatic stress debriefing, community empowerment

## *COMMUNITY TRAUMA: A CASE EXAMPLE*

An 18-year-old high school graduate is fatally shot while walking to a bus stop near the housing development where he grew up.[1] Across the street, several young children are playing in a neighborhood playground. Nearby, a group of city officials are meeting with a gathering of elderly residents, and, within earshot of the shooting, employees and customers of a neighborhood grocery store quickly become terrified witnesses to the chaos that follows: the sirens, the panic and confusion, and the terror that, for some, vividly recalls other violent events.

According to neighborhood residents, this young man and his family were well known and well liked. He had been a varsity athlete at his high school and since graduating had been coaching neighborhood youngsters from all segments of this ethnically and linguistically diverse community. He was related to a former city council member, and his grandmother was an active participant in housing and neighborhood development programs.

This was the fourth of five murders that occurred within a two-month period in a city where crime is on the rise but homicide is still a rare event. In its wake, a number of community groups were profoundly affected: members and friends of the victim's large and extended family, neighborhood residents and workers, children on the playground when the shooting occurred, their families and friends; teachers and school administrators who feared that at least some of these children had witnessed the shooting; and the victim's own friends, coaches, and teachers. Also affected was a community group unknown to the victim, namely, a group of high school seniors who were about to begin running summer camp programs for children in the neighborhood. Many of these students felt completely unprepared to assist children who may have been present at or affected by the shooting. Some feared for their own physical safety.

Violent crime can have traumatic impact on entire communities and on many different segments of affected communities. In the aftermath of violence, any number of community settings may become focal points of intervention. Crisis teams may enter a school or workplace following a shooting that has been witnessed by students or co-workers, for example, and trauma experts may meet with various at-risk and affected community groups. Indeed, community crisis response has become rather standard fare in the experience of communities affected by catastrophic events (Dyregrov, 1997; Kaplan, Iancu, & Bodner, 2001; Norris & Thompson, 1995; Paton, 1995; Raphael, 1986). Despite the best efforts of many crisis respondents, however, an increasingly divided literature cautions that even the most well meaning community interventions can have harmful rather than helpful effects (Bisson & Deahl, 1994; McNally, Bryant, & Ehlers, 2003; Raphael, Meldrum, & MacFarlane, 1995). Moreover, communities differ considerably in their need for and receptivity to outside intervention.

## *RESPONDING TO COMMUNITY TRAUMA*

In the days and weeks following this homicide, during which time no suspect was named and no assailant apprehended, many affected communities learned of and sought assistance from the Community Crisis Response Team (CCRT)[2] of the Victims of Violence (VOV) Program. Each request was assessed and responded to by the team's core administrative staff who, in turn, worked with community representatives to consider if and how the CCRT might be helpful, to plan interventions tailored to the needs, resources, values, and traditions of each "client community," and to consider who among the team's many volunteer members might participate. Team members familiar with the neighborhood were asked about community demographics and relationships among various segments of the community, for example. Team members fluent in Spanish, Portuguese, and Haitian-Creole and those who were licensed mental health professionals with expertise in working with children or the elderly were asked to be available for interventions on behalf of specific groups.

Over time, the CCRT implemented several responses. Soon after the event, for example, the CCRT Coordinator consulted with city officials, the manager of the housing development, and leaders of its tenants' association to plan a timely and informative community meeting. Team members fluent in various languages later attended that meeting as translators and support personnel. Over the next several weeks, some staff and team members conducted a traumatic stress debriefing with employees of the neighborhood grocery, while others met with a group of Central American immigrants who had experienced significant violence in their homelands. At these events, licensed clinicians provided support to particularly distressed individuals and, as needed, made referrals to clinical care. Finally, a series of workshops on children and traumatic stress was offered to students preparing to work with neighborhood children.

## THE COMMUNITY CRISIS RESPONSE TEAM

The array of interventions that followed this young man's death is illustrative of the work of the CCRT, a service of the VOV Program. VOV services are designed to foster recovery through the promotion of choice, self-determination, and social action (see Harvey, this volume). Within VOV, the aims of community intervention post-trauma are to address the community's vulnerability, augment and enhance existing community resources, and promote community-wide coping and healing. An outcome goal of every CCRT interventions is its ownership by the client community.

### The Team

The CCRT was established by VOV in 1988, in recognition of the devastating impact that violent crime can have on affected communities. Through the CCRT, a small coordinating staff organizes the work of more than 40 volunteer members drawn from mental health, criminal justice, religious, educational, social service, and victim advocacy agencies and organizations throughout Boston, Cambridge, and the surrounding four-county area. Together, CCRT staff and team members extend confidential crisis response and consultation to communities and community settings affected by violent crime

*The CCRT staff.* Staff of the CCRT includes a full-time coordinator who is a licensed clinical social worker and two part-time community liaison staff: an emergency mental health worker with a local hospital and a senior community police officer, both former volunteer members of the CCRT. The Coordinator is a member of VOV's core staff and a key participant in hospital and departmental crisis response planning forums.

*CCRT volunteers.* Volunteer members of the CCRT include specialists in such areas as victimization, crisis intervention, and the treatment of psychological trauma; people with experience and expertise in working with specific populations (e.g., children, the elderly, recent immigrants); and individuals with longstanding records of neighborhood activism and community leadership. Team members are recruited not only from diverse agencies and organizations but also from racially, culturally, and linguistically diverse communities, further enhancing the CCRT's ability to respond to a wide variety of groups and situations. In addition, team members are recruited from particularly vulnerable communities (e.g., high crime neighborhoods, immigrant and ethnic minority communities) and often from more than one agency or organization in urban neighborhoods afflicted by recurrent episodes of violent crime. A goal of this "cluster recruiting" is to contribute to the long-term development of a given community's crisis response capabilities, first by helping to develop the crisis response skills of community members, and secondly by facilitating their exchange of ideas and expertise and encouraging them to network with one another and utilize their CCRT training in off-team situations.

*The CCRT contract.* CCRT staff limit their recruitment of team members to individuals whose organizations contract with VOV to sponsor a volunteer member for a term of at least one year. CCRT volunteers are salaried by their sponsoring agencies and receive release time from their workplaces to participate in CCRT interventions and training. The contract specifies that those team members who are licensed mental health professionals will be covered by the sponsoring agency's professional liability insurance. Team members commit to being available for 8 to 10 hours of community crisis response activity during a membership year.

## Team Training and Team Building

Entry into the CCRT begins with an intensive two-day training that includes both didactic presentations and experiential exercises covering a range of topics, including the nature of acute and chronic trauma, crisis intervention skills, principles of community-level intervention, working with special populations, and the CCRT's community empowerment model.

Following the initial training, team members participate in monthly team meetings where CCRT interventions are reviewed and additional training and support is provided. These meetings serve many purposes: skill development, supervision, evaluation of recent interventions, and the ongoing development of the CCRT itself. Through their involvement in these meetings, team members become active participants in a unique network of community resources–agencies, groups, and individuals–that they may call upon off-team in many capacities, including their work-related capacities. Not surprisingly, the CCRT has evolved into its own kind of community: a community with a diverse and now multi-generational membership joined by common purpose, shared values, and well-established traditions (Yassen, 1995).

## Precipitating Events and Client Communities

The kinds of incidents that result in requests for CCRT assistance are varied. They include:

- Incidents occurring in communities in which people are strongly affiliated with one another (e.g., a school, a workplace, a church, or a neighborhood);
- Incidents in which there are multiple direct victims and/or eyewitnesses;
- Incidents in which the victims (or perpetrators) have a special significance to the affected community, as might happen with the violent death of a child or community leader;
- Incidents involving numerous emergency or rescue workers; and
- Incidents that attract a great deal of media attention.

Since the CCRT's inception in 1988, events precipitating requests for CCRT assistance have included catastrophic events like the terrorist attacks of September 11th, when representatives from host settings called upon the team for crisis response, consultation, and training. More often, however, the CCRT is called upon when more familiar crimes of violence–rape, family violence, child abuse, elder abuse, hate crime, or murder–send shock waves through one community setting after another. During one 24 month period, for example, over half of the more than 40 intervention requests received were precipitated by acts of homicide, double homicide, or homicide suicide. Other precipitating events included sexual assault, physical assault, school violence, and the distress of service providers working with victims of extreme violence. Requests for CCRT assistance following these events were made from a wide range of communities, agencies and educational institutions; from public schools to large private universities; social service agencies to community health centers. CCRT responses to these requests involved large community gatherings and small groups of neighborhood residents.

### The Services of the CCRT

Responding to requests from affected communities, the CCRT offers a range of confidential and time-limited crisis response services. Depending upon the needs and resources of a client community, these may entail any/all of the following:

- *Consultation to community settings as they plan and implement their own crisis response activities.* The CCRT Coordinator may meet with school administrators, workplace managers, or neighborhood representatives to help them think through what they want to do, when, and for whom. These meetings often involve considerations such as how to deal with the media, how to handle "rumor control," and if, when, and how to structure community meetings and group interventions. Community consultation encourages community representatives to step back from the crisis at hand, slow the response process down a bit, and take the time needed for developing thoughtful, well-considered interventions, making use of familiar resources whenever possible. The goal is to help communities mobilize and direct their own crisis response resources. Often, community consultation is the only–or, at least, the primary–service provided by the CCRT.
- *Direct assistance to affected community members and groups.* Direct services of the CCRT are offered only after an initial period of consultation and collaborative needs assessment, and rarely occur within the first 24 to 72 hours of an incident. These services may include: co-leadership of large or small community meetings, coordination of CCRT interventions with those of other crisis response groups, mental health needs assessment and clinical referral, group interventions, traumatic stress debriefings for small groups of individuals who are usually well-known to one another, or other modes of direct assistance. CCRT volunteers typically participate as members of two-to-three person intervention teams organized and supervised by CCRT staff. Virtually all direct interventions include the participation of a licensed clinician.
- *The CCRT's approach to traumatic stress debriefing.* The CCRT regularly reviews and modifies its direct service approaches. Initially, for example, the team's approach to traumatic stress debrief-

ings borrowed both structure and intent from Mitchell's (1983) critical incident stress debriefing model, a model designed to prevent posttraumatic stress disorder among first-responders (i.e., police, firefighters, emergency medical personnel) to tragic events. Over the ensuing years, with a diversification of debriefing models (Dyregrov, 1997; Paton, 1995), an increasingly divided research literature concerning the preventive efficacy of post-incident debriefings (see, e.g., Robinson & Mitchell, 1993; Deahl & Bisson, 1995; Kaplan et al., 2001; McNally et al., 2003) and the CCRT's own increasing involvement with chronically traumatized communities, this approach has been modified. Today, the emphasis is on creating a safe and containing forum where participants are supported as they review both personal and community reactions to one or a series of violent events, given information about normal reactions to psychologically traumatic events, helped to identify resources that have proven useful in the past, and encouraged to construct personally meaningful, affiliative strategies for future self-care. The focus is less on preventing PTSD among community residents than on educating community members about the impact of potentially traumatic events on themselves, their families, and friends, heightening their awareness of available resources, and confirming their collective membership in a caring community. CCRT debriefings are never mandatory, are preceded by considerable attention to issues of privacy, confidentiality, choice, and safety, and often result in the self-identification of participants who are having a particularly difficult time, at which point CCRT respondents are able to provide timely referrals to appropriate clinical and/or community resources.

• *Secondary traumatic stress workshops and peer support interventions on behalf of service providers impacted by violence.* When communities are impacted by crimes of violence, caregivers in these communities can become overwhelmed by a seemingly unbearable sense of responsibility and concern (McCann & Pearlman, 1990; Yassen, 1995). Among those who may be most severely affected by acts of violence are caregivers who live and work in what we have come to refer to as "chronically traumatized" communities. These individuals serve on the front lines of community engagement with violence. They remind us that even the most seasoned among us can feel immobilized by the prospect of offering care in the wake of one more tragedy. So it is both in the immediate aftermath of a violent crime and in a sometimes ominous "lull" between one incident of violence after another that the CCRT may be called upon to meet with mental health providers, first responders, and others who themselves are involved in the "heat" of crisis response. Typically, the work takes the form of secondary traumatic stress workshops that combine peer support with didactic presentations on the nature of secondary trauma and signs of vicarious traumatization (McCann & Pearlman, 1990; Yassen, 1995; Yassen & Harvey, 1998).

- *Follow-up support and assistance.* CCRT's services are always time limited. They have a beginning and an end, and are implemented and concluded in collaboration with the client community. Follow-up support and assistance is always available, however. This may take the form of checking in with a community representative when new information about a criminal case is in the news, or when a trial is about to begin. It may also involve an offer of support when a new incident has occurred within the same client community.

All services of the CCRT are offered free of charge and with guarantees of confidentiality. Moreover, while representatives of client communities may choose to introduce CCRT members at public gatherings, these team members are always present as guests of the community. They do not speak for a community and will generally decline media exposure. At other times and in other contexts, CCRT staff may well consult with media representatives about CCRT services and/or how they might better educate the public about psychological trauma. However, such consultations do not occur in the midst of a CCRT crisis response, when issues of community safety, trust, and privacy predominate.

## THE COMMUNITY EMPOWERMENT MODEL

Figure 1 depicts the community empowerment model that guides the design, conduct, and evaluation of all CCRT interventions.

### Community Entry

As indicated in Figure 1, the CCRT's involvement begins when a request for assistance is received from an affected community and when a legitimate point of entry into the community has been established. Initial conversations between CCRT staff and community representative

FIGURE 1. The Community Empowerment Model

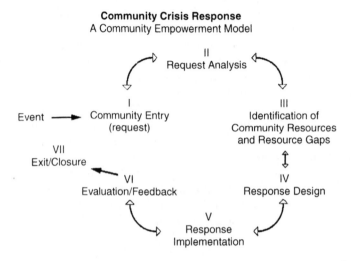

**Community Crisis Response**
A Community Empowerment Model

Community Crisis Response Team–Victims of Violence Program, The Cambridge Hospital, MA

focus on the nature of the event that has occurred, what (if anything) the representative knows about the CCRT, and determining if s/he is in a position to speak for the community in question. The inquiries and exchanges taking place at this early phase of the intervention process lay the foundation for shared ownership of any intervention that is subsequently initiated.

*A note about the CCRT's "pre-entry" activities with communities at risk.* Whatever services are ultimately offered to a client community, the work of the CCRT takes place year round as staff and team members reach out to organizations and groups throughout the metropolitan area. Outreach activities include distributions of CCRT literature, presentations to local agencies and community groups, year-round recruitment of new team members, on-going contact with sponsoring agencies, and week-in, week-out collaboration with anti-violence organizations and coalitions. It is noteworthy that over half of the requests received by the CCRT are initiated by individuals who had learned of the CCRT through an outreach presentation or who had knowledge of a previous CCRT intervention in their own or a nearby community.

## *Request Analysis*

Once a legitimate avenue of community entry and involvement has been established, the CCRT Coordinator (or designated staff) and client community begin the process of request analysis and mutual consultation. Questions considered during this phase include: What is the "trauma history" of the affected community? What individuals or groups are of greatest concern? How is the community's request changing as the request analysis process continues? What has been done thus far? What next steps have been planned? Request analysis with a community in crisis may last hours or days depending on any number of circumstances, including how rapidly things are changing within the community itself. Frequent telephone contact and face-to-face consultation give assurances of the CCRT's sustained concern and availability.

## *Identifying Community Resources and Resource Gaps; Clarifying CCRT Resources*

Request analysis typically moves rather seamlessly into a needs assessment phase in which existing community resources and resource gaps are identified, needs are prioritized, and participants consider if and how the CCRT might provide additional assistance. The CCRT's work with the community may end during this phase, as is the case when it becomes clear that the community is already doing and knows how to do all that can or should be done at the moment. In this event, the CCRT's contribution has been to serve as an outside source of reassurance and validation, providing support to the community's own crisis response planning and affirming the community's ability to address its own needs. In other cases, the process may highlight the need for continuing CCRT involvement.

## *Designing a CCRT Response*

When a community and CCRT coordinating staff agree that the team's continuing involvement could be a helpful element of the community's overall response, a response involving one or more direct CCRT services is formulated. If a traumatic stress debriefing or other group intervention is agreed upon, for example, or if the CCRT is to be present at or is to co-lead a community meeting, staff begins thinking about which team members to call upon, the roles they might play, and how they might be identified to the larger community. Questions raised and answered at this point include: What will be done by the CCRT and what by the community? How might an anticipated media presence be dealt with? How and where will CCRT and community participants meet to prepare for and discuss last minute changes? Response design is always a shared process, with both CCRT staff and community representative deciding together what will be done, when, where, and by whom.

It is during this phase of the empowerment model that the client community and CCRT staff begin to formally and informally identify desired outcomes. For example, outcome goals might include the hope that a community meeting will be well attended by particular groups, that particularly at-risk community members will give voice to their concerns and become more aware of and likely to make use of important community resources, and/or that members of an affected group will feel greater cohesion with one another following a CCRT intervention. These outcome goals, while relatively global in the early stages of involvement, become more refined as the process continues and are visited again after the intervention is concluded by all involved: community representative/s, CCRT staff, team members who have been directly involved in the intervention, and the team as a whole.

### Implementing the Response(s)

As client community and CCRT staff become clearer about ways in which the CCRT might be helpful, the two entities begin planning the logistics of it all. The emphasis during this phase is always on maximizing the community's ownership of and responsibility for the intervention. When the composition of the CCRT's intervention team is established, its members are convened by the Coordinator, who designates which team member will do what (e.g., give a presentation, serve as a translator, lead a group intervention, provide support, or act as an observer of the intervention process). Licensed mental health clinicians involved in the intervention will include among their responsibilities the job of noticing individuals who seem severely distressed and, as appropriate, extending to them on-site crisis care and follow-up referrals. As CCRT staff prepare team members for their work, the community representative manages the logistics back home–identifying the setting in which the intervention will occur, securing the involvement of other community members, preparing the environment, and, later, being on hand to welcome and introduce the CCRT respondents.

Many steps and considerations are involved in implementing and preparing to implement a CCRT response. These steps–from community entry to response implementation–can actually be carried out in very brief span of time: typically, a few days to one or two weeks, but, if needed, within a few hours. Particularly when the timing is short and emotions are running very high, it is the framework provided by the community empowerment model that "holds" the CCRT and, by extension, the community.

### Evaluation and Feedback

CCRT interventions come to a close with a multi-layered and collaborative evaluation process. As soon as possible, members of the intervention team meet, first, with one another and then with the CCRT Coordinator to evaluate how they think the intervention was conducted and received; how they are feeling about their own participation; what, if anything, they might have done differently; and where things were left with the community. This part of the evaluation process enables an assessment not only of the way in which a given intervention was conducted, but also of the developing skills and working relationships of intervention team members.

While the intervention team is reviewing its work, the community representative gathers feedback from community participants and meets with the CCRT Coordinator to review each intervention, determine whether or not previously agreed upon goals were or were not achieved, and consider what next steps should be taken, if any. These might include checking in with one another about particularly distressed community members or developing additional services as new segments of the community register their concerns. For the CCRT, a major concern is with assessing the quality of the relationship that has been achieved with the client community.

A final part of the evaluation process involves both staff and team review. When the intervention (or a series of related interventions) is reviewed at a monthly CCRT meeting, the discussion will integrate feedback from the community and from team members involved in the intervention. Topics will include a consideration of the intervention's impact on the CCRT itself and implication for the evolving relationship between CCRT and client community.

### Exit/Closure

CCRT involvement with a client community ends with a final follow-up by the CCRT Coordinator and an expression of appreciation for the community's interest in the CCRT as a resource. At this point, the intervention is considered "over" and the relationship with a client community concluded. This final step is a key element of the empowerment model, one that reminds team members and community representatives alike that CCRT members are invited guests and that, as such, they are outsiders who need not and should not overstay their welcome. Leaving the community is as important a step as gaining entry into it. Leaving a community whose resources and strengths have been affirmed and engaged builds and reinforces community resilience. Among the most gratifying outcomes of the CCRT's work to date has been the number of individuals who have joined the team precisely because of the way in which the CCRT intervened in–and exited from–their own communities.

## THE EMPOWERMENT MODEL IN ACTION

Returning to the case example with which we began this article, we know now that at the time of this homicide the CCRT was a resource known to some and unknown to others in the various communities impacted by the crime. The outreach and "pre-entry" work of the team had made some inroads into the community, and the recruitment of team members from diverse community settings had set the stage for legitimate community entry. Thus, a public health administrator who was herself a former team member encouraged the manager of the housing development to contact the CCRT. Her department, along with the police and other city officials, was trying to help the housing manager organize a community meeting at which this homicide and other recent violent events would be discussed. After speaking with CCRT staff, she encouraged the housing manager to seek a consultation with the CCRT Coordinator on how to structure and conduct the meeting and how to address the concerns and contain the emotions of an anticipated audience of over 100 multi-lingual community residents. The CCRT was invited to be present as a support to the housing manager, and to provide residents with information about the CCRT, the VOV Program, and other mental health resources in the community. Because of its diverse membership, the CCRT was able to provide bilingual translators and printed materials in several languages.

As additional requests came in, CCRT interventions also included crisis response planning sessions with city officials and neighborhood task forces, traumatic stress debriefings and other group interventions with neighborhood residents, and a series of interventions with the high school students who were about to begin the summer camp program with neighborhood children. In this instance, the request came from an official of the high school program who had learned of the CCRT from an outreach presentation by the CCRT Coordinator earlier in the year. After an initial period of request analysis and consultation, this official and the Coordinator agreed that the students could benefit most from an educational intervention to inform them about children's reactions to traumatic events–how they are affected, what is a normal reaction, and what to look for–and to remind them that their job was to provide the children with a positive camp experience, not to try and serve as therapists or crisis counselors. Thus, the intervention also provided the students with information about clinical resources for children and the CCRT Coordinator identified team members who would be available to provide support to any of the students who became concerned about a child in their care.

As each of these responses was implemented, the CCRT Coordinator and liaison staff stayed in close touch with representatives of the various client communities. Plans were discussed and revised up until the last minute–as the expected number and demography of participants changed, for example, and as various community leaders weighed in on what might be the most helpful response to changing circumstances. During this time, outcome goals associated with the planned interventions changed as well. At one point, for example, a police presence was considered an important element of the community meeting. Later, because some community planners felt that a police presence might have an intimidating effect on some segments of the desired audience, a decision was made for the police to provide updates to identified community leaders who would, in turn, hold smaller follow-up meetings for specific groups of neighborhood residents. An initial goal of creating police-community dialogue was replaced by that of enabling a possibly more open and vibrant dialogue among residents and community leaders. CCRT staff provided consultation to community members on some of these decisions and, in others, simply adapted to changes decided upon by the community.

As each response was completed, feedback was gathered and reviewed with key participants. CCRT staff learned that a particularly valued element of the large community meeting was the CCRT Coordinator's ability to address those in attendance in both Spanish and English, and that the CCRT's multi-lingual written materials had been readily consumed by persons attending the meeting. On the other hand, some CCRT team members felt the meeting had gone on way too long, and some community residents were upset that the police had not been in attendance. Clearly, leaders of this meeting had not successfully conveyed to participants the plan for smaller, follow-up sessions. The workshops conducted with the high school seniors were reviewed in a particularly positive light by all involved. The students reported feeling less personally fearful, more prepared to work with the children, and strongly supported by both their advisors and CCRT members.

In the weeks that followed this young man's murder, the CCRT Coordinator stayed in touch with representatives of each client community until the CCRT's work was done and then conducted a review and evaluation of each intervention with community representatives and participating team members. A final step in the process involved review all interventions arising from this one event by the CCRT membership at their regularly scheduled monthly meeting.

## *DISCUSSION*

Both the CCRT and the community empowerment model that guides its work trace their origins and theoretical rationale to the ecological perspective of community psychology (Harvey, this volume). An ecological view of psychological trauma (Harvey, 1996) assumes that human reactions to adverse and traumatic events are best understood in the ecological context of human community and that effective community interventions post-trauma are those that enhance the ecological relationship between community and community member. In the case of community crisis response, this perspective suggests that the efficacy of interventions undertaken post-trauma by outside experts and professionals will be realized (or not) in the extent to which they utilize, enhance, conserve, and help to restabilize community resources (Hobfall, 1991; Hobfall & Lilly, 1993; Hobfall, 1998).

Consistent with this perspective, the CCRT can be viewed as an on-going effort to develop and enhance the diverse resources of traumatized communities. An act of extreme violence or shared community disaster can sorely tax and threaten to overwhelm existing community resources. In the face of such threat, some community members may reach beyond the boundaries of local community in search of new resources, including outside consultation and assistance. Others, however, will resist outside influence and try to shield the community from the intrusions of media representatives, curiosity seekers, and/or "outside experts" who may have arrived uninvited only to be perceived as overbearing, inconsiderate, and/or ill-informed (Koss & Harvey, 1991). Within this ecological mix of reactions to tragic events, each intervention launched in a community becomes part of its history and identity. One aim of empowering community intervention must be to make a positive contribution to a traumatized community's crisis response resources and evolving identity. Since the early 1970s, research by community psychologists has examined the aims, nature, forms, and efficacy of community level interventions (see, e.g., Glidewell, 1976; Heller & Monahan, 1977; Harvey, 1985; Durlak & Wells, 1997; see also Harvey, this volume). One way to conceptualize community crisis response is in terms of its preventive possibilities. Preventive interventions have aimed at health-promotion and risk reduction with vulnerable populations, the promotion of social change and environmental reform in social organizations and institutions, and, apropos to the work of the CCRT, the promotion of resilience in individuals and communities affected by adverse events (Cowen, 1994; Durlak & Wells, 1997; Harvey, this volume; Norris & Thompson, 1995; Trickett, 1997).

An early study of preventive interventions (Paster, 1977) found that effective preventive intervention efforts (i.e., those that realized their intended benefit and were adopted by the communities into which they were introduced) were distinguished by five attributes: (a) early and ongoing participation of community members in planning and carrying out the intervention; (b) a high assumption of responsibility for the intervention among community members served by it; (c) the ability of the interveners to see themselves as resources to the intervention activity, rather than as person deserving "credit" for it; (d) a focus on the strengths of individuals and settings identified as the targets of intervention; and (e) the creation of on-going and self-renewing social supports to help build and maintain the competencies of community members involved in the intervention effort.

The first four of these attributes also describe core elements of the CCRT's Community Empowerment Model–a model that borrows its goals, form, and substance from the ecological analogy of community psychology (Kelly, 1987) and from the premise that community intervention in the aftermath of violence must have as a primary goal that of enhancing the relationship between affected individuals and the communities from they draw identity, belongingness, and meaning (Harvey, 1996, this volume; Norris & Thompson, 1995). Every CCRT intervention, however configured and however rapidly initiated, is guided by this model: it has been designed to ensure that CCRT members always pay attention not only to the task of initiating particular interventions, but also to the crucial importance of securing and maintaining on-going community engagement. The fifth of these attributes describes the fundamental rationale for the CCRT's annual training, monthly team meetings, and team member recruitment strategies. Together they ensure to team members and their sponsoring agencies recurrent opportunities for skill-development, social support, and self-renewal.

In recent years, a number of community psychologists have turned their attention to the importance of creating evaluation tools and approaches that engage, educate, and empower the communities that serve as host environments for community intervention (Fawcett et al., 2003; Fetterman, 2002; Suarez-Balcazar, Orellan-Damacela, Portillo, Sharma, & Lanum, 2003). Among these authors, Suarez-Balcazar et al. suggest that participatory and empowerment approaches to the evaluation of interventions enhance the likelihood that a client community will take ownership of the intervention and make use of the evaluation findings.

The empowerment evaluation literature has important implications for the CCRT. Currently, the evaluation of CCRT activities takes place at two levels. One is that required by the funding agency[2] and begins with an annual articulation of specific program goals and objectives, followed by a delineation of the number of communities served in a given year, the services provided, and the communities prioritized for CCRT outreach and team member recruitment. A second level of evaluation is participatory and collaborative and is embedded in the community empowerment model. Indeed, participatory evaluation of CCRT interventions is anticipated by each element of the empowerment model. At the very earliest phases of community engagement CCRT staff and community representatives mutually assess the needs of a community in crisis and consider what, if any, CCRT interventions are likely to benefit to community members. These discussions ensure the collaborative design and implementation of targeted interventions and for the identification of mutually agreed upon outcome goals. They also give shape and content to a final series of intervention reviews that aim to engage client communities in an empowering evaluation process (Fawcett et al., 2003; Suarez-Balcazar et al., 2003). A future goal will be to make more explicit the connection between the empowerment model and the evaluation strategies recommended by these and other empowerment evaluation authors.

## CONCLUSIONS

An ecological view of communities and community intervention suggests that we need to look not only at the helpfulness or harmfulness of specific interventions (e.g., critical incident stress debriefings) but also, and perhaps more importantly, at the ways in which trauma-informed interventions are initiated and carried out in and with affected communities. To paraphrase community psychologist Jim Kelly's (1979), maybe "'taint [only] what you do, but the way that you do it." *How* professionals intervene in communities is as essential to the outcome of their efforts as *what* they do. The CCRT's community empowerment model is a guide to the "how" of community crisis response–and to the "how" of staff and team member behavior with representatives of traumatized client communities.

Since its beginnings in 1988, the CCRT has developed in size and complexity, with many more members than originally intended and certainly more experience in the realm of trauma response than originally anticipated. Particularly unanticipated was the extent to which the team would be working with what we have come to call "chronically traumatized" communities (i.e., urban communities in which recurrent violence may have devastating impact on already vulnerable community ecosystems). To achieve what community psychologists refer to as "ecological fit" between our interventions and the needs of our client communities, we have recruited and learned from team members within those communities about the meaning of events, the groups most severely impacted by them, and the values, traditions, and expectations that should inform CCRT behavior in these communities. These lessons are embodied in the community empowerment model, which not only guides the design, conduct, and evaluation of all CCRT interventions but also links the task of time-limited community crisis response to the larger and longer-term goal of community development.

## NOTES

1. This case typifies the kinds of events that prompt requests for CCRT assistance. Attributes of the case have been altered to ensure the anonymity of the victim, his family, and his community.

2. The Community Crisis Response Team is supported by federal Victims of Crime Act funds, awarded to the Victims of Violence Program by the Massachusetts Board of Victim Assistance

# REFERENCES

Bisson, J., & Deahl, M. (1994). Psychological debriefing and prevention of post-traumatic stress. More research is needed. *British Journal of Psychiatry, 165,* 717-720.

Cowen, E. L. (1994). The enhancement of psychological wellness: Challenges and opportunities. *American Journal of Community Psychology, 22*(4), 149-177.

Durlak, J.A. and Wells, A.M. (1997) Primary prevention mental health programs for children and adolescents: A meta-analytic review. *American Journal of Community Psychology, 25*(2), 115-152.

Dyregrov, A. (1997). The process in psychological debriefings. *Journal of Traumatic Stress, 10*(4), 589-606.

Fawcett, S. B., Boothroyd, R., Schultz, J. A., Francisco, V. T., Carson, V., & Bremby, R. (2003). Building capacity for participatory evaluation within community initiatives. *Journal of Prevention and Intervention in the Community, 26*(2), 21-36.

Fetterman, D. M. (2002). Empowerment evaluation: Building communities of practice and a culture of learning. *American Journal of Community Psychology, 30,* 89-102.

Glidewell, J. (1976). A theory of induced social change. *American Journal of Community Psychology, 4,* 227-242.

Harvey, M. R. (1985). *Exemplary rape crisis programs: A cross-site analysis and case studies.* Washington, DC: U.S. Department of Health and Human Services.

Harvey, M. R. (1996). An ecological view of psychological trauma and trauma recovery. *Journal of Traumatic Stress, 9*(1), 3-23.

Harvey, M. R. (2007). Towards an ecological understanding of resilience in trauma survivors: Implications for theory, research, and practice. *Journal of Aggression, Maltreatment & Trauma, 14*(1/2), 9-32.

Heller, K., & Monahan, J. (1977). *Psychology and community change.* Homewood, IL: The Dorsey Press.

Hobfoll, S. (1991). Traumatic stress: A theory based on rapid loss of resources. *Anxiety Research, 4,* 187-197.

Hobfall, S.E. (1998). *Stress, culture and community: The psychology and philosophy of stress.* New York: Plenum.

Hobfoll, S., & Lilly, R. (1993). Resource conservation as a strategy for community psychology. *Journal of Community Psychology, 21,* 128-148.

Kaplan, Z., Iancu, I., & Bodner, E. (2001). A review of psychological debriefing after extreme stress. *Psychiatric Services, 52*(6), 824-827,

Kelly, J. G. (1979). "Taint what you do, it's the way that you do it. *American Journal of Community Psychology, 7,* 244-261.

Kelly, J. G. (1987). An ecological paradigm: Defining mental health consultation as a preventive service. *Prevention in Human Services, 4*(3/4), 1-36.

Koss, M., & Harvey, M. (1991). *The rape victim: Clinical and community interventions* (2nd ed.). Newbury Park, CA: Sage.

McCann, L., & Pearlman, L. A. (1990). Vicarious traumatization: A contextual model for understanding the effects of trauma on helpers. *Journal of Traumatic Stress, 3*(1), 131-149.

McNally, R. J., Bryant, R. A., & Ehlers, A. (2003). Does early psychological intervention promote recovery from posttraumatic stress? *Psychological Science in the Public Interest, 4*(2), 45-77.

Mitchell, J. T. (1983). When disaster strikes: The critical incident stress debriefing process. *Journal of Emergency Medical Services, 8,* 36-39.

Norris, F. H. and Thompson, M.P. (1995) Applying community psychology to the prevention of trauma and traumatic life events. In J. Freedy & S. Hobfall (Eds.), *Traumatic stress: from theory to practice.* New York: Plenum Press.

Paster, V. B. (1977). Organizing primary prevention programs with disadvantaged community groups. In D. C. Klein & S. E. Goldston (Eds.), *Primary prevention: An idea whose time has come* (pp. 85-89). Washington, DC: Government Printing Office.

Paton, D. (1995). *Dealing with traumatic incidents in the workplace: Management and organizational strategies for preparation and support.* Perth: Curtin University.

Raphael, B. (1986). *When disaster strikes: How individuals and communities cope with catastrophe.* New York: Basic Books.

Raphael, B., Meldrum, L., & MacFarlane, A. C. (1995). Does debriefing after psychological trauma work? *British Medical Journal, 310,* 1479-1480.

Robinson, R. C., & Mitchell, J. R. (1993). Evaluations of psychological debriefings. *Journal of Traumatic Stress, 6,* 367-382.

Suarez-Balcazar, Y., Orellan-Damacela, L., Portillo, N., Sharma, A., & Lanum, M. (2003). Implementing an outcomes model in the participatory evaluation of community initiatives. *Journal of Prevention and Intervention in the Community, 26*(2), 5-20.

Trickett, E. J. (1997). Ecology and primary prevention: Reflections on a meta-analysis. *American Journal of Community Psychology, 25*(2), 197-206.

Yassen, J. (1995). Preventing secondary traumatic stress disorder. In C. Figley (Ed.), *Compassion fatigue: Coping with secondary-traumatic stress disorder in those who treat the traumatized* (pp. 178-209). New York: Bruner-Mazel.

Yassen, J., & Harvey, M. (1998). Crisis assessment and interventions with victims of violence. In P. M. Kleespies (Ed.), *Emergencies in mental health practice: Evaluation and management* (pp. 117-114). New York: Guilford Publications.

doi:10.1300/J146v14n01_14

# Resilience and Post-Traumatic Recovery in Cultural and Political Context: Two Pakistani Women's Strategies for Survival

Shahla Haeri

**SUMMARY.** Violence against women has been conceptualized in terms of controlling female sexuality, restricting women's autonomy, humiliating and keeping women out of sight, maintaining male control and dominance, and dishonoring other [male] enemies. This paper discusses situations where the violation of women's bodies becomes the site for political rivalries and thus incurring masculine/national honor. The etching of political rivalries onto women's bodies for national honor or to inflict dishonor has a long history and is not unique to Pakistan. Within the theoretical frameworks of ecological psychology and cultural anthropol-

---

Address correspondence to: Dr. Shahla Haeri, Boston University, Women's Studies Program, 704 Commonwealth Avenue, Boston, MA 02215 (E-mail: shaeri@bu.edu).

The author would like to express appreciation to Dr. Mary Harvey and Dr. Pratyusha Tummala for their helpful comments on an earlier draft of this paper. The author also wishes to thank the three anonymous reviewers for their constructive suggestions and comments.

[Haworth co-indexing entry note]: "Resilience and Post-Traumatic Recovery in Cultural and Political Context: Two Pakistani Women's Strategies for Survival." Haeri, Shahla. Co-published simultaneously in *Journal of Aggression, Maltreatment & Trauma* (The Haworth Maltreatment & Trauma Press, an imprint of The Haworth Press, Inc.) Vol. 14, No. 1/2, 2007, pp. 287-304; and: *Sources and Expressions of Resiliency in Trauma Survivors: Ecological Theory, Multicultural Practice* (ed: Mary R. Harvey, and Pratyusha Tummala-Narra) The Haworth Maltreatment & Trauma Press, an imprint of The Haworth Press, Inc., 2007, pp. 287-304. Single or multiple copies of this article are available for a fee from The Haworth Document Delivery Service [1-800-HAWORTH, 9:00 a.m. - 5:00 p.m. (EST). E-mail address: docdelivery@haworthpress.com].

ogy, this paper highlights the resiliency shown by two Pakistani women in their efforts toward posttraumatic recovery as they situate their traumatic experiences within their immediate structural, political, and cultural contexts, which in turn influence their behavior and shape the specific choices they make. doi:10.1300/J146v14n01_15    *[Article copies available for a fee from The Haworth Document Delivery Service: 1-800-HAWORTH. E-mail address: <docdelivery@haworthpress.com> Website: <http://www.HaworthPress.com> © 2007 by The Haworth Press, Inc. All rights reserved.]*

**KEYWORDS.** Resilience, trauma, violence against women, Pakistan, cultural anthropology

The etching of political rivalries onto women's bodies for national honor–or to inflict dishonor–has a long and shameful history and is not unique to any particular society.[1] A global glance at the ways political and ethnic conflicts are expressed across cultures reveals the symbolic significance of violating women's bodies as a means for dishonoring the enemy while underscoring the assailant's national pride and masculine honor. One may refer to the Serbian atrocities and gang-rape of Bosnian and Croat women, and the Rwandan mass rape and slaughter of Tutsis, to name only a few, where women's bodies become the site for masculine, ethnic, and national rivalries.

Theoretically, violence against women has been conceptualized in terms of controlling female sexuality, restricting women's autonomy, humiliating and keeping women out of sight,[2] and in terms of maintaining male control and dominance. Although these ideas are relevant to understanding of rape and rape trauma in any society, this article focuses on specific structural relations, cultural meanings, and political rivalries that shaped the choices and influenced the behavior of two Pakistani women whose responses to rape and allegations of rape drew considerable public attention in their home communities. One woman, Rahila, who had been tortured for her political activities while in police custody, insisted to public and private audiences that she had not been raped. The second woman, Veena, not only acknowledged her rape and identified her assailants, but also consented to her father's arranging a press conference to publicize her plight–an act almost unprecedented in her society until then. These and other similar cases, which were extensively covered in the local media,[3] heightened the public's awareness of rape and violence against women. They also led many politicians to take public stands against rape, at least rhetorically.[4] While each woman made a different choice, when considered within the cultural, religious, and political contexts that influenced the women's behavior, the resiliency expressed in their choices becomes evident.

A rash of incidents of politically motivated violence against women in Pakistan galvanized the public, and mobilized women's and human rights organizations to stage demonstrations on behalf of the victims and to demand justice for the perpetrators. Rahila and Veena were both politically, and in the case of Veena socially, associated with Pakistan People's Party headed by Benazir Bhutto, Pakistan's twice elected Prime Minister (1989-1990, 1993-1996). Both cases took place in Karachi, the capital of Sindh province, in late 1990 and 1991, when Benazir Bhutto had been dismissed from her position by the President but was campaigning hard for a new term.[5] While both women showed moral courage and personal stamina in the face of extreme brutality, they used different strategies to deal with their calamity. Both underwent intensive psychiatric help, and both had the support of their immediate family, but not necessarily that of their communities, which though sympathetic by and large, exhibited ambivalence and uncertainty in the face of the highly contested publicity surrounding these cases. Such cultural ambivalence seemed to be more pronounced in the case of Rahila, whose public political activities potentially left her vulnerable to community suspicion (i.e., "she was asking for it"). Veena's high-class pedigree, on the other hand, kept her relatively immune to gossip, innuendos, or community reproach.

The ethnographic information presented in this article is based on my field research during 1991-1993, when I lived in Pakistan. I traveled extensively in the country and had formal and informal talks and discussions with many Pakistani women, including Rahila. Formally, I interviewed Rahila intensively and extensively in May of 1993,[6] and I collected data on Veena from newspapers, magazines and journals, and interviews with Pakistani journalists and others who were familiar with her case.[7] Although trained as a cultural anthropologist, in this article I also wish to incorporate psychological insight into my discussion of rape and violence against women in Pakistan. Cultural anthropology and psychology represent complementary approaches to understanding human responses to trauma and torture. Both take into consideration a multiplicity of factors, concentrating on particular constellations of structural constraints, and on opportunities and choices available to individuals in specific family settings and within a particular cultural and political environment. The analysis of Veena's and Rahila's survival

strategies that follows employs the theoretical perspective and research methodology of cultural anthropology and utilizes the ecological framework, which community psychologists (Harvey, 1996, this
volume; Harvey, Mishler, Koenen, & Harney, 2002) have posited as a
means of understanding responses to violence. The ecological perspective of community psychology, similar to that of cultural anthropology,
situates individuals and their responses to trauma and crisis within broader
sociocultural contexts, emphasizing the interdependence of person, event,
and environment (Harvey, 1996).

## CASE STUDY APPROACH

In the following pages, I describe the cases of Rahila and Veena in
some detail, highlighting the specific events that traumatized them and
the culture/environment within which violence was committed against
these women, or from which they drew support. Next, each woman's response to crimes of sexual assault and allegations of rape are considered
with a focus on better understanding their choices, their behaviors, and
their attempts at recovery in the aftermath of extreme cruelty.

### Rahila: In Police Custody

Rahila was a devoted 24-year-old political activist who belonged to
the Pakistan Student Federation, the student wing of the Pakistan People's Party, headed by the former Pakistan Prime Minister, Benazir
Bhutto.[8] Rahila's father is a civil servant, living with his wife, their four
daughters, of whom Rahila is the eldest, and one son in a comfortable
state-owned house in a colony just outside Karachi. Like Rahila, all her
family members were devotees of Benazir Bhutto and activists on behalf of her People's Party. Repeatedly, Rahila described how much she
loved Benazir Bhutto and how worried she was for her leader's life because while in jail she heard her interrogators threatening to kill Benazir
Bhutto.[9] For Rahila, Benazir Bhutto was clearly an idol, a leader, and a
role model par excellence.

Rahila was arrested, tortured, and later hospitalized in a psychiatric
ward for over nine months in 1990. Before Rahila's arrest, her house
was searched, and she was arrested on the pretext that she had received
weapons and ammunition and had passed secret messages to Indian
agents. When she refused to cooperate with the Sindh[10] authorities to

fabricate charges of sexual misconduct and national security allegations against Benazir Bhutto and her husband, her interrogators turned sadistic.[11] So severely was she beaten and tortured that at some point she lost consciousness and subsequently had to be hospitalized and placed in psychiatric care. It was the media publicity surrounding her torture in police custody and her psychiatric hospitalization that fueled the culturally over-productive gossip mills regarding her "rape" while in police custody. Faced with culturally potent shame of rape, Rahila adamantly denied having been raped.

## *Veena: Political Rape*

At the time of her ordeal (November 1991), Veena was a self-employed divorced woman living in a prosperous neighborhood of Karachi. She had two sons, one of whom was studying in the United States at the time, and the other was at a friend's house. Her ordeal began with an evening raid by masked men who gagged and tied her two servants, then waited to ambush her when she arrived home. When Veena's car drew up, they pulled her out of it, beat her, and pulled her by the hair to the top floor of her house where they humiliated and raped her. Significantly, the masked men did not steal much, but stayed in her house for 12 hours, terrorizing, taunting, and torturing Veena and her domestic workers. Clearly, they were not ordinary thieves, as was later claimed by the Sindh authorities. The gang rape of Veena, a woman of landed aristocracy and close friend of Benazir Bhutto and her husband, shattered the belief that only poor and peasant women get raped and that women of the elite are safe. In the words of an observer, "The Veena Hayat case had literally come to knock at the very gates of power" (Yusuf, 1992, p. 41).

What followed this horrific incident of gang rape was nothing short of an unprecedented social drama. On December 7, 1991, Veena's aging father held a press conference, during which time he, obviously in pain and at times weeping, publicly revealed that his daughter had been gang raped a fortnight ago. His action was all the more powerful socially and politically because he was a member of the political elite, and an old colleague of Pakistan's foremost leader, Muhammad Ali Jinnah (d. 1948). No "dishonoring" of women had ever been made public, at least not in this dramatic fashion and in such a public forum, let alone broadcast via electronic and print media. He pointed his finger at the highest political leaders, accusing them of masterminding politically motivated violence against his daughter. She was punished, he charged, because she was a close friend of the opposition leader, who happened to be Benazir Bhutto at that time. He demanded swift justice and retribution.[13] Similar to Rahila, in her legal suit, Veena asserted that she was repeatedly asked by her assailants questions regarding Benazir Bhutto, and was pressured to state–untruthfully–that she had had illicit relations with Benazir's husband.

These women's narratives bring into focus individually specific responses to trauma, while highlighting yet again the painful reality of rape as a highly gendered political weapon. The violence perpetrated against Rahila while in police custody and the terror unleashed at her to oblige her to do the bidding of the state is an improvisation on the theme of "feudal" rape, which often has the knowledge and the support of feudal lords. "Feuds are settled," writes Khalid Ahmed (1991), "through 'rape.' Men avenge themselves on each other by raping each other's mothers, wives, daughters, and sisters. A brave adversary is supposed to break down under the grief and dishonor of the violation of his womenfolk" (p. 1).

Likewise, the politically motivated gang rape of Veena, in its modern context, has the tacit, and at times explicit, legitimization of the state, just as honor rape has continued to have cultural support and collective sanctions. Symbolically, political rape in Pakistan draws on its feudal heritage,[14] and becomes particularly meaningful within the context of Pakistani society's overlapping political structures, lineage solidarity, feudal patronage, and the deeply entrenched moral codes of honor and shame (H. Ahmed, 1992, p. 3). It is in this sense that political rape and rape in police custody manifest their cultural specificity. The target of humiliation and shame is not necessarily a specific woman. Indeed, the individuality of the violated woman seems to be irrelevant in the eyes of the perpetrators.[15] She is a "stand-in" for a political rival–an enemy–on whom revenge is to be taken. In the cases under discussion here, the "enemy," the political rival, was none other than Benazir Bhutto, herself a woman.[16] Although out of office at the time, Benazir Bhutto was a powerful rival with whom the opposition had to contend. When female members of her party were tortured and raped, it was not only the individual women who were dishonored, but it was Benazir Bhutto herself–the leader of the opposition, a woman of feudal lineage, a notable citizen, and the model of womanhood–who was "raped" symbolically by association.[17]

Feminism, however, has brought a paradigm shift in the perception and symbolism of honor, gender relations, and patriarchy in Pakistan. Feminism is, of course, a dynamic and contested phenomenon, and is far from being monolithic in Pakistan or anywhere else for that matter. Women's strategies diverge and their interests differ depending on their class, ethnicity, profession, education, and lineage. Nonetheless, a majority of women I met and interviewed, and many more about whom I read, share clear objectives about improving women's lives and liberty. Active in public, professional Pakistani women such as Veena and Rahila defy the traditionally sanctioned central tenets of cultural beliefs and practices that require women's seclusion, invisibility, and deference to men. On the contrary, as citizens of a postcolonial and modern nation-state, such women challenge the perception of women as the embodiment of purity and as repository of their husbands' or their lineages' honor. Exorcizing honor from their bodies, they empower themselves accordingly and embody their individuality. At the same time, women's agency in the public domain and the gender competition over utilization of public space (Low 1996, p. 390) provoked violent reaction in Pakistan and elsewhere, and thus confronts the state with inherent contradictions[18] (Haeri, 2002, pp. 40-41).

As more and more women become politically active, they too become the specific targets of violence and humiliation, not only for whom they are related to, but for who they are. They bear the multiple burdens of being violated physically, shamed culturally, and dishonored publicly. Their public humiliation and personal violation is highlighted as a warning to other women: quit politics and the public domain or else.

## RESILIENCY: STRATEGIES FOR SURVIVAL

> In the aftermath of victimization, the . . . actions and understandings of family and friends, caregivers, and other significant individuals and groups constitute important elements of the victim's recovery environment. (Harvey, 1996, p. 8)

Pakistani women have for centuries buried in their hearts the rage and anguish of rape. In the interests of family honor and from fear of ostracism, they were–and still are–forced to keep quiet or face humiliation and abandonment by their families.[19] Pakistani families customarily hide the "shame" of their women whose honor has been "looted." Traditionally, this society, like many other, actively discouraged public disclosures of rape, and until recently it preferred not to know (Haeri, 1995).

## Rahila: Denial

Aware of her culture's prevailing attitude, Rahila denied adamantly that she had been raped while in police custody. Registering strong objections to the persistence of rape allegations, Rahila stressed frequently that, "nothing like that [rape] happened!" She insisted that she was "telling the truth," and that she was still "clean." For Rahila, this was "a very hard period" (Haeri, 2002, pp. 107-68). Her mother, though supportive, also worried that because of the prevalence of the rape rumor her daughter may "never get married."[20]

Potentially, she faced the dilemma of many raped victims who are shunned socially and whose family honor is jeopardized by the rape of a family member. They may be banished by their families, mistreated, or even killed, in some instances. Determined to avoid these outcomes, and notwithstanding the lingering doubt in the public mind, Rahila categorically denied having been raped, and so acted "appropriately." Her denial secured her social acceptance–ambivalent though it might have been–and her honorable return to her family. It also saved her family from the shame of living with a "raped" daughter. She supported her claim to purity on the basis of her family pedigree and lineage, insisting that the police did not dare to touch her, even though they often rape women in custody.[21]

Rahila herself ironically seemed to have internalized the state's projection of sexuality and dishonor onto Benazir Bhutto. She clearly identified her persona with that of Benazir Bhutto and appeared to imagine herself as Benazir's "double" (Doniger, 1999). She repeatedly denied accusations of sexual misconduct made against Benazir Bhutto and appealed to Muslim female religious figures to underscore her own honorable intent and conduct. Rahila perceived herself as not "an ordinary woman," like Benazir Bhutto, and argued that Benazir (and, by implication, she herself) was a "savior" of the nation and that, above all, she had managed to become a woman leader in a Muslim state, something Rahila aspired to in her highly patriarchal society.[22] By steadfastly denying any possibility of rape, Rahila protected not only her own honor, but also that of her leader/double, and thus of her nation as well. Saving her leader, for whom she repeatedly proclaimed love, Rahila refused to substantiate allegations of sexual misconduct against her. In turn, she ensured her own salvation, not only psychologically but also politically.

Benazir Bhutto publicly acknowledged Rahila's plight by arranging for her to be sent to America for rehabilitation and gave her a party ticket to run for an Assembly seat.

Moreover, Rahila's persistent refusal to implicate Benazir Bhutto in the face of extreme brutality saved her and her leader from being trapped in a cultural and political "no-win" situation (Doniger, 1999, p. 283). She escaped the possibility of being rejected by her family (and the nation, in Benazir Bhutto's case) as well as of being destroyed by her own and Benazir's enemies. She upheld her honor, izzat, as a member of the Rajput tribe and as a pure (sexually unspoiled) woman.[23] Her public stands for social justice and her categorical denial of rape, in turn, denied her tormentors and Benazir's "enemies" the satisfaction of having broken or dishonored her. In fact, it did the opposite, and allowed her to gain a degree of self-respect. It enabled her to run for a political seat and restored a degree of honor to her family.

## *Veena: Speaking Out*

Shielded and supported by her family and having their full moral support, Veena, unlike Rahila, did not deny or hide the sexual crime directed at her. Indeed, her father publicized it to a degree unprecedented in Pakistani society.[24] Veena's younger sister participated in demonstrations organized by Pakistani lawyers, judges, and human rights and feminist associations, and demanded retribution against some members of the political elite who were alleged to have perpetrated the crime. The State, however, was unsympathetic. In one instance, when Veena's family attempted to stage a day-long fast in Islamabad, the capital, they were initially prevented by a police contingency who took her younger sister to police custody. Her family was eventually able to go ahead with the hunger strike (*The Frontier Post*, 1991, p. 3). Joining Veena's family in their hunger strike in another instance, a leader of the Pakistan's People's Party "strongly slated the indifferent behavior of the president, the prime minister, and the interior minister" (*The Frontier Post*, 1991, p. 3; Zaman, 1991).

Despite such strong shows of family support, Veena hardly appeared in public and did not give many interviews, though her family, particularly her many siblings, aggressively pursued the alleged perpetrators of the gang-rape crime. In one of her interviews, however, Veena said, "I know that a lot of dirt is going to be flung at me. But I have decided to take them on. And I hope I have the courage to see it through to the end or I will kill myself" (*Herald*, 1992, p. 42). Identifying her tormentors as high-level political operatives, she demanded redress from Pakistan's justice system, and when dissatisfied with the judiciary's verdict, she appealed to her feudal lineage's consultative assembly for retribution.

## SELF-EMPOWERMENT

In Pakistan, as in many other societies, religion articulates with cultural practices and local structures of power to manifest itself in widely different rituals and ceremonies. In this sense, Geertz (1973) views religion as a "cultural system" (pp. 124-25), where although religious beliefs render the mundane world of social relationships and psychological events graspable, they also provide a template for people to conduct their daily secular lives. In his view, all religions articulate with cultural practices and local traditions to create moods and motivations for culturally meaningful symbolic action (Geertz, 1973).

Religion presently does appear omnipresent in Pakistan, and the state cloaks many of its actions and intentions, in particular those related to gender relations and women, in the garb of Islam. Many religious beliefs and rituals are filtered through the local practices as they have evolved historically and within the context of Pakistan's multilayered social organizations, class structures, lineage systems, and feudalism. From this perspective, Pakistani Islam is neither the hegemonic discourse nor is it the only source of women's oppression and victimization. On the contrary for many women, including for Rahila, religion provides the comfort and solace needed to give meaning to one's action and to shore up one's resiliency.

### Rahila: Religious Symbolism

Rahila had a mystical sense of her religion, and frequently invoked religious imagery to underscore the justice of her political objectives and the propriety of her actions as well as to rationalize the personal consequences of her imprisonment. In dreams and in wakefulness, she identified herself with the prominent religious female leaders such as Zainab (Prophet Muhammad's granddaughter), whose political courage and purity while held in captivity by her enemies became legendary and exemplary.[25] Rahila upheld leading Muslim women as models of womanly conduct and moral courage. She conjured up images of martyrdom and invoked the moods and ambience of the massacre of the Prophet's grandson in Karbala (680 AD)[26] to calm down her brother[27] who was also jailed with her, and to reassure themselves of the justice of their political action. The spiritual power she received from Islam intimidated her male captors while providing her with the means to cope with her ordeal psychologically and culturally: "There is this hell, this fire inside me," said Rahila to me, "fire as big as a volcano. This is what moved me and gave me strength. . . . Once Marwat[28] said, 'We'll kill you in the CIA Center.'[29] I said, 'Fine! If I am dead in the CIA Center, this is your triumph, this is your reward. But if I go outside, I am your death. This is my promise.' He said, 'You are a crazy woman.' I said, 'Yes, because you think women are very delicate and weak. I am a student leader, I am a Muslim woman. I show you who I am, what is my character.' They were all so scared [smiling]. They were scared of what I could be able to do, so they tried to be alternatively compromising or strict with me."

Rahila's active political participation and agitation for democracy and civil society, and Veena's campaign on behalf of Benazir Bhutto, challenge many an outsider's view of "Muslim women"–a meaningless mega-category in its extreme generality–who are imagined to be generally passive and without social visions. Their actions also threaten a radicalized segment of their transitional and patriarchal society that has increasingly felt compromised by the politically and professionally active women's autonomy and independence. This "radicalized traditionalists," whom Riesebrodt (1993, p. 177) identifies as fundamentalists, see women's public appearance and activism as contrary to the ideal of women's role and gender relations, and thus as an infringement on the male privileges that, in their view, are sanctioned by divine command.

Rahila had her parents' blessing for political activism, but emotionally did not seem to be sure how to behave as a young political leader in her society or how to justify her conduct in Pakistan's ornately multilayered cultural and political contexts. Her active political involvement put her in a potentially precarious position vis-à-vis the cultural ideal of female vulnerability, chastity, and modesty. Her wish to safeguard her honor at all costs simultaneously underscored both her determination not to seem like a woman of easy virtue and her ambivalence regarding women's political mobility and right to control her own body. Her close associations with men in her party, however, riddled her claim to propriety with contradictions and made these claims culturally suspect.

Religion simultaneously granted Rahila yet another strong link with Benazir Bhutto. Intellectually, she downplayed religious differences between Shi'a and Sunni,[30] and claimed not to have much tolerance for the religious schism. But because she, like Benazir, happened to be a

Shi'a Muslim, she found another emotionally meaningful way to empower herself and to find her "double" in the latter. Her heroic refusal to cooperate with Benazir's enemies not only saved her leader/double–and thus herself, professionally at least–but also redeemed her religiously. In the last day of our interviews and conversations, Rahila said, "My ordeal took a long time, while I am telling you the whole story in two or three days. Now I feel I am in the last stages [of recovery]. I listen to music. I like Sufi [mystical] music. When I listen to this kind of music, I feel, yes, we are humans and must be ready for sacrifice. I read a book, which is about the life of the Prophet Muhammad [Peace Be Upon Him]. When he would go for missionary work, he would confront very bad behavior and hardship. Then I feel comforted. When I remember how I was insulted, I think about the great women leaders such as Hazrat Bibi Zainab, Hazrat Bibi Sakina and Hazrat Bibi Ayesha,[31] when she was accused of wrong doing.[32] When people say bad things about me, I think about these women and I feel very comforted. This is my will power [smiling]. I know one thing: we are our own doctors at all times. When I feel sad I don't cry. I become very quiet. I rest and I think. I will try to find a solution. You know, after Najib's death[33] I was very puzzled. I was sick, mentally sick. But I now realize the meaning of life. This time I have an aim in my life" (Haeri, 2002, pp. 159-160).[34]

### Veena: Gender Justice

Veena, on the other hand, made no appeal to religion and religious figures in order to find solace from the pain of brutality directed at her, or justifications for her public political involvement. Hers and her family's vociferous and protracted public protests against her gang rape provided the right environment and gave her the protective shield she needed for recovery. What distinguishes Veena's reaction to trauma from that of Rahila's can be attributed to at least two major factors. One is that of class differences between these two women, which set apart their immediate family's standing in the community, and two, that of the unequivocal backing of Veena's father, the "patriarch," who was willing to personally take a public stand against the gang rape of his daughter. With her father unambiguously on her side, Veena was able to publicize the plight of violated and abused women, and to help break through the heavily fortified wall of silence.

Veena's public and publicized demand for social and gender justice struck a familiar chord in Pakistani society, releasing century old anger and pent up frustration. Her cry for justice and retribution was echoed by numerous NGOs and other human rights organizations. It also provided the right context for community activists and professional women to come together and create organizations in order to help victims of violence and rape. Further, the publicity surrounding these women's cases as well as heightened public awareness and expectations motivated some high-ranking politicians to take note of crimes of violence against women and to take stand against it.

## *DISCUSSION*

Cultural anthropology and the ecological framework of community psychology, as I have tried to discuss in this article, call for a closer and more nuanced look at the relationship between and interdependence of individuals and their social, political, and cultural contexts. By "ecologically" situating individuals' trauma, we are able to understand what is and is not resilient, what is and is not "normal." The cases of Rahila and Veena highlight multiple sources within their immediate community environment that assisted each woman to empower herself, to engage with families and friends, to seek solace from religion and politics, and to pursue an individually meaningful course of action to overcome unspeakable brutality.

Rahila said that she was "not an ordinary woman." Having spent several intensive days with her, this author found herself in agreement with this statement. Recalling her experience of imprisonment, torture, and potentially devastating gossip, she demonstrated an ability to distance herself from her horrifying ordeal, to reflect on it philosophically, and to speak about it analytically. More important, her powerful imagination–and her determination–helped her to develop vital survival skills during both her torture and her recovery, and to maintain her sanity and enhance her budding political career. By denying being raped[35] while identifying her plight and her conduct in jail with those of the leading religious women of her society, she situated her ordeal within familiar and sanctified cultural, moral, and religious contexts. Triumphant, in a sense, Rahila thus laid claim to her honor unambiguously.

Veena, however, spoke out. Her daring action, backed by her father and her family, revealed the darker side of their society's political structure. Her action also problematized a well-entrenched cultural assumption that associates purity and family honor with women's sexuality and conduct, which in turn leaves them vulnerable as targets of political rivalries and feudal vendettas. In Pakistan, women, feminists, and human rights organizations are no longer willing to bite their tongues and be shamed into silence in the face of rape, violence, and brutality that have been unabashedly directed at women. The mounting literatures on such topics attest to a shift of paradigms of shame and silence in this society.

Helped and supported by their parents, immediate families and friends, and by their caring therapists, both Rahila and Veena were assisted to shore up their personal strength and resiliency, to make specific choices, and pursue their course of recovery. This seems to be particularly true in the case of Rahila, who made a healthy comeback to the public and political life, as her highly prestigious position of the Deputy Speaker of Sindh Assembly demonstrates.

## NOTES

1. Sexual abuse of women in police custody is evidently cross-culturally perpetrated and is not peculiar to the developing or underdeveloped societies. For a comprehensive report on the issue, see Human Rights Watch (1996).

2. Kakar (1989, p. 33), a noted Indian psychoanalyst, has argued that one way of making women unagentic is to humiliate them sexually or, worse yet, subject them to the violence of rape, which sends a double message: stay out of sight and behave or else pay the consequences.

3. One must distinguish between English and other local language print media in Pakistan because the intensity and focus of coverage on issues such as rape and violence against women can, and often do, vary in these languages. The cases referenced here were mostly, though not exclusively, covered in the English newspapers, where English is spoken by less that 2% of the population of over 150 million people.

4. Several Pakistani feminist organizations demanded transparency from their high-ranking politicians. Women Against Rape (1993), editorialized: "Where the (erstwhile) Prime Minister's compassion towards rape victims is appreciated, it is a matter of grave concern that the victim and her family's plight is reduced to a farce by television and print media exposure. WAR continues to question the rationale behind the Prime Minister's high profile visits including offering yellow cabs to the victim's family as a compensation" (p. 4).

5. On August 6, 1990, Ghulam Ishaq Khan, Pakistan's President from 1988 to 1993, dismissed the democratically elected Prime Minister Benazir Bhutto by invoking the Eighth Amendment, which was passed under the military regime of General Mohammed Zia ul-Haq (1977-88). It gave a president the right to dissolve the parliament and to dismiss the elected prime minister. Ghulam Ishaq Khan exercised his power twice during his presidency, once in 1990, and the second time in 1993 to dismiss Prime Minister Nawaz Sharif's government.

6. I lived in Pakistan from 1991-1993, learned Urdu, and participated in the day to day life of the people. In addition to being a participant observer by the virtue of living for so long in Pakistan, I conducted formal and informal interviews with as many women–and some men, particularly the religious leaders–as I could. Most of my interviews were in English, though Rahila preferred to switch back and forth between English and Urdu. She was highly articulate and at times sounded philosophical in her

native language. For a fuller description of her life story and interview, see Haeri (2002), chapter 3.

7. Veena Hayat's plight and her father's public denunciation of Pakistani authorities as the perpetrators of his daughter's gang rape attracted much publicity both in print and electronic media. Being a member of Pakistani elite, Veena and her family were known to many of the women with whom I associated.

8. Rahila's life story forms a chapter in my book (Haeri, 2002). A slightly revised version of this book is published by Oxford University Press in Karachi, Pakistan (2004). Rahila and the other five Pakistani women whom I interviewed for my book all knew that their life stories were being published in my book under their real name. I had their permission to do so.

9. Pakistan's political landscape has much changed since then. With the military coup of General Parvez Musharraf in October of 1999, Benazir was forced into exile. With several allegations of financial corruption pending against her, she has lost much of her support in Pakistan.

10. Pakistan is divided into four major provinces, each of which enjoys its own distinct language, ethnicity, and cultural heritage, though of course they also share national identity. These include Punjab, the most populous and prosperous province; Sindh, from where Benazir Bhutto hails; Baluchistan; and North West Frontier Province. At the time of Rahila and Veena's ordeals, the president was a Pathan from North West Frontier, and Prime Minister Nawaz Sharif was an industrialist from Punjab.

11. See also Malik (1997, pp. 112-113). Two of Pakistan's most prestigious monthly magazines, the *Herald* and *Newsline*, as well as many daily newspapers at the time (1990-1991) also published numerous articles regarding Rahila's plight.

12. Many Pakistani feminists and human right activists have written extensively on rape, honor killing, and violence against women, some of which were published in the *Frontier Post*, an English language Pakistani daily. See the many articles by Sarwar (1991, 1992), Hoodbhoy (1989), Rahman (1989), Zaman (1990), Ahmed (1991), and Shirkat Gah's *Newsheets*.

13. This particular case attracted much international attention (Sarwar, 1992, p. 8).

14. By "feudal," I mean a relatively small group of big, politically active, and powerful landowners.

15. Ward (1996, p. 261) similarly argues that in gang rapes the identity of women assaulted is irrelevant.

16. The "enemy" is usually another man whose humiliation through the rape of his womenfolk is publicized and so is made all the more unbearable. Benazir Bhutto had clearly "usurped" an exclusively male privilege. The shame of rape was therefore to humiliate her both in her official capacity as the head of the state *and* as a woman.

17. "All nationalist discourse," argue Breckenridge and van der Veer (1993), "appeal to primordial images of blood, of kinship, of soil, and of sexuality–to imbibe the nation with the force of bodily self-interest" (p. 11).

18. H. Ahmed (1992, p. 1) sees the rise in rape and violence against women as the result of deprivation created by rising expectations, which then lead to anger and aggression.

19. In the aftermath of the partition of the Indian subcontinent into India and Pakistan in 1947, writes Jalal (2001), "The gift of independence in 1947 came like shroud of death for the vulnerable, weak and infirm. Women from the lower social classes were the primary victims of a horrific carnage in which Muslims, Hindus and Sikh men fell

upon them as well as on each other with staggering brutality and murderous hatred" (pp. 564-565). Many of these women were never claimed by their families.

20. In a telephone conversation I had with Rahila sometime in the summer of 2002, the first thing she told me was that she was still unmarried, but that, adding laughingly, she was the Speaker of Sindh National Assembly, a politically powerful and prestigious position.

21. See Human Rights Watch (1992, 1999).

22. As of 2005, Rahila continues to maintain the prestigious position of the Deputy Speaker of Sindh Assembly.

23. The Rajputs are "a group of clans of the Kshatriya (warrior) caste, who fall just beneath the Brahman intellectual-priests. . . [T]heir harsh code of honor and their code of chivalry have often been compared to those of medieval European knights. The Rajputs would fight against all odds" (Weaver, 2000, p. 52). Or, in Caroe's (1958/1983) view, "In many ways the Rajput bears such a strong resemblance to the Highlanders of Scotland with some trifling differences of names and costumes. They had the same reckless daring, the same loyalty to a chief they trusted, they same love of sport, the same readiness to take offence and quarrel among themselves when they could find no enemy to give them employment" (p. 87).

24. Unlike the father, it is interesting to note his sons and sons-in-law were initially "reluctant to go public," whereas his daughters and daughters-in-laws "were in agreement with his decision to make public indictment" (Ahmed, 1991, p. 8).

25. See note below.

26. Karbala is in present-day Iraq, where the Prophet's grandson and the Shi'is' third Imam. Husain, and a small number of his companions were massacred in 680 AD. In the aftermath of this tragedy, the Imam's sister, Zainab, was taken to the court of Yazid, the reigning caliph, where she delivered a historic speech against the caliph and his tyrannical regime. See also Pinault, 1998.

27. Rahila's younger and the only brother, Afzal, was also arrested, jailed, and tortured, primarily to put pressure on Rahila to bring [false] charges against Benazir Bhutto. I interviewed both of them together.

28. Marvat was President Ghulam Ishaq Khan's son-in-law and one of Rahila's tormentors. He was also the same man accused by Veena of having masterminded her gang rape.

29. CIA stands for Crime Investigation Agency in Pakistan. It "has acquired ill repute not only through violations of human rights but also by becoming an active party in organized crime in the turbulent province of Sindh. During its hey day [in the 1980s and early 1990s], the CIA practiced victimization, personal vendetta, forgery, car theft, kidnapping, torture of innocent citizens including gang-rape against women and operated as a parallel organization pursuing its own kind of interrogation. The CIA was originally intended to help the police in its criminal investigation, but political patronage and the exclusive nature of its leadership helped the agency to run a reign of terror in Sindh until the death of [Chief Minister] in early 1992" (Malik, 1997, p. 112).

30. Dispute over who should succeed Prophet Muhammad as the leader of the nascent Muslim community split Muslims into various factions after the Prophet's death in 632 A.D.

31. These women are, respectively, the sister and daughter of the Shi'ites third Imam. Hussain, and the Prophet's favorite wife. "Hazrat" is an honorary term of address, essentially meaning 'Her Presence.'

32. Ayesha, the Prophet's favorite wife, became embroiled in a controversy of "proper conduct" for a wife of the Prophet, and was left vulnerable to wrongful accusations. While The Prophet agonized over how to respond to these accusations and how to treat her, he received a Quranic revelation (24:11-20), in which it is stated that women are presumed innocent until proven guilty by testimony of four male eye-witnesses. See also Spellberg (1994).

33. Najib was Rahila's fellow student activist and comrade-in-arms, for whom she evidently had strong feelings, but she never admitted it to him, at least not in so many words. In April 1990, shortly before her arrest, police shot him to death. At the time of his death, he was 25 years old.

34. Toward the end of our intensive and long interview, Rahila said, "you know, this is my first complete interview. I don't give many interviews, but this is very, very deep. I am very happy because this is very important" (Haeri, 2002, p. 162, n.104).

35. I must stress here that I am not arguing that Rahila *was* raped. The point I am making is the resourcefulness and resiliency she exhibited in the face of relentless gossip.

# REFERENCES

Ahmed, H. (1992, February 20). *Effects and trends of rape in Pakistan.* Paper presented at Human Rights Commission in Pakistan (HRCP), Karachi, Pakistan.

Ahmed, K. (1991, December 13). Gang-rape as an instrument of oppression. *Weekend Post,* p. 8.

Breckenride, C. A., & van der Veer, P. (1993). *Orientalism and the postcolonial predicament perspectives on South Asia.* Philadilphia: University of Pennsylvania Press.

Caroe, O. (1958/1983). *The Pathans: 350 B.C.-A.D.* Karachi: Oxford University Press.

Doniger, W. (1999). *Splitting the difference: Gender and myth in Ancient Greece and India.* Chicago: University of Chicago Press.

*Frontier Post,* an English language Pakistani daily. (1991, December 20). p. 3.

Geertz, C. (1973). *The interpretation of cultures.* New York: Basic.

Haeri, S. (1995). Politics of dishonor: Rape and power in Pakistan. In M. Afkhami (Ed.), *Faith and freedom: Women's human rights in the Muslim world* (pp. 129-149). London: I.B. Tauris.

Haeri, S. (2002). *No shame for the sun: Lives of professional Pakistani women.* Syracuse, NY: Syracuse University Press.

Harvey, M. (1996). An ecological view of psychological trauma and trauma recovery. *Journal of Traumatic Stress, 9*(1), 3-24.

Harvey, M. R. (2007). Towards an ecological understanding of resilience in trauma survivors: Implications for theory, research, and practice. *Journal of Aggression, Maltreatment & Trauma, 14*(1/2), 33-53.

Harvey, M. R., Mishler, E. G., Koenen, K., & Harney, P. A. (2002). In the aftermath of sexual abuse: Making and remaking meaning in narratives of trauma and recovery. *Narrative Inquiry, 10*(2), 291-311.

*Herald.* (1992, January). Article of unknown title appearing in a Pakistani monthly magazine, p. 42.

Hoodbhoy, N. (1989, October). Corridors of fear. *Herald*, pp. 147-150.

Human Rights Watch. (1992). *Double jeopardy: Police abuse of women in Pakistan.* New York: Author.

Human Rights Watch. (1996). *All too familiar: Sexual abuse of women in the U.S. state prisons.* New York: Author

Human Rights Watch. (1999). *Crime or custom? Violence against women in Pakistan.* Available from, www.hrw.org/reports/1999/Pakistan.

Jalal, A. (2001). *Self and sovereignty: Individual and community in South Asian Islam since 1850.* Lahore, Pakistan: Sang-e Meel Publications.

Kakar, S. (1989). *Intimate relations: Exploring Indian sexuality.* Chicago: University of Chicago Press.

Low, S. M. (1996). The anthropology of cities: Imagining and theorizing the city. *Annual Review of Anthropology, 25*, 383-409.

Malik, I. (1997). *State and civil society in Pakistan: Politics of authority, ideology, and ethnicity.* London: McMillan.

Rahman, I. A. (1989, September). Of female bondage. *Newsline*, pp. 66-68.

Pinault, D. (1998). The place of the women of the household of the First Imam in Shi'ite devotional literature. In C. B. Hambly (Ed.), *Women in the Medieval Islamic World: Power, patronage, and piety* (pp. 69-98). New York: St. Martin Press.

Riesebrodt, M. (1993). *Pious passion: The emergence of modern fundamentalism in the United States and Iran.* Berkeley, CA: University of California Press.

Sarwar, B. (1991, December 9). Politically motivated rape. *The Frontier Post*, p. 16.

Sarwar, B. (1992, January 10). No one to turn, nowhere to go. *The Weekend Post*, p. 8.

Shirkat Gah. (1992). *Newsheet*, a quarterly on women, laws, and society produced by the Shirkat Gah for the international solidarity network Women Living Under Muslim Laws.

Spellberg, D. (1994). *Politics, gender, and the Islamic past: The legacy of A'isha Bint Abi Bakr.* New York: Columbia University Press.

Ward, M. (1996). *A world full of women.* Boston: Allyn and Bacon.

Weaver, M. A. (2000, January 10). Gandhi's daughters: India's poorest women embark on an epic social experiment. *The New Yorker*, 52-54.

Women Against Rape. (1993, April). Newsletter.

Yusuf, Z. (1992, January). A rising graph? *Herald*, pp. 47-48.

Zaman, R. (1990, June). Rape is violence against a woman in which sex is the weapon. *Newsline Special Issue*, pp. 121-122.

doi:10.1300/J146v14n01_15

# Epilogue

The articles presented here give testimony not only to the enormous resilience that trauma survivors and traumatized communities may evince in the aftermath of suffering, but also to the range and scope of atrocities that human beings worldwide suffer and impose on one another. As this volume goes to press, there is no evidence that the violence will abate or suffering end. Therefore, as we recognize and honor the capacities that enable human beings, their communities and cultures to survive and, one hopes, to thrive, it is imperative that we also acknowledge the terrible harm that human beings seem prone to. Nothing about a focus on resilience should in any way diminish our recognition of–or our attentiveness to–the many and complicated ways in which violence and abuse compromise psychological functioning, undermine individual and public health and threaten the sometimes fragile ecosystems of human community. While we may celebrate the resilient capacities that trauma survivors and their communities may develop without professional help, that celebration should not divert our attention from the need for more in the way of culturally attuned professional assistance and more in the way of ecologically-informed, multiculturally relevant practice. As psychotherapists who work with trauma survivors, we are both proud of and humbled by the role we are called upon to play as witnesses to the harm our clients have endured and the healing they are able to achieve. We have learned from them and with them a great

[Haworth co-indexing entry note]: "Epilogue." Harvey, Mary R., and Pratyusha Tummala-Narra. Co-published simultaneously in *Journal of Aggression, Maltreatment & Trauma* (The Haworth Maltreatment & Trauma Press, an imprint of The Haworth Press, Inc.) Vol. 14, No. 1/2, 2007, pp. 305-306; and: *Sources and Expressions of Resiliency in Trauma Survivors: Ecological Theory, Multicultural Practice* (ed: Mary R. Harvey, and Pratyusha Tummala-Narra) The Haworth Maltreatment & Trauma Press, an imprint of The Haworth Press, Inc., 2007, pp. 305-306. Single or multiple copies of this article are available for a fee from The Haworth Document Delivery Service [1-800-HAWORTH, 9:00 a.m. - 5:00 p.m. (EST). E-mail address: docdelivery@haworthpress.com].

Available online at http://jamt.haworthpress.com
doi:10.1300/J146v14n01_16

deal about the repairative possiblilities of safe and empowering human relationships. We have also learned that our role as witnesses requires us to act outside the therapeutic milieu, to speak out against the violence and oppression our clients have suffered and to join with others in a spirited search for social justice and political reform.

*Mary R. Harvey*
*Pratyusha Tummala-Narra*

# Appendix A:
# Multidimensional Trauma Recovery and Resiliency Scale (MTRR-99) Clinical Rating Form

Harvey, M.R., Westen, D., Lebowitz, L., Saunders, E., Avi-Yonah, O, & Harney, P.A. (1994 version, MTRR-135), plus Liang, B. & Tummala-Narra, P. (MTRR-99, 2000 version)

### DOMAIN 1: AUTHORITY OVER MEMORY

| Item No. | | Circle [1 = Not at all descriptive to 5 = Highly descriptive] | Score |
|---|---|---|---|
| 3. | Has relatively continuous memory for adulthood. | . 1 2 3 4 5 | = _____ |
| 4. | Has difficulty recalling events from the very recent past. | 1 2 3 4 5 | = 6 − __ = __ __ |
| 15. | Can remember and can relate to others a relatively complete story of his or her life, from childhood to present. | 1 2 3 4 5 | = _____ |
| 17. | Can recall painful events, including traumatic events, with detail and clarity. | 1 2 3 4 5 | = _____ |
| 26. | Has relatively continuous memory for events in childhood and adolescence. | 1 2 3 4 5 | = _____ |
| 27. | Can recall both positive and negative experiences from childhood and adolescence. | 1 2 3 4 5 | = _____ |
| 33.* | Has nightmares or night terrors in which traumatic experiences are relived. | 1 2 3 4 5 | = 6 − __ = _____ |

Reprinted with permission.

[Haworth co-indexing entry note]: "Appendix A: Multidimensional Trauma Recovery and Resiliency Scale (MTRR-99) Clinical Rating Form." Co-published simultaneously in *Journal of Aggression, Maltreatment & Trauma* (The Haworth Maltreatment & Trauma Press, an imprint of The Haworth Press, Inc.) Vol. 14, No. 1/2, 2007, pp. 307-313; and: *Sources and Expressions of Resiliency in Trauma Survivors: Ecological Theory, Multicultural Practice* (ed: Mary R. Harvey, and Pratyusha Tummala-Narra) The Haworth Maltreatment & Trauma Press, an imprint of The Haworth Press, Inc., 2007, pp. 307-313. Single or multiple copies of this article are available for a fee from The Haworth Document Delivery Service [1-800-HAWORTH, 9:00 a.m. - 5:00 p.m. (EST). E-mail address: docdelivery@haworthpress.com].

Available online at http://jamt.haworthpress.com
doi:10.1300/J146v14n01_17

## APPENDIX A (continued)

| Item No. | | Circle<br>[1 = Not at all descriptive to<br>5 = Highly descriptive] | Score |
|---|---|---|---|
| 52.* | Unwanted thoughts, memories or images intrude on consciousness. | 1 2 3 4 5 | = 6 − __ = ____ |
| 62.** | Functions adaptively after retrieving painful memories, including memories of traumatic events. | 1 2 3 4 5 | = ____ |
| 89.* | At times behaves as if a past event (specifically a past traumatic event) is happening when it is not. | 1 2 3 4 5 | = 6 − __ = ____ |
| 97. | Can choose to recall or to put aside memories of painful events, including traumatic events. | 1 2 3 4 5 | = ____ |

Sum of Scores = ____

* Item Assesses PTSD Sx      No. of Items = ____

**Optional Item at Intake Assessment      Mean Score = ____

### DOMAIN 2: INTEGRATION OF MEMORY AND AFFECT

| | | | |
|---|---|---|---|
| 11. | When recalling painful or traumatic events s/he is able to remember feelings experienced at the time. | 1 2 3 4 5 | = ____ |
| 12. | When recalling painful or traumatic events, s/he is able to feel emotions experienced at the time. | 1 2 3 4 5 | = ____ |
| 53.* | When recalling painful or traumatic events, s/he vacillates between feeling flooded with emotion and experiencing no emotion at all. | 1 2 3 4 5 | = 6 − __ = ____ |
| 60. | Memories for painful or traumatic events integrate feelings from the past with new (and possibly different) feelings about the past. | 1 2 3 4 5 | = ____ |
| 94. | Can reflect upon painful events, including traumatic events, with varied and appropriate feeling. | 1 2 3 4 5 | = ____ |

Sum of Scores = ____

* Item Assesses PTSD Sx      No. of Items = ____

**Optional Item at Intake Assessment      Mean Score = ____

### DOMAIN 3: AFFECT TOLERANCE AND REGULATION

| | | | |
|---|---|---|---|
| 18. | Is able to regulate unpleasant affects without resorting to self-harming, self destructive behaviors (e.g., substance abuse, cutting etc.) | 1 2 3 4 5 | = ____ |
| 21.* | Daily functioning is compromised by the avoidance of thoughts or situations that might elicit difficult or unpleasant emotions. | 1 2 3 4 5 | = 6 − __ = ____ |
| 24. | Is able to experience a wide range of emotions, specifically: Anger, fear/anxiety, sadness, pleasure, anticipation, joy and hope. | 1 2 3 4 5 | = ____ |
| 25. | Is able to experience each of these emotions in a range of intensities. | 1 2 3 4 5 | = ____ |
| 28. | Often feels intense anger and rage. | 1 2 3 4 5 | = 6 − __ = ____ |
| 30.* | Often feels emotionally numb. | 1 2 3 4 5 | = 6 − __ = ____ |

| | | | |
|---|---|---|---|
| 37. | Often experiences feelings of helplessness. | 1 2 3 4 5 | = 6 − __ = ____ |
| 38. | Experiences impulses to abuse drugs or alcohol whether or not s/he acts on these impulses. | 1 2 3 4 5 | = 6 − __ = ____ |
| 39. | Abuses drugs or alcohol. | 1 2 3 4 5 | = 6 − __ = ____ |
| 40.* | Seldom re-experiences extreme trauma-related affects such as terror, rage, overwhelming arousal, or utter helplessness. | 1 2 3 4 5 | = ____ |
| 67. | Is troubled by feelings of shame and guilt. | 1 2 3 4 5 | = 6 − __ = ____ |
| 78. | Often feels hopeless or depressed. | 1 2 3 4 5 | = 6 − __ = ____ |
| 88. | Often feels anxious. | 1 2 3 4 5 | = 6 − __ = ____ |
| 93. | Maintains a realistic view of situations even when emotions are strong. | 1 2 3 4 5 | = ____ |
| 98. | Is troubled by feelings of loss and grief. | 1 2 3 4 5 | = 6 − __ = ____ |

Sum of Scores = ____

\* Item Assesses PTSD Sx    No. of Items = ____

\*\*Optional Item at Intake Assessment    Mean Score = ____

**DOMAIN 4: SYMPTOM MASTERY AND POSITIVE COPING**

| | | | |
|---|---|---|---|
| 7. | Uses humor appropriately and effectively to manage stress. | 1 2 3 4 5 | = ____ |
| 10. | Is able to accept help and experience help as helpful. | 1 2 3 4 5 | = ____ |
| 13.* | Is readily startled. | 1 2 3 4 5 | = 6 − __ = ____ |
| 44. | Practices and makes effective use of one or more stress management techniques (e.g., relaxation, meditation). | 1 2 3 4 5 | = ____ |
| 47. | Enjoys work and is able to be task involved despite outside stressors. | 1 2 3 4 5 | = ____ |
| 51. | Utilizes imaginative capacities to manage distress. | 1 2 3 4 5 | = ____ |
| 54. | Has panic attacks. | 1 2 3 4 5 | = 6 − __ = ____ |
| 61.** | Responds empathetically to other peoples' needs. | 1 2 3 4 5 | = ____ |
| 65. | Recognizes and avoids anxiety provoking situations. | 1 2 3 4 5 | = ____ |
| 73.** | Is preoccupied with or distracted by fears of danger. | 1 2 3 4 5 | = 6 − __ = ____ |
| 82.* | Is troubled by disturbed sleep. | 1 2 3 4 5 | = 6 − __ = ____ |
| 85.** | Is excessively preoccupied with medical concerns or stress related physical ailments. | 1 2 3 4 5 | = 6 − __ = ____ |

Sum of Scores = ____

\* Item Assesses PTSD Sx    No. of Items = ____

\*\*Optional Item at Intake Assessment    Mean Score = ____

**DOMAIN 5: SELF ESTEEM (SELF CARE & SELF REGARD)**

| | | | |
|---|---|---|---|
| 2. | Takes unnecessary risks with her or his physical safety. | 1 2 3 4 5 | = 6 − __ = ____ |
| 9. | Exhibits self-care by maintaining healthy sleeping and eating routines. | 1 2 3 4 5 | = ____ |

## APPENDIX A (continued)

| Item No. | | Circle [1 = Not at all descriptive to 5 = Highly descriptive] | Score |
|---|---|---|---|
| 20. | Ascribes a number and range of positive and valued qualities to self (e.g., sees self as compassionate and caring, empathic, competent, hardworking, creative). | 1 2 3 4 5 | = _____ |
| 22. | Experiences self as evil, stigmatized or alien. | 1 2 3 4 5 | = 6 − __ = _____ |
| 29. | Exhibits self care by engaging in a well balanced variety of personally meaningful activities. | 1 2 3 4 5 | = _____ |
| 35. | Feels worthy of care and nurturance from others. | 1 2 3 4 5 | = _____ |
| 41. | Experiences suicidal **thoughts or impulses**, whether s/he acts on these or not. | 1 2 3 4 5 | = 6 − __ = _____ |
| 42. | At times **acts** on suicidal thoughts or impulses. | 1 2 3 4 5 | = 6 − __ = _____ |
| 45. | Experiences **impulses** to behave in self abusive ways, such as cutting, burning, whether or not s/he acts on these impulses or not. | 1 2 3 4 5 | = 6 − __ = _____ |
| 46. | **Behaves** in ways that are physically self-abusive, such as cutting, burning, etc. | 1 2 3 4 5 | = 6 − __ = _____ |
| 64.** | Experiences self as mentally, emotionally or or physically damaged. | 1 2 3 4 5 | = 6 − __ = _____ |
| 71. | Experiences self as "special" in worrisome ways (e.g., as selected for victimization, or as especially powerful or endowed with uncanny powers and attractions) | 1 2 3 4 5 | = 6 − __ = _____ |
| 72. | Recognizes and avoids situations that are demeaning, humiliating or unnecessarily painful. | 1 2 3 4 5 | = _____ |
| 75.** | Is comfortable with her or his sexual orientation. | 1 2 3 4 5 | = _____ |
| 84. | Has an occupation appropriate to her or his abilities and talents. | 1 2 3 4 5 | = _____ |

Sum of Scores = _____

\* Item Assesses PTSD Sx          No. of Items = _____

\*\*Optional Item at Intake Assessment          Mean Score = _____

**DOMAIN 6: SELF COHESION**

| | | | |
|---|---|---|---|
| 14. | Experiences strange or intense bodily sensations that seem to come from nowhere. | 1 2 3 4 5 | = 6 − __ = _____ |
| 16. | Experience of self shifts markedly with change of mood or situation. | 1 2 3 4 5 | = 6 − __ = _____ |
| 34. | Appears to have multiple personalities that compete for control of consciousness and may have little awareness of each other. | 1 2 3 4 5 | = 6 − __ = _____ |
| 57. | Experiences dissociative states (e.g., feels like s/he leaves her/his body or that her/his feelings are somewhere else). | 1 2 3 4 5 | = 6 − __ = _____ |

| | | | |
|---|---|---|---|
| 63.** | Leads a carefully compartmentalized life characterized by secrecy and duplicity. | 1 2 3 4 5 | = 6 − __ = ____ |
| 69. | Has assumed control over dissociative capacities that once compromised psychological status and daily functioning. | 1 2 3 4 5 | = _____ Or NA (not applicable) |
| 79. | Feels like an integrated person whose actions and emotions fit together coherently. | 1 2 3 4 5 | = _____ |
| 99. | Appears to enter an altered or dissociative state when recounting traumatic experiences. | 1 2 3 4 5 | = 6 − __ = ____ |

Sum of Scores = _____

* Item Assesses PTSD Sx  No. of Items = _____

**Optional Item at Intake Assessment  Mean Score = _____

## DOMAIN 7: SAFE ATTACHMENT

| | | | |
|---|---|---|---|
| 5. | Gets involved in emotionally, physically or sexually abusive relationships in the role of perpetrator. | 1 2 3 4 5 | = 6 − __ = ____ |
| 6. | Gets involved in emotionally, physically or sexually abusive relationships in the role of victim. | 1 2 3 4 5 | = 6 − __ = ____ |
| 19. | Is comfortable with current relationship (and level of contact) with family of origin. | 1 2 3 4 5 | = _____ |
| 31. | Is able to enter into and maintain safe and mutually satisfying relationships with intimate partners. | 1 2 3 4 5 | = _____ |
| 36. | Is unusually sensitive to (or is preoccupied with) issues of power and control in relationships. | 1 2 3 4 5 | = 6 − __ = ____ |
| 43. | Has generally positive experiences with members of the opposite sex. | 1 2 3 4 5 | = _____ |
| 55. | Experiences aggressive impulses towards others. | 1 2 3 4 5 | = 6 − __ = ____ |
| 56. | Acts on aggressive impulses towards others. | 1 2 3 4 5 | = 6 − __ = ____ |
| 68. | Forms and maintains safe and mutually satisfying friendships. | 1 2 3 4 5 | = _____ |
| 76. | Experiences altruistic inclinations towards others. | 1 2 3 4 5 | = _____ |
| 77. | Acts on altruistic inclinations towards others. | 1 2 3 4 5 | = _____ |
| 80. | Avoids sexual contact. | 1 2 3 4 5 | = 6 − __ = ____ |
| 81. | Engages in compulsive or indiscriminate sexual activity. | 1 2 3 4 5 | = 6 − __ = ____ |
| 83.* | Avoids relationships. | 1 2 3 4 5 | = 6 − __ = ____ |
| 86. | Has generally positive experiences with members of own sex. | 1 2 3 4 5 | = _____ |
| 87.** | Engages in safe, pleasurable and consensual sex. | 1 2 3 4 5 | = _____ |
| 95.** | Is distrustful even when trust is warranted. | 1 2 3 4 5 | = 6 − __ = ____ |
| 96. | Is overly trusting when caution is warranted. | 1 2 3 4 5 | = 6 − __ = ____ |

Sum of Scores = _____

* Item Assesses PTSD Sx  No. of Items = _____

**Optional Item at Intake Assessment  Mean Score = _____

## APPENDIX A (continued)

| Item No. | | Circle<br>[1 = Not at all descriptive to<br>5 = Highly descriptive] | Score |
|---|---|---|---|
| **DOMAIN 8: MEANING** | | | |
| 1. | Has developed a coherent, personally meaningful and realistic narrative of her/his life, including painful and traumatic events. | 1 2 3 4 5 | = _____ |
| 8. | Is preoccupied with issues of trauma and abuse. | 1 2 3 4 5 | = 6 – __ = _____ |
| 23. | Understanding of painful or traumatic past is marked by excessive and unreasonable self-blame. | 1 2 3 4 5 | = 6 – __ = _____ |
| 32. | Understanding of painful or traumatic past incorporates conflicting and ambiguous aspects of reality. | 1 2 3 4 5 | = _____ |
| 48. | Understands the nature and origins of her/his psychological difficulties or vulnerabilities. | 1 2 3 4 5 | = _____ |
| 49. | Draws meaning from membership in a larger community. | 1 2 3 4 5 | = _____ |
| 50. | Appears to have come to terms with painful or traumatic events of the past. | 1 2 3 4 5 | = _____ |
| 58. | Is able to feel a realistic sense of hope and optimism about the future. | 1 2 3 4 5 | = _____ |
| 59. | Engages in creative pursuits and artistic endeavors as a way of making meaning of past trauma. | 1 2 3 4 5 | = _____ |
| 66. | Engages in educational, philanthropic or altruistic activities as a way of making meaning of past trauma. | 1 2 3 4 5 | = _____ |
| 70. | Is involved in (or draws meaning from) activities aimed at helping victims of trauma. | 1 2 3 4 5 | = _____ |
| 74. | Engages in social or political action as a way of making meaning of past trauma. | 1 2 3 4 5 | = _____ |
| 90. | Is able to draw comfort and meaning from a coherent set of religious, spiritual beliefs and/or moral values. | 1 2 3 4 5 | = _____ |
| 91. | View of self incorporates but is not dominated by painful or traumatic experiences. | 1 2 3 4 5 | = _____ |
| 92. | Finds meaning in life (and in past suffering or trauma) | 1 2 3 4 5 | = _____ |

**Sum of Scores = _____**

\* Item Assesses PTSD Sx   **No. of Items = _____**

\*\*Optional Item at Intake Assessment   **Mean Score = _____**

### SCORING THE MTRR RATING FORM

*Instructions:* The rating form you have completed is designed to help you calculate item scores and domain scores. If you wish, you may calculate these and plot the domain scores on the bar graph in order to construct a multidimensional profile of the subject or patient you have rated.

### Scoring the Items

The score for any item which is stated as a positive recovery attribute (e.g. "has relatively continuous memory for adulthood") is equal to the rating which was given to the subject on that item. If, for example, you felt that this item was quite descriptive of the subject, then you might have given a rating of "4" on this item. Therefore the score for this item would be "4."

The score for any item which is stated as a problematic attribute (e.g. "had difficulty recalling events from the very recent past") is equal to the score of 6 minus the rating given the subject on that item. Thus, if you felt that this statement was not at all descriptive of the subject, you would have given a rating of "1." The score for the item would be 6 minus 1 . . . or "5."

### Calculating the Domain Scores

Each domain is comprised of a number of items. To calculate the domain score, you must add the scores of the individual items in that domain and then divide by the number of items. If, for example, the scores for Domain Number One–Authority Over Memory add up to 44, and the domain is comprised of 11 items, all of which were given a rating and a score, then the domain score would be 44 divided by 11, or "4."

If you were unable to rate a subject on one or more items within a domain, then divide the sum of scores in that domain only by the number of items that were actually scored. Thus, if the scores assigned to items in Domain Number One add up to 40, but you were only able to rate the subject on 8 items, then the domain score would be 40 divided by 8, or "5."

## CONSTRUCTING A PROFILE

When you have calculated the domain scores for your subject, you may plot them on a bar graph. The resultant "profile" will give you some indication of the strengths this individual brings to the challenge of recovering from trauma and of the areas of impairment that may require clinical attention. Items you were unable to rate may represent areas of functioning that remain to be explored. This information, too, can assist you in formulating a multi-dimensional treatment for your patient.

# Appendix B:
# Multidimensional Trauma Recovery and Resiliency Interview (MTRR-I) (Short Form, 2000 Version)

Harvey, M.R., Westen, D., Lebowitz, L., Saunders, E., Avi-Yonah, O. and Harney, P. (1994)

## INTRODUCTORY REMARKS

### Time One Introductory Remarks

Thank you so much for giving us your time today. The purpose of this interview is to help us learn more about the impact of traumatic experiences on the lives of individual survivors and, more importantly, to learn something about how people survive, cope with and recover from these experiences. The interview will take about 90 minutes and will cover many topics–your history, your memory for events, difficulties you may have and ways in which you cope, your relationships with others, your feelings about yourself and how you make sense of your experiences and your life. I may move us along from one topic to another in the interest of time; if this ever makes you feel uncomfortable, please let me know. Also, please know that you are free to decline to answer any question I may ask you. Again, thanks so much. Are you ready to begin?

### Time Two (or more) Introductory Remarks

Thank you so much for giving us your time today and for agreeing to let us interview you once again. As you know, the purpose of this interview is to help us learn more about the impact of traumatic experiences on the lives of individual survivors and, more importantly, to learn something about how individuals survive, cope with and recover from these experiences. We are particularly interested in learning how things may have changed for you since the last interview–e.g., as applicable: what VOV (or other designated) services

Reprinted with permission.

[Haworth co-indexing entry note]: "Appendix B: Multidimensional Trauma Recovery and Resiliency Interview (MTRR-I) (Short Form, 2000 version)." Co-published simultaneously in *Journal of Aggression, Maltreatment & Trauma* (The Haworth Maltreatment & Trauma Press, an imprint of The Haworth Press, Inc.) Vol. 14, No. 1/2, 2007, pp. 315-317; and: *Sources and Expressions of Resiliency in Trauma Survivors: Ecological Theory, Multicultural Practice* (ed: Mary R. Harvey, and Pratyusha Tummala-Narra) The Haworth Maltreatment & Trauma Press, an imprint of The Haworth Press, Inc., 2007, pp. 315-317. Single or multiple copies of this article are available for a fee from The Haworth Document Delivery Service [1-800-HAWORTH, 9:00 a.m. - 5:00 p.m. (EST). E-mail address: docdelivery@haworthpress.com].

Available online at http://jamt.haworthpress.com
doi:10.1300/J146v14n01_18

you may have utilized, what community resources you may have accessed, what new things have happened in your life. Like the original, this interview will take about 90 minutes and will cover many topics–your history, your memory for events, your difficulties and your coping strategies, your relationships, how you feel about yourself and how you make sense of your experiences and your life. As before, I may move us along from one topic to another in the interest of time; if this ever makes you feel uncomfortable, please let me know. Also, if you do not wish to answer any question I ask you, please know that you are free to decline. Again, thanks so much. Are you ready to begin?

1. I'd like to begin by asking you some questions about your history. Could you begin by telling me about your childhood, starting as early as you can remember, and working your way up through your teenage years–almost as if you were telling the story of your life, or writing an autobiography.
2. Now, if you can, please tell me about a really painful or traumatic experience from when you were growing up.
3. Now, can you tell me about your adult life–like what you do or have done for work; who are, and have been, the important people in your life; and any other events that have been particularly significant to you, either good or bad.

*Probe the following domains as appropriate, letting the personal narrative determine order of inquiry:*

- *Ability to tell a coherent and continuous life story.*
- *Work History*
- *Family History and Relationships*
- *Social Life and Friendships*
- *Romantic & Sexual Relationships.*
- *Relationships Generally*

4. Have there been changes in the nature or quality of your relationships over time? *Probes: For second and other follow-up interviews, also ask:* have there been any changes in the nature or quality of your relationships since we last interviewed you or *(if applicable)* since you entered treatment in VOV (or other designated clinical setting)?
5. Now I'd like you to tell me, if you can, about a painful or traumatic experience you've had as an adult. Prompts: When you recall painful events like these, do you have feelings? For example, do you remember what you felt at the time, or actually reexperience the feelings when you recall the events?
6. You've told me about some very painful experiences–*[mention what the person has told about painful childhood and adult experiences].* Do memories of this or other painful events ever jump into your mind and prevent you from thinking about or doing something else? *(If yes, probe how often and how recently.)*
7. Have you experienced any changes in what you remember about your past or in how you remember–like how vividly, or with how much detail? *(Again, if this is a second or other follow-up interview, ask about changes since the last interview and if applicable changes since entering VOV or other designated treatment.)*
8. Are there ways you think the painful or traumatic events you've experienced affect your day-to-day your life?
9. What kinds of things do you do to cope or to manage when you get stressed or distressed? *Probe for both adaptive and maladaptive coping strategies.*
10. Have you changed in the way you manage your distress or cope with your problems? *Explore changes since the last interview and, if applicable, since entering VOV or other designated treatment.*
11. Now, I'd like to ask you some questions about your feelings and how you handle them. What is your normal mood–that is, how do you usually feel?
12. Has there been any change in what you feel, how intensely you feel things, or your ability to deal with difficult feelings? *(If so, probe what has changed and what caused the changes.) (Again ask about changes since last interview and if applicable since receiving treatment in VOV or in other context.)*
13. Now I'd like to ask you some questions about how you see, feel about, and take care of yourself. Let's start with feelings. How do you generally feel about yourself? Do your feelings about yourself change a lot from day to day or moment to moment?

14.  Have your feelings about yourself, the way you see yourself, or the ways you treat yourself or your body changed in any way? *Explore changes since last interview and if applicable since entering VOV (or other designated) treatment.*
15.  Does life feel meaningful to you? Does it ever feel meaningless? *(If yes, probe for details re: intensity and pervasiveness.)*
16.  How do you understand the painful and traumatic experience/s of your life?
17.  Has your understanding of these experiences changed over time? How? Does life seem more or less meaningful to you than it used to? *(Ask about changes since last interview and entering VOV or other designated treatment).*
18.  How do you feel about the future?
19.  *If this is a second or later interview and if the subject is a current or former VOV patient or a patient in another treatment of interest, ask:* How do you think the treatment you've received in VOV (or elsewhere) has affected your recovery? What, if any, changes have resulted from your work with us in VOV (or in another designated treatment)?

*Closing Question:* I really appreciate the time you've taken to answer these questions. How has this interview been for you? Are there any other areas of difficulty or sources of strength that we haven't talked about? Is there anything you'd like to add, or anything you'd like to ask?
*Close the interview by thanking the participant, inviting future questions, and assuring her/him of the value and contribution s/he has made to us, to the field, and to other survivors.*
*Assess mental status and emotional well-being of interviewee, offer support and, as needed, provide appropriate referrals and follow-up.*

---

This interview can be rated quantitatively by means of the MTRR-99.

Interviewer(s) should complete the rating immediately following the interview itself.

Note: This is a short form of the MTRR-I. For more information about the measure and/or to obtain a copy of the longer form, which includes specific prompts and probes, please contact: Mary Harvey, Ph.D. at haverymr@comcast.net or BLouis@challiance.org. In addition, information about the Spanish, French, and Japanese language versions of the MTRR-I can be obtained from Angela Radan, Ph.D. at ARadan@challiance.org., Isabelle Daigneault at isabelle.daigneault@sympatico.ca, and Kuniko Muramoto at kunikomura@mub.biglobe.ne.jp, respectively.

# Index

Abram, K.M., 125
Abuse
  physical
    in adults, in study of
      interpersonal violence,
      recovery, and resilience in
      incarcerated women, 130
    of children, in study of
      interpersonal violence,
      recovery, and resilience in
      incarcerated women, 130
  sexual
    characteristics of, 171
    of children, in study of
      interpersonal violence,
      recovery, and resilience in
      incarcerated women, 129-130
Adolescent(ies), sexually abused,
    recovery trajectories in,
    exploration of, 165-184. *See
    also* Sexually abused
    adolescents, recovery
    trajectories in, exploration of
Adult physical abuse (APA), in study
    of interpersonal violence,
    recovery, and resilience in
    incarcerated women, 130
Adult sexual assault (ASA), in study of
    interpersonal violence,
    recovery, and resilience in
    incarcerated women, 130
Advocacy
  in aftermath of violence, client
    example, 247-250
  as individual and social justice, 247
Advocacy practices, individual and
    social, on behalf of trauma
    survivors, 245-263. *See also*
    Trauma survivors, individual

and social advocacy practice
  on behalf of
Ahmed, K., 291
Aldrich, H., xix,6,265
Allen, S.N., 230
Andrews, B., 35
Angelou, M., 48
APA. *See* Adult physical abuse (APA)
Aron, A., 150
Artistic creation, trauma and, 47-48
ASA. *See* Adult sexual assault (ASA)
Asian Pacific Islander Women's Social
    Justice Project, xx
Assertiveness, in early recovery of
    trauma survivors, 90-91
Ataques de nervios, 161
Ayesha, H.B., 298


Bank Street College, xxii
Belief(s), cultural, resilience and,
    37-38
Best, C.L., 128
Bhutto, B., 289-295,297
Bias, cultural, in resiliency research,
    35-36
Bloom, S.L., 47,230
Bonanno, G., 14,15
Boston Area Rape Crisis Center, xxiii
Boston College, xxii
  Lynch School of Education at, xxi
Boston University, xx
Bradley, R., xix,4,5,55,123
Brewin, C.R., 35
Brown University, xxi
Browne, A., 124
Bukowski, L.T., xix,4,75
Burke, M.J., 172

Burstow, B., 48,118

Caddell, J.M., 125
Cambridge Health Alliance (CHA),
    xxi,xxii
    South Asian Mental Health Clinic
        at, xxvi
    VOV Program of. *See* Victims of
        Violence (VOV) Program, of
        Cambridge Health Alliance
Cambridge Hospital, xix,231
CCRT. *See* Community Crisis
    Response Team (CCRT)
Center for Homicide Bereavement
    (CHB), xix,21
Center for Middle Eastern Studies, xxi
Center for Research on Gender and
    Sexuality, at San Francisco
    State University, xxii
Central America, women survivors in
    exposure to violence and
        expressions of resilience in,
        147-164
    ecological perspective on,
        149-150
    future research in, 162-163
    study of, 152-163,157t,158t
        comparisons of Guatemalan
            and El Salvadoran
            women in, 155-156
        discussion of, 158-162
        exposure to traumatic events
            in, 156,157t
        limitations of, 162
        measures in, 153-154
        methods in, 152-155
        multidimensional profiles of
            resilience in,
            156-158,157t,158t
        participants in, 152-153
        procedures in, 154-155
        results of, 155-158,157t,158t
    war and post-war experiences of,
        150-152

Centre de recherche interdisciplinaire
    sur les problèmes conjugaux
    et les agressions sexuelles
    (CRIPCAS), xix,xx,xxiii
CHA. *See* Cambridge Health Alliance
    (CHA)
Channer, E.G., xix,4,75
CHB. *See* Center for Homicide
    Bereavement (CHB)
Child physical abuse (CPA), in study
    of interpersonal violence,
    recovery, and resilience in
    incarcerated women, 130
Child Protective Services (CPS), 166
    mental health impacts of, 166-167
Child sexual abuse (CSA), in study of
    interpersonal violence,
    recovery, and resilience in
    incarcerated women, 129-130
Chronic interpersonal trauma, effects
    of, 229
CIA Center, 297
Clarence Thomas–Anita Hill hearings,
    40-41
Cohen, J., 172
Community(ies)
    new, for trauma survivors, group
        therapy as ecological bridge
        to, 227-243
    racially diverse, trauma in, 38-43.
        *See also* Trauma, in racially
        diverse communities
    in resiliency, 37
    traumatized, resilience in, fostering
        of, 265-285. *See also*
        Traumatized communities,
        resilience in, fostering of
Community Crisis Response Team
    (CCRT), xix
    of VOV Program, xxi,xxii,6,21,
        265,267-268
        described, 268-269
        precipitating events and client
            communities, 270-271
        services of, 271-273

team building, 269-270
team training, 269-270
Community empowerment model of
    intervention, 273-278,274f
in action, 278-280
clarifying CCRT resources in, 275
community entry in, 273-274,274f
described, 280-282
designing CCRT response in,
    275-276
evaluation of, 277
exit/closure, 277-278
feedback for, 277
identifying community resources
    and resource gaps in, 275
implementing responses in,
    276-277
request analysis in, 275
Community psychology
    brief history of, 16
    contributions of, 15-20
    ecological perspective of, 16-20
    VOV Program and, 25-26
Community trauma
    case example of, 266-267
    responding to, 267-268
"Complex PTSD," 12
Conflict Tactics Scale, 128,129
Coping, in early recovery of trauma
    survivors, 89-90
Corbin, J., 136
Cortina, J.M., 172
Costa Rican Psychological
    Association, Distinguished
    Service Award from, xxii
Cousineau, M., 35
Cowen, E.L., 17,18,26
CPA. *See* Child physical abuse (CPA)
CPS. *See* Child Protective Services
    (CPS)
CRIPCAS (Centre de recherche
    interdisciplinaire sur les
    problèmes conjugaux et les
    afressions sexuelles), xix,xx,
    xxiii

CSA. *See* Child sexual abuse (CSA)
Csikszentmihalyi, M., 14
Cultural and political contexts,
    resilience and post-traumatic
    recovery in, Pakistani
    women's strategies for
    survival, 287-304. *See also*
    Resilience, in cultural and
    political context, Pakistani
    women's strategies for
    survival
Cultural and racial contexts,
    psychotherapeutic
    relationship and, 219-221
Cultural beliefs, resilience and, 37-38
Cultural bias, in resiliency research,
    35-36
Cultural contexts, resilience within and
    across, defined, 36-38
Cultural identity, individual, reshaping
    of, resilience and, 43-45
Cyr, M., xix.5,165

Daigneault, I., xx,5,165
Daniel, J.H., 40,41
Dansky, B.S., 128
Davino, K., xx,5,123
*Diagnostic and Statistical Manual of
    Mental Disorders* (DSM-III),
    56,100,190
Distinguished Service Award, from
    Costa Rican Psychological
    Association, xxii
Downs, W.R., 168
DSM-III. *See Diagnostic and
    Statistical Manual of Mental
    Disorders* (DSM-III)
Dunlop, W.P., 172

EFI. *See* Enright Forgiveness
    Inventory (EFI)
Emory University, xix,xx

Enright Forgiveness Inventory (EFI), 190

Fairbank, J.A., 125
Family support, in healing from trauma, 46-47
Fielding Graduate Institute, xxii
Foy, D.W., 230
Freire, P., 261
Fulbright Scholarship, xxi,xxii
Functioning, eight domains of, 216-218

Geertz, C., 296
Gender justice, in Pakistani women's strategies for survival, 298-299
Gomez, C., xx,6,245
Governor's Commission on Domestic Violence and Sexual Assault, xx
Graduate School of Education, of Harvard University, xxii
Group movements, social change and, 47
Group therapy
    as ecological bridge to new community for trauma survivors, 227-243. *See also* Victims of Violence (VOV) Program, group treatment at
    for survivors of interpersonal trauma, 230-231
Guatemalan women, war and post-war experiences of, 150-152

Haeri, S., xx,7,287
Hall, G.C.N., 209
Hall, J., 94
Harney, P.A., xxi,36,227
Harvard Divinity School, Women's Studies in Religion Program of, xxi

Harvard Medical School, xix,xxi,xxvi, 231,246
Harvard Trauma Questionnaire (HTQ), 147,153-154,156,159-161
Harvard University, xxi
    Graduate School of Education of, xxii
Harvey, M.R., xxix,xxvi,1,3,4,6,9,36, 43,55,57,72,79,125-127,131, 143,149,152,171,186,208, 209,216,218-219,233, 265,306
Healing
    as revolutionary act, 261-262
    from trauma in diverse contexts, 46-49
Health, defined, 252
Herman, J.L., xxv,2,3,12,207,229, 230,232
Higgins, G.O., 78,93
Hobfoll, S.E., 19,38
Hollingstead, A.B., 40
Hope
    collective resilience and, 46-48
    in early recovery of trauma survivors, 92
HTQ. *See* Harvard Trauma Questionnaire (HTQ)
Huberman, A., 136,137
Human suffering, epidemiology of, 11-12

ICITE! Women of Color Against Violence, xx
Idaho State University, xxi
Identity, cultural, individual, reshaping of, resilience and, 43-45
Incarcerated women
    interpersonal violence, recovery, and resilience in, MTRR-I in determination of impact of, studies of, 126-144,132t,134t, 136t,137f,138t,139f,141f,142t
    adult sexual assault in, 130

*Index* 	*323*
background information in,
135-136,137f
child physical abuse in, 130
child sexual abuse in, 129-130
data display in, 138-140,139f,
141f,142t
data reduction in, 136-138,138t
discussion of, 140,142-144
measures in, 127-129
method in, 126-129,
135-136,136t,137f
MTRR scores in,
130-131,132t,134t
participants in, 127
patient history in, 129-130
procedure for, 126
profiles of resilience in,
131-135,132t,134t
results of, 129-140,132t,
134t,138t,139f,141f,142t
PTSD in, 125
Individual advocacy practice, on
behalf of trauma survivors,
245-263. *See also* Trauma
survivors, individual and
social advocacy practice on
behalf of
Individual justice, advocacy as, 247
Individual psychotherapy, in
multicultural context,
205-225. *See also*
Psychotherapy, individual, in
multicultural context
International Society for the
Prevention of Child Abuse
and Neglect, xxii
Internet, 256
Interpersonal trauma
chronic, effects of, 229
survivors of, group therapy for,
230-231
Interpersonal violence, recovery from,
resilience to, in incarcerated
women, 123-146. *See also*
Incarcerated women,

interpersonal violence,
recovery, and resilience in

Jinnah, M.A., 292
Jordan, B., 125
Justice
individual, advocacy as, 247
social, advocacy as, 247

Keasler, A.L., xxi,4
Kelly, J.G., 10,283
Kesler, A.L., 75
Kilpatrick, D.G., 128
Koenen, K., 36

Lahiri, J., 48
Latin American psychologists,
contributions to context of
war, 148-149
Latino Mental Health Program, xxii
*Law of Desire: Temporary Marriage,
Mut'a, in Iran*, xxi
LemonAid Fund, xxii
Liang, B., xxi,4,55
Limitations, in early recovery of
trauma survivors, 90-91
Loo, C.M., 42
Luthar, S.S., 168
Lynch School of Education, at Boston
College, xxi
Lynch, S.M., xxi,4,75

Maguin, E., 124
Martín-Baró, I., 148-149,160
Massachusetts Office of Victim
Assistance, 246
Masten, A.S., 95-96,115-116
MataHari–Eye of the Day, xx
Maton, K., 20,26
McClelland, G.M., 125

McGloin, J.M., 77
Mendelsohn, M., xxi,6,227
Mental health, CPS impact on,
    166-167
Miles, M., 136,137
Miller, B., 124
Mishler, E.G., 36
Mitchell, J.T., 272
Mondesir, A.V., xxii,6,265
Moos, H., 25
Moos, R., 18
Morrison, T., 48
MTRR-99. *See* Multidimensional
    Trauma Recovery and
    Resiliency Scale
    (MTRR-135)
MTRR-135. *See* Multidimensional
    Trauma Recovery and
    Resiliency Scale
    (MTRR-135)
MTRR-I. *See* Multidimensional
    Trauma Recovery and
    Resiliency Instrument
    (MTRR-I)
MTRR-Q. *See* Multidimensional
    Trauma Recovery and
    Resiliency Q-sort (MTRR-Q)
Multicultural expressions of resilience,
    43-45
Multicultural influences, in trauma
    research, 13
Multidimensional Trauma Recovery
    and Resiliency, domains of,
    definitions of, 57,58t
Multidimensional Trauma Recovery
    and Resiliency Interview
    (MTRR-I), 55-74,79,165,
    170,185,186,315-317. *See
    also* Multidimensional
    Trauma Recovery and
    Resiliency Scale
    (MMTR-135)
abridged version of
    development of, 57-59,58t

preliminary examination of,
    55-74
in assessment of violence and
    expressions of resilience in
    women in Central America,
    147-164. *See also* Central
    America, women survivors in
Q-sort of, 56
Multidimensional Trauma Recovery
    and Resiliency Q-sort
    (MMTR-Q), 56
Multidimensional Trauma Recovery
    and Resiliency Scale
    (MMTR-135), 55-74
Multidimensional Trauma Recovery
    and Resiliency Scale
    (MTRR-135), 55-74,79,170,
    185,186,208
in assessment of violence and
    expressions of resilience in
    women in Central America,
    147-164. *See also* Central
    America, women survivors in
clinical rating form, 307-313
construction and evaluation of,
    study of, 59-73,60t,64t,65t,
    70t,71t
    construct validity of, 63-66,65t
    item analysis in, 62-63,64t
    measures in, 59-60,60t
    method in, 59-61,60t
    participants in, 59
    procedure for, 60-61
    reliability in, 62-63
    results of, 61-66,64t,65t
discussion of, 69,71-73
future directions for, 72-73
limitations of, 72-73
psychometric studies leading to,
    57-59
psychometrics of, study of, 66-69
    goal of, 66
    measures in, 68
    method in, 66-68
    participants in, 66-67

preliminary psychometric properties in, 69,71t
procedure for, 67-68
reliability in, 68-69,70t
results of, 68-69,70t
Multidimensional Trauma Recovery and Resiliency Scale (MTRR-99) and Interview (MTRR-I), 4,5,23
Multidimensional Trauma Resilience and Recovery Interview (MTRR-I), in determination of impact of interpersonal violence, recovery, and resilience in incarcerated women, 126-135,132t,134t. *See also* Incarcerated women

Narratives, of trauma survivors early in recovery, 75-97. *See also* Trauma survivors, early in recovery, narratives of
National Resources Center on Domestic Violence, 253,260
Nazi Holocaust, 41,47
*No Shame for the Sun: Lives of Professional Pakistani Women*, xx
Northern Illinois University, xix

Oxford University, xxi

Pakistan People's Party, 289,290
Pakistani women, strategies for survival of, 287-304. *See also* Resilience, in cultural and political context, Pakistani women's strategies for survival
Passageways, 234
Peddle, N., xxii,6,185,197

Pembroke Center for Teaching and Research on Women, xxi
Pentagon, terrorist attacks on, 43
Physical abuse
in adults, in study of interpersonal violence, recovery, and resilience in incarcerated women, 130
of children, in study of interpersonal violence, recovery, and resilience in incarcerated women, 130
Plaza de Mayo, 47
Political Trauma Services Network, xxii
Post-traumatic recovery, in cultural and political context, Pakistani women's strategies for survival, 287-305. *See also* Resilience, in cultural and political context, Pakistani women's strategies for survival
Post-traumatic stress disorder (PTSD), xxv
complex, 12
in incarcerated women, 125
Post-war experiences, of Guatemalan and Salvadoran women, 150-152
Powell, T.A., 125
Prevent Child Abuse America, xxii
Psychological aftermath of trauma, 12
Psychological trauma, ecological view of, 21-22
Psychology, community. *See* Community psychology
Psychotherapy
individual, in multicultural context, 205-225
study of
discussion of, 215-221
domains of functioning in, 216-218

patient history and
background in,
210-211
presenting problem in, 210
racial and cultural context in,
219-221
treatment course in, 212-215
in trauma healing, 48-49
with trauma survivors, theoretical
framework for, 207-209
PTSD. *See* Post-traumatic stress
disorder (PTSD)

QIS. *See* Quebec Incidence Study of
Reported Child Abuse,
Neglect, Abandonment, and
Serious Behavior Problems
(QIS)
Quebec Incidence Study of Reported
Child Abuse, Neglect,
Abandonment, and Serious
Behavior Problems (QIS),
xxiii

Race, in complexity of trauma, 99-121.
*See also* Trauma, complexity
of, race, resiliency and
Racial and cultural contexts,
psychotherapeutic
relationship and, 219-221
Racial trauma, 38-43
Racially diverse communities, trauma
in, 38-43. *See also* Trauma,
in racially diverse
communities
Racism, trauma and, 110-114
Radan, A., xxii,6,147,188,196
Reaves, R.C., xxii,4,75
Recovery trajectories, in sexually
abused adolescents,
exploration of, 165-184. *See
also* Sexually abused

adolescents, recovery
trajectories in, exploration of
Redlich, F.C., 40
Refugees of war, trauma impact,
recovery, and resiliency in,
assessment of, 185-204
future directions in, 199-200
study of, 188-200,189t,193t,194t
discussion of, 195-200
instrumentation in, 190-191
limitations of, 199-200
methods in, 188-192,189t
participants in, 188-190,189t
procedures in, 191-192
psychometric characteristics in,
195
results of, 189t,192-195,193t,
194t
Religious symbolism, resilience and,
296-298
Research
resiliency, cultural bias in, 35-36
trauma. *See* Trauma research
at VOV, 22-23
Resilience
within and across cultural contexts,
defined, 36-38
collective, hope and, 46-48
in cultural and political context,
Pakistani women's strategies
for survival, 287-304
case study, 290-293
discussion of, 299-300
gender justice, 298-299
religious symbolism, 296-298
self-empowerment, 296-299
cultural beliefs and, 37-38
defined, 34-36
ecological view of, 21-22
in incarcerated women, 123-146.
*See also* Incarcerated women,
interpersonal violence,
recovery, and resilience in
multicultural expressions of, 43-45
multicultural perspective of, 33-53

profiles of, in study of interpersonal violence, recovery, and resilience in incarcerated women, 131-135,132t,134t
relational context and, 105-110
reshaping of individual cultural identity and, 43-45
trauma and, individual psychotherapy in multicultural context, 205-225. *See also* Psychotherapy, individual, in multicultural context
trauma recovery and, cultural definition of, 218-219
trauma research related to, 14-15
defined, 34-36
in trauma survivors, ecological understanding of, 9-32
premises of, 24-25
in traumatized communities, fostering of, 265-285
of women survivors of violence in Central America, 147-164. *See also* Central America, women survivors in, exposure to violence and expressions of resilience in
Resiliency
community in, 37
in complexity of trauma, 99-121. *See also* Trauma, complexity of, race, resiliency and
of refugees of war, after trauma, assessment of, 185-204. *See also* Refugees of war, trauma impact, recovery, and resiliency in, assessment of
strategies for survival and, 293-296
Resiliency research, cultural bias in, 35-36
Resnick, H.S., 128
Responsibility, in early recovery of trauma survivors, 91-92
Riesebrodt, M., 297

Rondeau, G., 35
Russell, D.E.H., 128

SAATH. *See* South Asian American Theater (SAATH)
Safety and Self-Care (SSC) Group, 234
SafetyNet Program, xx
Sakina, H.B., 298
Salvadoran women, war and post-war experiences of, 150-152
San Francisco State University, Center for Research on Gender and Sexuality at, xxii
Saunders, B.E., 128
Schlenger, W.E., 125
Second National Family Violence Survey, 129
Self-care, in early recovery of trauma survivors, 89-90
Self-change, process of, in early recovery of trauma survivors, 88-92
Self-empowerment, in Pakistani women's strategies for survival, 296-299
Seligman, M.E.P., 14
Sense of self, racial trauma effects on, 42-43
September 11, 2001, 43
Sexual abuse
characteristics of, 171
of children, in study of interpersonal violence, recovery, and resilience in incarcerated women, 129-130
Sexual Assault Nurse Examiners, 254
Sexually abused adolescents, recovery trajectories in, exploration of, 165-184
factors in, 168-169
resilient or adaptive outcomes, 167-168
study of, 169-180,173t,175t,177t

analyses in, 172
discussion of, 178-180
measures in, 170-172
participants in, 169-170
procedures in, 169
results of, 172-178,173t,
175t,177t
TSCC in, 171
Shalev, A.Y., 100
SIDES. *See* Structured Interview for
Disorders of Extreme Stress
(SIDES)
Social advocacy practice, on behalf of
trauma survivors, 245-263.
*See also* Trauma survivors,
individual and social
advocacy practice on behalf
of
Social change, group movements and,
47
Social justice, advocacy as, 247
Social Science Research Council, xxi
Sorsoli, L., xxii,4-5,99
South Asian American Theater
(SAATH), 48
South Asian Health Board, xx
South Asian Mental Health Clinic, at
Cambridge Health Alliance,
xxvi
SSC Group. *See* Safety and Self-Care
(SSC) Group
St. Anthony's College, xxi
Stage-based matching of patients, in
group therapy, of VOV
Program, 234-235
Stages-by-dimensions approach, in
group treatment, of VOV
Program, 231-234
Strauss, A., 136
Stress Management Group, 234
Structured Interview for Disorders of
Extreme Stress (SIDES), 167
Suffering, human, epidemiology of,
11-12

Survival, strategies for, resiliency and,
293-296
Surviving, as revolutionary act,
261-262
Survivor(s), trauma. *See* Trauma
survivors
Swampscott, 16
Symbolism, religious, resilience and,
296-298

Tan, A., 48
Tatum, B.D., 114
Teplin, L.A., 125
Terrorist attacks
on Pentagon, 43
on World Trade Center, 43
The Trafficking Victims Outreach and
Services network, xx
Tourigny, M., xxiii,5,165
Trauma
community
case example of, 266-267
responding to, 267-268
complexity of, race, resiliency and,
99-121
study of
discussion of, 114-117
method in, 102-103
racism and trauma in,
110-114
resilience and relational
context in, 105-110
results of, 103-114
in diverse contexts, healing from,
46-49
healing from
artistic creation and, 47-48
in diverse contexts, 46-49
family support in, 46-47
psychotherapy in, 48-49
interpersonal
chronic, effects of, 229
survivors of, group therapy for,
230-231

psychological, ecological view of, 21-22
psychological aftermath of, 12
in racially diverse communities, 38-43
  effects of, 41-43
  experience of, 39-40
  misdiagnosis, 40-41
  sense-of-self effects of, 42-43
racism and, 110-114
in refugees of war, impact of, assessment of, 185-204. *See also* Refugees of war, trauma impact, recovery, and resiliency in, assessment of
resilience and, individual psychotherapy in multicultural context, 205-225. *See also* Psychotherapy, individual, in multicultural context
resilient or adaptive outcomes after, 167-168
Trauma Information Group, 234
Trauma recovery, ecological view of, 21-22
Trauma recovery and resilience, cultural definition of, 218-219
Trauma Recovery and Resiliency Research Project, of VOV, 4
Trauma research
in multicultural influences, 13
new directions in, 12-15
resilience in, 14-15
  defined, 34-36
role of context in, 13
in untreated survivors, 12-13
Trauma survivors
early in recovery, narratives of, 75-97
analysis of, method of, 81-83,84t
discussion, 93-96
inspiration through connection, 84-87

interview, 81-83,84t
opportunities to be successful, 87-88
participants, 80
procedure for, 80-81
processes of self-change, 88-92
results, 83-92
individual and social advocacy practice on behalf of, 245-263
community response, 251-252
guidelines for, 254-261
actively learn about and integrate different theoretical approaches, 257-259
address historic mistrust between mental health clinicians and community-based advocates, 260
advocate for clients in community settings, 255-256
advocate for systemic change, 259
become knowledgeable about systems with which victims of violence may interface, 254-255
evaluate program, 260-261
expand and enhance training and education curriculum, 257
facilitate collaboration, communication, and coordinated response, 256
move beyond clinical walls, 260
provide and get support from other providers, 256

implications for practice,
254-261
needs assessment, 250-251
risk assessment, 250-251
safety planning, 250-251
interpersonal trauma-related, group
therapy for, 230-231
new community for, group therapy
as ecological bridge to,
227-243
psychotherapy with, theoretical
framework for, 207-209
Trauma Symptoms Checklist for
Children (TSCC), 171
Traumatized communities. *See also*
Community trauma
case example of, 266-267
resilience in, fostering of, 265-285.
*See also* Community
empowerment model of
intervention
Trickett, E.J., 10,19
Truth and Reconciliation Commission
of South Africa, 47
TSCC. *See* Trauma Symptoms
Checklist for Children
(TSCC)
Tufts University, xxii
Tummala-Narra, P., xxix,xxvi,1,3,4,6,
19,33,55,205,306


United States Holocaust Memorial
Museum, 47
Université de Montréal, xix,xx
Université du Québec à Montréal, xx
University of Massachusetts Medical
School, xx
University of Michigan, xxi,xxvi
University of Sherbrooke, xxiii
University of South Carolina, xix,xx
U.S. Department of Justice, 124


Valentine, J.D., 35
Vaslow, J.B., 172

VAST. *See* Victim Advocacy and
Support Team (VAST)
Victim Advocacy and Support Team
(VAST), xx,6,21,23,246-251
Victims of Crime Act, 246
Victims of Violence (VOV) Program,
of Cambridge Health
Alliance, xix,xx,xxi,xxiii,
xxvi,3,10
CCRT of. *See* Community Crisis
Response Team (CCRT), of
VOV Program
described, 20-23
ecological perspective of
community psychology and,
25-26
ecologically informed intervention
at, 22-23
group treatment at, 231-236
case study, 236-239
co-leadership in, 236
focus on individual goals in, 235
relational focus in, 235
stage-based matching of patients
in, 234-235
stages-by-dimensions approach,
231-234
research at, 22-23
services and service components of,
21
Trauma Recovery and Resiliency
Research Project of, 4
Victims of Violence (VOV) Research
Project, xxi
Vietnam War, 42
Violence
advocacy in aftermath of, client
example, 247-250
interpersonal, recovery from,
resilience to, in incarcerated
women, 123-146. *See also*
Incarcerated women,
interpersonal violence,
recovery, and resilience in

of women in Central America,
expressions of resilience
following, 147-164. *See also*
Central America, women
survivors in, exposure to
violence and expressions of
resilience in
VOV Program. *See* Victims of
Violence (VOV) Program


War
context of, contributions of Latin
American psychologists,
148-149
refugees of, trauma impact,
recovery, and resiliency in,
assessment of, 185-204. *See
also* Refugees of war, trauma
impact, recovery, and
resiliency in, assessment of
War experiences, Guatemalan and
Salvadoran women, 150-152
Western Illinois University, xix,
xxi,xxii
Widom, C.S., 77
Wilks Criterion, 69
WinMax, 82
Women, incarcerated, interpersonal
violence, recovery, and
resilience in, 123-146. *See
also* Incarcerated women,
interpersonal violence,
recovery, and resilience in

Women survivors, in Central America,
exposure to violence and
expressions of resilience in,
147-164. *See also* Central
America, women survivors
in, exposure to violence and
expressions of resilience in
Women's Studies in Religion Program,
Harvard Divinity School,
xx,xxi
Women's Time-Limited (WTL) group,
236-239
World Health Organization, 252
World Trade Center, terrorist attacks
on, 43
World War II, 41
WTL group. *See* Women's
Time-Limited (WTL) group
Wyatt, G.E., 128


Yassen, J., xxiii,6,245
Yehuda, R., 15


Zachary, R.S., xxiii,6,227
Zainab, H.B., 298

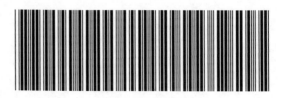